COOK
THIS
NOT
THAT!™

EASY & AWESOME
350-CALORIE MEALS

The No-Diet Weight Loss Solution

BY DAVID ZINCZENKO
AND MATT GOULDING

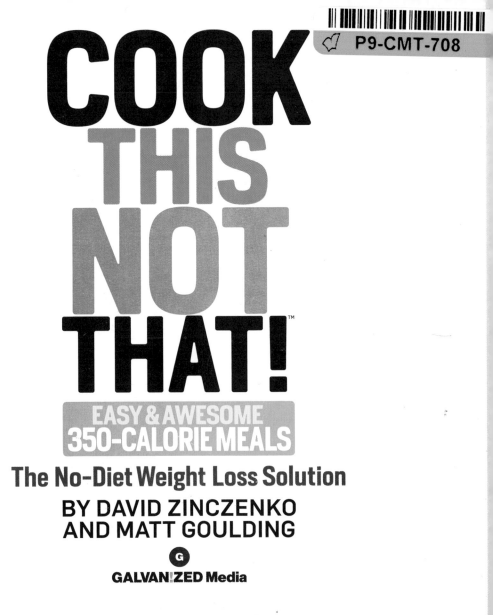

GALVANIZED Media

Notice
This book is intended as a reference volume only, not as a medical manual.
The information given here is designed to help you make informed decisions about your health.
It is not intended as a substitute for any treatment that may have been prescribed by your doctor.
If you suspect that you have a medical problem, we urge you to seek competent medical help.

Mention of specific companies, organizations, or authorities in this book does not imply endorsement
by the author or publisher, nor does mention of specific companies, organizations, or authorities imply
that they endorse this book, its author, or the publisher.

Eat This, Not That!, Cook This, Not That!, and Drink This, Not That!
are registered trademarks of Galvanized Media, LLC.
© 2018 by Galvanized Media.

Printed in the United States of America.
Galvanized Media. makes every effort to use acid-free, recycled paper.

Book design by George Karabotsos

Photo direction by Tara Long

Cover photographs by Jeff Harris, and food styling by Ed Gabriels for Halley Resources

All interior photos by Mitch Mandel and Thomas MacDonald
and food styling by Diane Simone Vezza and Melissa Reiss

ISBN 978–1–940358-33-8 paperback

DEDICATION

For those who'd rather not "stay hungry."
Here's to staying happy, healthy, and satisfied.
—Dave and Matt

ACKNOWLEDGMENTS

Plenty of charred burgers and fallen soufflés went into making this book. So did a lot of long days and nights spent designing pages, checking facts, correcting punctuation, buying ingredients, crunching numbers, grating cheese, taking photos, and countless other efforts, both big and small. This book is the product of all those efforts—and all those people behind them that make this team the finest in the publishing industry. Thanks to all of you who were a part of this project, especially:

To George Karabotsos and his crew of rock star designers, including Courtney Eltringham, Laura White, Elizabeth Neal, Rob Campos, and Mark Michaelson. If these past 10 books have proved anything, it's that this design team has no equal.

To our brigade of fearless sous chefs, including Rusty Goulding, James Perry, Michael Tsai, and Katie Kennedy. The food in this book wouldn't be nearly as delicious without your collective culinary chops. And to Clint Carter and Andrew Del-Colle, for whom no factoid or calorie count is too obscure to unearth.

To Debbie McHugh: It's hard to imagine how we ever did these books without you.

To Tara Long, who could make peanut butter smeared on a rice cake look like a four-star feast: Thank you for being so good at what you do.

And to our friends, family, and loved ones: There's no one we'd rather cook for.

—Dave and Matt

Check out the other informative books in the *EAT THIS, NOT THAT!* series:

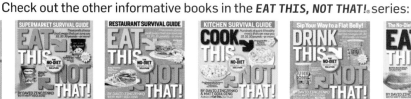

Eat This, Not That! for Kids! (2008)

Eat This, Not That! Supermarket Survival Guide (2009)

Eat This, Not That! Restaurant Survival Guide (2009)

CookThis, Not That! (2010)

Drink This, Not That! (2010)

Eat This, Not That! 2011 (2010)

CONTENTS

Hunger is making you fat.

That may sound counterintuitive, but it's true, and it's why this book is essential for anyone who wants to enjoy delicious food while also losing weight quickly, safely, and effectively. See, this may be a cookbook, but it's not necessarily a book for people who love to cook.

This is a book for people who love to eat.

The goal of this book is to help you get from "hmm, I'm hungry" to "yum, that's good" in as little time as possible. It's designed to help you keep hunger—and weight gain—at bay by keeping your belly filled with smart, lean versions of all your favorite foods and letting you eat to your heart's content whenever you want. Especially if you want it fast.

Now, that doesn't mean there isn't plenty of joy to be found in the process of planning, shopping, and prepping a meal. Plenty of people just love to pore through their recipe collection, selecting the ultimate creation for that night's meal and improvising like a jazz artist over the stove. They love sorting through the kitchen shelves to ensure they have just the right colander and the perfect gauge of grater for their next pasta masterpiece. They love to linger in the supermarket, rapping on the melons and sniffing the peaches and poking the beef and talking shop with the fishmonger. And they're happiest of all when they're watching the yellow-blue flame of the stovetop lap at the steel bottom of their designer cookware.

But you don't have to be one of those people to get the most out of this book. I've got nothing against the pleasures of chefdom myself, but I'm happiest when all that's done, and the food is on its way to my mouth. And I'm even happier when I can eat all I want, when I want, and know that my indulgence isn't going to cost me on the bathroom scale.

That makes me especially fortunate to have a recipe-shuffling, melon-rapping, cookware-rattling, James Beard Award—nominated writer and chef as a coauthor. Because while everybody wants AWESOME food, people who don't like to feel hungry also want EASY food. And people who want to eat all they want, when they want, are looking for food they can enjoy without the fat, sugar, and calories that have forced too many of us food lovers onto diets—the food-lover's purgatory. We want easy and awesome foods that we can eat lots of, whenever we want, without having to spend hours at the gym or wasting our time watching our waists. And that's where this book comes in.

Easy & Awesome 350-Calorie Meals is the ultimate cookbook for people who want to eat great food—and lots of it—and never have to worry about gaining weight. In fact, learning to cook fast and lean—and cutting down the time between the first hunger pangs and the first bite of smart, healthy food—is just about the best thing you can do to start losing weight more effectively. Why? It's simple:

The 350-Calorie Rule

You are going to find a handful of recipes in this book that drift north of the 350-calorie border. Truth is, we could have followed the lead of other low-calorie cookbooks and shrunk down entrées to Lilliputian portions, turned to scary food anomalies like fat-free half-and-half, and played funny math games with the nutritionals, but we wanted to feed you, not deceive you. The recipes in this book are for real food, the kind of seemingly decadent plates that won't just tickle your taste buds, but also keep you from raiding the pantry an hour later. Even if you ate the "worst" dish in this book, the 410-calorie Baked Ziti, every night of the week, we're positive you'd still shed pounds and you'd still save plenty of cash.

Hunger is making you fat.

Seriously. When your body gets hungry, it starts doing two things that are bad for your belly:

• ***It goes foraging for fast calories.*** When your body senses hunger, it goes into stress mode. Since there's no telling how long this food shortage will last, your instinct—diet be damned—is to try to get calories, fast. In primitive times, that meant climbing trees to find fruit or turning over boulders to find worms. Today, it means climbing kitchen shelves to find Fruity Pebbles and turning to Burger King to find Whoppers. Hunger sets the stage for cravings, and cravings set the stage, inevitably, for unhealthy calories. And that's why dieting doesn't work: One moment you're "being good," "sticking to your diet," and "maintaining discipline," and the next moment you're chewing through the freezer door and diving into an ill-advised love triangle with two guys named Ben and Jerry. But there's something else your body does when it gets hungry that's even worse.

• ***It starts burning body tissue.*** Since your body needs energy to do things like pump your heart, fill your lungs, think great thoughts, keep up with the Kardashians, and all the myriad other projects it has going on right now, shutting down when you run out of gas simply isn't an option. So when you get hungry, your body starts looking around for stored calories to burn. At first, that sounds great: I'm feeling fat, so I'll just skip some meals and let my body burn off my flab. But as anyone who's tried to starve themselves slim knows, losing weight that way is hard, and once you start eating again, you gain it all back—and more! (See Alley, Kirstie.)

Why? Because it's not fat that your body wants to burn first, it's muscle. You see, your body stores fat to protect itself in times of severe hardship. When you get peckish for a few hours, your body senses that, hmmm, maybe all is not well in the food supply chain, and it instinctively starts to store and protect flab. And because it's counting on that stored flab for the future, when hunger strikes, it looks elsewhere for quick calories—to the protein stored in your muscles. Put it another way: Every time you feel hungry, what you're really feeling is your body burning away muscle and preserving fat. And worse, when you start eating again, your body—having now been taught that starvation might just be a threat—is even more prone to storing fat, just in case.

Hunger is robbing your wallet.

The fastest, most effective way to drop pounds is to pick up a cookpot, because always having something healthy and delicious to eat will keep your body running at its best, burning food and belly fat (and not muscle) for energy. But cooking your own food will do more than make you look better in clothes— it'll help you afford better clothes. (And with all the weight you're going to lose, believe me, you're going to need new clothes!)

For example: Let's say you love Olive Garden's Spaghetti and Italian Sausage. That meal will cost you about $14.75—and 1,270 calories—per person. Feeding a family of four? Good-bye, $59. Now, feed those same four family members our Spaghetti with Spicy Tomato Sauce—a lusty bowl of noodles goosed with hunks of smoky bacon—and your cost per person goes down by nearly $12.74 (and you'll save 900 calories as well). That's $50.96 back in your pocket.

And the savings are everywhere: Our Bloody Mary Skirt Steak will save you $13.05 (and 740 calories) per person over T.G.I. Friday's Flat Iron Steak. Stay home and whip up our Sea Bass Pockets instead of driving to P.F. Chang's for the Oolong Marinated Sea Bass, and ring up $15.07 (and 380 calories) in savings per person. Even a simple Reuben sandwich at Applebee's costs nearly 16 bucks; we'll save you $13.05 (and 740 calories) with our fast and easy home recipe.

Now, imagine a family of four saving just $10 per person once a day. At the end of the year, they'd have amassed an extra $14,600! For that kind of money, you could buy a brand-new Toyota Yaris; pay most of the yearly mortgage on a $200,000 home; splurge on a 2-week stay at a luxury Caribbean resort; or, if you're crazy, buy one bottle of 55-year-old Macallan single-malt Scotch. Regardless of what you choose, it's not the kind of money you sniff at.

Hunger is ruining your fun.

If you're concerned about eating right, then you've probably tried a bunch of "healthy" foods, "diet" foods, "low-fat" or "low-carb" (or as I might call them, "low-fun") foods. And you've probably discovered that eating gimmicky diet foods is about as enjoyable as watching *Iron Man* in black and white, with the sound turned off. Something's missing!

Too many "diet" plans insist that eating healthy must mean eating blandly. Too many recipe books and health foods call on flavorless concoctions like fat-free cheese or ask you to perform illogical hocus-pocus like using mashed beans instead of butter or applesauce in place of ice cream. Sorry, but I don't want to feel like I'm eating my dinner with a rubber glove wrapped around my taste buds—I want real food!

That's why **Easy & Awesome 350-Calorie Meals** uses plenty of the freshest, healthiest ingredients out there: real meat, real cheese, real butter, great produce, tangy spices, and none of the cheap, bland filler that adds calories (but not much else) to restaurant versions. And we perfectly portion out these great foods, so you not only enjoy what you're eating, but you stay full, satisfied, and happy for hours—so you can go out and have some fun. (Maybe by spending that 14 grand you just found in your kitchen!)

By the way: Isn't it more fun to have dinner with the people you choose, the lighting you choose, and the music you choose, than be surrounded by cranky strangers, dismissive waiters, fluorescent bulbs, and piped-in tunes from 1979? (Do you really need to hear "Boogie Wonderland" ever again? Ever?)

4 Reasons to Spend More Time in the Kitchen Than You Do in the Gym

Here are two things that have roughly doubled over the past 20 years: the number of gym memberships and the number of obese people. Wait—what? Our gym sweat is being rewarded with cellulite? It certainly would appear that way. But don't go burning your gym card just yet—the treadmill isn't the problem. Also during the past 20 years, we've seen countless meals move from the stovetop to restaurant kitchens and commercial food labs. That means bigger portions, more oils and sweeteners, and heightened emphasis on desserts, appetizers, and cocktails. So if you want to get serious about getting in shape, you've got to realign your priorities. It's all about the food.

Cutting calories has a bigger impact than burning calories

In a meta-analysis of 33 clinical trials, Brazilian scientists determined that diet controls about 75 percent of weight loss. Working out helps, of course, but a smart eating plan will get you three-fourths of the way there without you ever having to break a sweat. (That's the difference between six-pack and eight-pack abs!) Another study published by the Public Library of Science found that women who worked out with a trainer for 6 months lost no more weight than those who merely filled out health forms—in other words, those who started thinking about what they were eating. You can do that easily. As soon as you start cooking, you become instantly aware of everything on your plate.

Forcing yourself into the gym increases your likelihood of indulging later

Some researchers have compared willpower to muscle—once you work it hard, it becomes weak. So by forcing yourself into the gym today—when you don't really have the time—you're setting yourself up to fail tomorrow when you're confronted with milk shakes, French fries, and chimichangas. Unfortunately, it takes only one slip to negate an entire sweat session. Ever reward a trip to the gym with some food outside your normal eating regime? Sure, we all have. But the truth is, we're probably better off sticking to home-cooked food and skipping the gym.

It takes less time to cook in than it does to work out

You can eat a 1,000-calorie fast-food burger in 5 minutes, but you'll spend an hour or more burning it off at the gym. And that's if you're busting your butt. Now imagine that you decided instead to skip the burger and forego the gym. You could head home and, in about 20 minutes, you could have a juicier, tastier, 350-calorie cheeseburger made with the finest ingredients and seasoned just the way you like it. Will the portion be smaller? Probably, but so what? Cornell University research shows that eating satisfaction is derived from the flavor intensity and visual impact of a meal, not necessarily the amount served. Plus, you're left with extra cash in your wallet, you've saved 45 minutes, and you've "burned" more than 600 calories.

You can work exercise into your daily routine

Think of all the opportunities you have to be active throughout the day. Do you take advantage? Try taking the stairs over the elevator, walking across the office instead of sending an e-mail, or riding a bike instead of taking a cab. In essence, you can cheat your gym session. But food? There's no cheating there; it's only good when it's made fresh. Researchers at the University of Minnesota determined that compared with cooking for yourself, consuming more restaurant and ready-made meals—think frozen dinners and carryout—could have a negative impact on your overall health. So food should come first, and dedicated gym time second.

Hunger is hurting your family life.

Okay, so maybe basking in the cold, blue, fluorescent light of your local chain restaurant actually is your idea of fun. And maybe you really, really like the musical selections at your local Red Robin. But there's one more factor to consider: Hunger messes up our mealtimes.

Think about it. If Jimmy is hungry at 3 and snacks on some junk food, and Susie is hungry at 4 and runs out to McDonald's, and Uncle Fester is hungry at 5 and defrosts a Pizza Pocket, who's joining you for dinner at 6? Kinda lonely at the table, isn't it? (Now "Boogie Wonderland" really sounds sad . . .)

When we're driven by cravings, our family meals get disrupted because nobody's hungry at the same time. And that's just bad family policy. A 2000 Harvard Medical School study of more than 16,000 boys and girls ages 9 to 14 found that adolescents who frequently shared meals with their families ate more fruits and vegetables and less fried food, saturated fat, and trans fat. And a 2004 study found that families who regularly ate together were closer than those who ate separately.

And it's a lot easier to get the family to eat together when you're whipping up awesome food that's just as good—or better—than the stuff they'd find down at the mall. (And I'm not saying you need to make it a formal dinner every night—who has time to dust the chandelier, anyway? A University of Minnesota study focused on the eating habits of 5,000 middle and high school students and determined that even when families ate in front of the TV, as long as they were dining together, they still ate healthier.)

Bottom line: Hunger is bad for you, period. You know that phrase, "Stay hungry?" You know who came up with that? Neither do I, but my guess is that it was some rich guy who wanted to stay lean, wealthy, and happy by eating all our food.

Stay hungry? No way. Stay full, satisfied, and fit for life with **Easy & Awesome 350-Calorie Meals.**

The 350-Calorie Kitchen

The skills and ingredients
you need for amazing healthy meals

Cooking is not a chore.

At least, it shouldn't be. And yet, for so many people, the idea of coming home from a long day of work only to have to fire up the stovetop and find a way to put dinner on the table is only slightly more tolerable than, say, pulling weeds or changing the oil in your car. The main goal of this book isn't to make you skinnier and healthier; it's to make you a better, more enthusiastic cook. Once we do that, those other two admirable goals will fall into place easily enough.

We sincerely hope the abundance of delicious recipes—and the mouthwatering photos that accompany them—found within this book will provide plenty of inspiration and motivation for your time in the kitchen. But more than just concrete recipes intended for repetition, we hope that the mixture of simple cooking lessons and ingredient spotlights will help you build a set of skills and a well-stocked pantry that can be tapped into at any given moment to create magical meals in an instant. It's precisely at that moment, when you can put away the recipe and create something uniquely your own, that cooking ceases to be a chore and starts to become a lifelong passion.

Master the Techniques

Teach a man to fish, feed him for a day. Teach him to fillet that fish, pan-sear it, and serve it with a scoop of mango salsa, and you'll feed him for a lifetime. Combine these essential techniques with fresh ingredients and you'll eat well for the rest of your years.

Broiling

The broiler is the most underused appliance in the kitchen. Those blazing coils in your oven are nothing more than an inverted grill, capable of delivering big blasts of heat—and deep, flavorful caramelization— to your food in a short period of time.

BEST FOR:
Burgers, steaks, fish fillets, chicken breasts

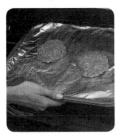

Step 1: *Preheat the broiler and allow it to warm up for at least 5 minutes before cooking. Line a broiling pan or baking dish with foil (because of the high heat, cleanup can be a mess without the foil) and place the meat on top. Situate the pan or dish 6 inches below the heat source. This is close enough to help brown the food, but not so close it will char it before it's done cooking through.*

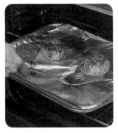

Step 2: *Since the heat is only coming from one direction, you'll need to flip the meat or fish at the halfway cooking point. Burgers and steaks will take about 10 minutes to cook to medium rare underneath the broiler; a fish fillet of medium thickness should be done in 7 to 8 minutes. Beyond cooking protein, the broiler is perfect for melting cheese, toasting a sandwich, and putting a crust on baked pasta dishes.*

Sautéing

Sautéing simply means cooking in a pan with butter or oil. Done slowly over low heat, sautéing cooks the excess water out of vegetables, concentrating their natural sugars and innate flavor. Done quickly over moderare to high heat, sautéing produce nicely browned exteriors on everything from mushroom and zucchini slices to shrimp and chunks of chicken.

BEST FOR:
Delicate fish, shellfish, nearly all vegetables

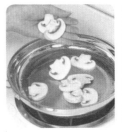

Step 1: *Preheat a pan or skillet with enough butter or oil to coat. Vary the heat depending on what you're going for: low heat for slowly caramelizing onions and cooking down tomatoes; high heat for browning mushrooms, peppers, and other vegetables. If you're doing the latter, don't crowd the pan. Too much butter or oil will make it impossible for the ingredients to properly brown.*

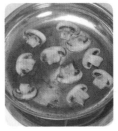

Step 2: *Stir as often as possible so that all sides of the food cook evenly. Season, but be mindful of when you do so: Salt draws out water, so if you add it early, the moisture will cause your food to steam in its own juices. For caramelizing onions, this is a good thing; for browning mushrooms, not so much. Thin fish fillets like sole and tilapia can also be sautéed, but this should be done in a nonstick pan.*

Braising

Braising is the technique responsible for the most tender meats and the most complex flavors. It's also the most effective way to stretch a dollar in the kitchen, as braising is all about turning tough, inexpensive cuts of meat into intensely flavored, deeply satisfying meals. After taking 10 minutes to put the dish into motion, braising requires little or no effort from you.

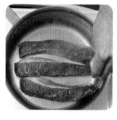

Step 1: *Heat a stainless steel pot or pan over medium-high heat and coat with enough oil to cover. Season meat with salt and pepper and add it to the pan. The goal is a deeply browned exterior, which will in turn flavor the braising liquid. Warning: If you crowd the pan, the surface temp will plummet and the food will not brown properly.*

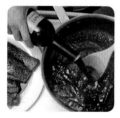

Step 2: *Once the meat has been fully browned, it's time to deglaze. Add wine or stock or a combination of both. As it simmers, use a wooden spoon to scrape up any bits stuck to the bottom of the pan. These little bits constitute the flavor that will ultimately infuse the entire braise, so be sure to work them off the pan.*

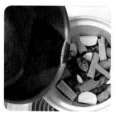

Step 3: *If braising on the stovetop or in the oven, return the meat to the pan, along with a mix of chopped onions, carrots, celery, and garlic. If you prefer a slow cooker, line the bottom with the meat, top with the vegetables, then pour the deglazing liquid over it all. Cook over low heat until the meat is fork-tender.*

Pan-Sear

Like sautéing on steroids, pan-searing concentrates the natural flavors in fish and meat. The high-heat technique is best for when you want to create a crust on your food, a caramelized layer that is not just big on flavor, but also provides important textural contrast to the soft meat within.

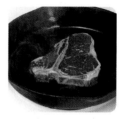

Step 1: *Heat a bit of oil in a pan over high heat. Because it requires such intense heat, pan-searing should be done in a cast-iron skillet or in a stainless steel pan. (High heat will eat away at the Teflon on nonstick pans.) When wisps of smoke rise from the pan, season the meat or fish and place in the pan.*

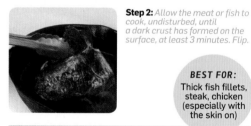

Step 2: *Allow the meat or fish to cook, undisturbed, until a dark crust has formed on the surface, at least 3 minutes. Flip.*

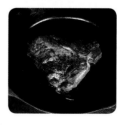

Step 3: *Place the pan in a preheated 400°F oven to finish cooking. If you try to finish on the stovetop, you're likely to burn the outside of the food before cooking it all the way through. The consistent, enveloping heat of the oven allows for even cooking, so your food will be uniformly cooked all the way through.*

Knife Skills

More than any other technique, sound knife skills will help you cook more quickly and efficiently. Not only that, there's something unbelievably thrilling about being to work your way through a pile of vegetables like a world-class chef.

The best piece of food you can learn to cut is an onion. That's because the same basic technique that goes into chopping, dicing, or mincing an onion can be applied to nearly any fruit or vegetable you'll find on your cutting board. See how it works in the first sequence.

The other critical knife technique is the rock, which gives you full control of the blade as you slice, dice, and mince your way through anything and everything. The far-right sequence lays the move out in full.

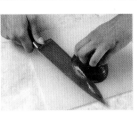

Step 1: *Holding the knife parallel to the cutting board, make horizontal cuts through the onion, stopping just short of cutting all the way through.*

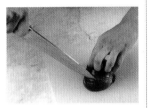

Step 2: *Use the tip of the blade to make vertical cuts, again being careful not to cut through the back of the onion (keeping it intact holds the onion together).*

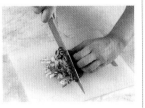

Step 3: *Tucking your fingertips in to protect them from the blade, slowly work your free hand toward the back of the onion, with the knife chopping closely in its wake. The more horizontal and vertical cuts you've made, the finer the cut.*

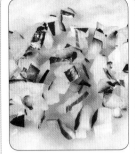

MINCED

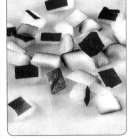

DICED

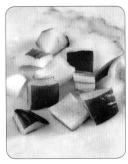

CHOPPED

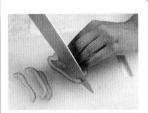

Step 1: *Plant the tip of the blade on the cutting board. Tuck the fingers of your free hand in and use it to stabilize the vegetable.*

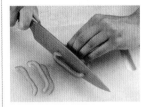

Step 2: *Bring the knife down in a steady motion. The heel of the blade should just come off the board.*

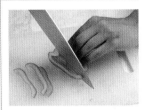

Step 3: *Pull the knife immediately back up, creating a seamless rocking motion. Repeat, using your free hand to guide the blade as you cut your way across the vegetable.*

5 Calorie-Cutting Techniques

We keep calories in check throughout this book by emphasizing lean protein and fresh fruits and vegetables over fat, sugar, and salt; by keeping portion sizes substantial but not elephantine; and by making smart substitutions that lighten a dish without compromising the taste or texture. But there are also a few basic techniques that you should add to your arsenal that will help eliminate some of the biggest caloric pitfalls of restaurant cooking. Learn the basics behind these five calorie-slashing skills and you'll be ready to add layers of flavor to your food without adding layers of fat to your body.

1. Béchamel

When making an Alfredo sauce or mac and cheese—dishes that traditionally rely on heavy cream as their base—this mixture of milk and butter, thickened with a bit of flour, could save you 300 or 400 calories per serving. Béchamel is also the basis of traditional Italian lasagna and can be turned into a cheese sauce that can stretch a handful of cheese into a rich topping for nachos or baked potatoes. Here's how you make it:

Step 1: Combine equal parts butter and flour in a saucepan set over medium heat. Cook for a minute or two, enough to get rid of the raw flour taste, but not enough to brown the butter.

Step 2: Slowly add milk, a few tablespoons at a time, whisking constantly to help keep the flour from forming lumps in the liquid.

Step 3: Season and simmer. Add salt and pepper to taste, plus any other flavors you like. Ground nutmeg, half an onion, or a few cloves of garlic (the latter of which should both be removed at the end) all boost the béchamel flavor.

2. Fresh Salsa

You'd be hard-pressed to find a healthier, more flavorful condiment than fresh-chopped salsa, especially when you experiment with different vegetables and fruit. The blueprint for every bowl of salsa is the same, so all you need to do is understand the basic three-step principle and you'll be ready to salsa your way through the produce aisle.

Step 1: Choose a base. Tomatoes are traditional, of course, but a variety of fruits and vegetables work perfectly here: mangoes, pineapple, papaya, corn, even black beans.

Step 2: Add the supporting cast. Chopped red onion, chopped fresh cilantro, and minced jalapeño are the standard and they work equally well for fruit- and vegetable-based salsas. Other options include chopped bell pepper, scallions, and finely minced garlic.

Step 3: Add acid. Usually that means the juice of a lemon or a lime, but a splash of red wine or apple cider vinegar will have a similar flavor-enhancing effect.

3. Pan Sauces

Why bother with fussy, high-calorie sauces and condiments when the best possible accompaniment to your steak or chicken breast is clinging to the bottom of the pan you just cooked it in? All you need is a bit of liquid to extract that flavor from the surface of the pan and you'll have a bold, beautiful sauce ready in a matter of minutes. (This same technique works in conjuction with pan-searing.)

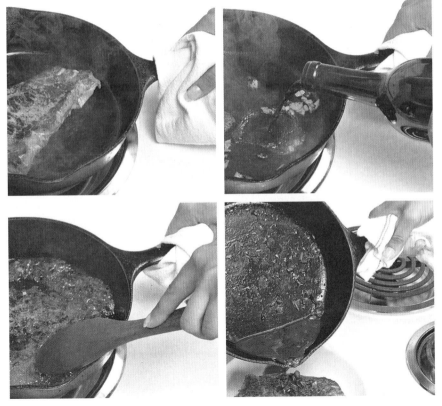

Step 1: Cook meat or fish in a stainless steel sauté pan or cast-iron skillet. Remove and return the pan on the flame.

Step 2: Add minced shallots or red onions and a ½ cup of either red (for beef, lamb, and duck) or white (for chicken, fish, and pork) wine and a ½ cup of chicken stock. Use a wooden spoon to scrape up any browned bits that cling to the bottom of the pan. Add any other flavoring elements now; Dijon mustard, chopped rosemary, capers, and balsamic vinegar are all welcome additions.

Step 3: Boil vigorously until the liquid has reduced by 75 percent, about 5 minutes. Season with salt and pepper and remove from heat. At the last moment, swirl in a pat of butter. Besides adding richness, it also gives the sauce a velvety texture.

Step 4: Pour the sauce over the meat or fish and dig in.

4. Spice Rubs

Sometimes the only thing to make a piece of meat or fish an exciting prospect on your plate rather than a boring afterthought is a simple but smart sheath of spices. Rather than bog down your food with excess calories, they infuse a dish with a variety of powerful antioxidants— potent micronutrients known to fight cancer, reduce inflammation, and even speed up metabolism, among other marvelous side effects.

The best rubs blend a spectrum of flavors into one seamless powder you can use to coat your favorite proteins. The whole idea is to tweak and refine your own blends, based on personal preferences, but as a general rule, it's best to incorporate one member of at least three of these groups below into your magical meat dust.

SALT	HEAT	SWEET	SMOKE	HERBAL
kosher salt	black pepper	sugar	cumin	oregano
garlic salt	cayenne	brown sugar	smoked paprika	thyme
onion salt	chili powder	cinnamon		rosemary
	mustard powder			basil
				dill

HERE ARE SOME OF OUR FAVORITE BLENDS:

- **FOR BEEF:** Salt and pepper, garlic salt, cayenne, cumin, pinch of cinnamon
- **FOR CHICKEN:** Salt and pepper, cumin, chili powder, brown sugar
- **FOR FISH:** Salt and pepper, smoked paprika, thyme

5. Oven Frying

Not only is deep-frying the quickest way to shackle your food with excess calories, it's also expensive, inconvenient, and potentially dangerous to have a vat of bubbling oil in a home kitchen. With the right oven temperature and technique, oven frying gives you the outside crunch and interior juiciness that we crave in fried foods without the hassle and the empty calories. Here's how you do it:

Step 1: Make sure your meat, fish, or vegetables are all similar in size and shape (that way they cook evenly in the same amount of time). Set up three separate dips: a plate with flour, a bowl of beaten eggs, and a plate of breadcrumbs.

Step 2: Dip the meat, fish, or vegetables first in the flour, then into the egg (the flour helps the egg adhere to the food). From the egg, dip them into the bread crumbs, tossing so that each piece is thoroughly covered. Note: It's best to keep one hand free for dry ingredients and the other for wet ones, otherwise things get messy.

Step 3: Place in a preheated oven. For larger pieces of meat such as whole chicken breasts, you'll want a lower temperature (350 to 375°F) to ensure the bread crumbs don't burn before the meat is cooked. For smaller pieces, a high temp (400 to 425°F) will help brown the bread crumbs into a crunchy crust before the meat or fish is overcooked. Chicken breasts will take about 15 minutes to cook through, fish fillets about 10 to 12.

The
50
Best Foods in the Supermarket

Every good meal starts with a properly stocked pantry and fridge. To ensure you have the best building blocks possible, we've taken years' worth of supermarket reconnaissance and distilled it down to our 50 favorite products in the aisles. Whether you're looking for the healthiest sliced cheese for sandwiches, the best flour for pancakes and baked goods, or the leanest, tastiest frozen pizza for the nights you want to stay out of the kitchen, this is the last grocery list you'll ever need to make.

Breads and Grains

1. BEST CEREAL

Post Spoon-Size Shredded Wheat

This box contains no added sugars, oils, or artificial colors. Inside is nothing but pure, unadulterated whole wheat. Liven it up with fresh blueberries.

Per cup: 170 calories, 1 g fat, 40 g carbs, 6 g fiber

2. BEST ENGLISH MUFFIN

Thomas' Light Multi-Grain English Muffin

You won't find a lighter English muffin. Nor will you find one with more fiber.

Per muffin: 100 calories, 1.5 g fat, 24 g carbs, 8 g fiber

3. BEST BREAD

Martin's Whole Wheat Potato Bread

Potato bread crowns a sandwich with a light touch of sweetness, and the heft of fiber in Martin's Whole Wheat makes it a guilt-free upgrade.

Per slice: 70 calories, 1 g fat, 14 g carbs, 4 g fiber

4. BEST BURGER BUN

Arnold Select 100% Whole Wheat Sandwich Thins

Bulging buns don't hold burgers any better, but they do saddle you with loads of superfluous calories.

Per roll: 100 calories, 1 g fat, 21 g carbs, 5 g fiber

5. BEST TORTILLA

La Tortilla Factory Smart & Delicious EVOO MultiGrain

La Tortilla Factory's wrap employs an arsenal of nutritional powerhouses such as sunflower seeds, oat fiber, and flax seed.

Per wrap: 100 calories, 3.5 g fat (0.5 g saturated), 18 g carbs, 12 g fiber

6. BEST PIZZA CRUST

Rustic Crust Organic Pizza Originale

No pizza is as healthy—or flavorful—as the one that sits atop a crust of basil and garlic-infused whole wheat. You won't find a pizza base with fewer calories.

Per 2-oz serving (about ⅙ of pie): 120 calories, 1.5 g fat , 25 g carbs, 1 g fiber

7. BEST PASTA

Ronzoni Healthy Harvest Whole Wheat Thin Spaghetti

Ronzoni manages to pack in all the fiber without the gritty texture of some of its whole-wheat competitors.

Per 2 oz (uncooked): 180 calories, 2 g fat, 41 g carbs, 6 g fiber

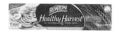

8. BEST GRAIN

Bob's Red Mill Organic Whole Grain Quinoa

Quinoa packs in about twice as much protein as the typical cereal grain, and it contains all the essential amino acids your body needs to function at its peak.

Per ¼ cup (uncooked): 170 calories, 30 g carbs, 3 g fiber, 2.5 g fat

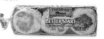

9. BEST FLOUR

King Arthur Traditional 100% Whole Wheat

The hard red wheat used to produce this flour provides bolsters your diet with vitamin E and manganese, among other vital nutrients.

Per ¼ cup: 110 calories, 0.5 g fat, 21 g carbs, 4 g fiber

Dairy and Deli

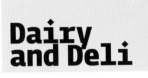

10. BEST MILK
Organic Valley Reduced Fat 2%

Thanks to new USDA regulations, cows used for organic milk are now guaranteed to spend at least a few months of every year grazing on natural pasture grasses.

Per cup: 130 calories, 5 g fat, 8 g protein

11. BEST SLICED CHEESE
Sargento Reduced Fat Swiss

Saving calories isn't the only boon: The other payoff is more protein in each slice.

Per slice: 60 calories, 4 g fat, 5 g protein

12. BEST SHREDDED CHEESE
Kraft Natural 2% Milk Mozzarella

The mild flavor and of mozzarella makes it the best utility player in the dairy cooler. Plus, no cheese comes with a lighter caloric toll.

Per oz: 70 calories, 4 g fat, 8 g protein

13. BEST CREAM CHEESE
Philadelphia Whipped

The whipping process introduces air to the cream, which reduces the calories per serving and makes it easier to spread.

Per 2 Tbsp: 60 calories, 6 g fat

14. BEST BUTTER
Organic Valley Sweet Cream Cultured Unsalted Butter

Don't be afraid of real butter. Research shows that the fat in a pat of butter helps you better absorb vitamins A, E, and K.

Per Tbsp: 100 calories, 11 g fat

15. BEST YOGURT
Fage Total 2% Greek Yogurt (7 oz container)

More than twice as much protein as standard American-style yogurt. Plus, the thicker consistency of Greek yogurt makes a prime base for sauces and marinades.

Per container: 130 calories, 4.5 g fat, 15 g protein

16. BEST EGGS
Eggland's Best

Each egg contains 115 milligrams of heart-healthy omega-3 fatty acids.

Per large egg: 70 calories, 4 g fat, 6 g protein

17. BEST COLD CUT
Hormel Natural Choice Pre-Sliced Turkey and Ham

Packaged without nitrates or nitrites, Natural Choice makes some of the freshest-tasting deli meats ever to come out of a package.

Per 4 slices Oven Roasted Deli turkey: 50 calories, 1 g fat, 10 g protein

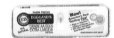

18. BEST BACON
Oscar Mayer Center Cut Naturally Smoked

When it comes to nationally available strips, these are tough to beat. Center cut bacon has a higher meat-to-fat ratio, making it less calorie dense.

Per 3 slices: 60 calories, 4 g fat, 6 g protein

Dairy and Deli cont.

19. BEST SAUSAGE

Al Fresco Sundried Tomato & Basil Chicken Sausage

Al Fresco's chicken sausages pack big flavor into a low-calorie package.

Per link: 140 calories, 7 g fat, 15 g protein

20. BEST HOT DOG

Applegate Farms Uncured Beef Hot Dogs

They're low in calories, sure, but they also taste like real beef—a huge improvement over the bologna-like dogs from Ball Park and Oscar Mayer.

Per dog: 70 calories, 4.5 g fat, 6 g protein

Packaged Foods & Snacks

21. BEST CANNED TOMATOES

Muir Glen Organic Whole Peeled Tomatoes

Muir Glen cans its tomatoes within 8 hours of harvest, giving them a far fresher flavor than the pallid out-of-season supermarket tomato.

Per ½ cup: 25 calories, 1 g fiber, 5 g carbs

22. BEST POTATO CHIP

Popchips All Natural Barbecue

The heat-compression technique developed by Popchips gives these spuds more flavor than a baked chip with fewer calories than a fried chip.

Per oz: 120 calories, 4 g fat, 20 g carbs, 1 g fiber

23. BEST TORTILLA CHIP

Food Should Taste Good Sweet Potato Tortilla Chips

They deliver more flavor than a typical tortilla chip, and each serving meets 20% of your day's vitamin A requirement.

Per oz: 140 calories, 6 g fat, 18 g carbs, 3 g fiber

24. BEST CRACKER

Triscuit Original

Perfect foods come in simple packages, and Triscuits are as simple as crackers can be.

Per 6 crackers: 120 calories, 4.5 g fat, 19 g carbs, 3 g fiber

25. BEST NUTS

Emerald Cocoa Roast Almonds, Dark Chocolate

This snack tastes like candy, but instead of bombarding you with sugar, it offers up a hearty dose of heart-healthy fats.

Per ¼ cup: 150 calories, 13 g fat, 6 g carbs, 3 g fiber

26. BEST SNACK BAR

Lärabar Pecan Pie

The only ingredients in this delicious snack bar are dates, pecans, and almonds. If only real pecan pie were so honest.

Per bar: 220 calories, 14 g fat, 24 g carbs, 4 g fiber

27. BEST CHOCOLATE BAR
Chocolove Strong Dark Chocolate 70% Cocoa
Enjoy all the health benefits of dark chocolate, but without the bitter taste.
Per ⅓ bar: 160 calories, 12 g fat, 15 g carbs, 4 g fiber

28. BEST COOKIE
Newman-O's Mint Creme Filled Chocolate Cookies
These cookies are organic, trans-fat free, and made with natural peppermint oil.
Per 2 cookies: 130 calories, 4.5 g fat, 20 g carbs, 1 g fiber

Drinks
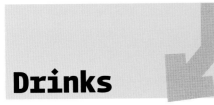

29. BEST BOTTLED TEA
Honest Tea Organic Honey Green Tea
This one has the highest antioxidant content of any tea we checked out. Plus, it's not overloaded with sugar.
Per 8 fl oz: 35 calories, 9 g carbs

30. BEST BEER
Guinness Draught
Good luck finding a more robustly flavored beer for 125 calories.
Per bottle: 125 calories, 10 g carbs
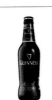

31. BEST LIGHT BEER
Amstel Light
It's lighter than Bud Select but tastes less watered down than most light beers.
Per 12 fl oz: 95 calories, 5 g carbs

Frozen Foods
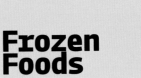

32. BEST PIZZA
Kashi Thin Crust Margherita
The pizza aisle is the nutrition badlands of the grocery store, but with a whole-wheat crust and veggie toppings, Kashi is giving other purveyors a hero to look up to.
Per ⅓ pizza: 260 calories, 9 g fat, 29 g carbs, 4 g fiber
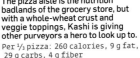

33. BEST FROZEN WAFFLE
Van's 8 Whole Grains Multigrain Waffles
The bevy of grains in this waffle makes it a laudable stand-in for toast in your morning breakfast sandwich.
Per 2 waffles: 180 calories, 7 g fat, 31 g carbs, 6 g fiber

HOW WE CHOSE THE WINNERS: We created this list by first comparing the nutrition labels of competing brands in each of our 50 categories. We gave bonus points to products with more protein and fiber and less added sugar and sodium. We also took calories per serving into consideration. Once we pared down our choices, we matched them in head-to-head taste tests to determine the victors. As for draws, the nod went to the product with the fewest ingredients—which happens to be a good rule of thumb, period.

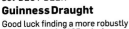

Frozen Foods cont.

34. BEST ICE CREAM

Breyers Natural Vanilla

With only five ingredients, it's as unadulterated as you'll get without churning it yourself.

Per ½ cup: 130 calories, 7 g fat, 14 g carbs

35. BEST FROZEN TREAT

Klondike Slim a Bear No Sugar Added Vanilla Bars

Individual packaging acts as a built-in portion monitor—as long as you limit yourself to just one.

Per bar: 170 calories, 9 g fat, 21 g carbs, 4 g fiber

Condiments & Cooking Extras

36. BEST KETCHUP

Heinz Organic

Perfectly balanced. And researchers found that organic ketchup has close to double the lycopene of regular ketchups.

Per Tbsp: 20 calories, 0 g fat, 5 g carbs

37. BEST MUSTARD

Inglehoffer Original Stone Ground Mustard

It's grainy and robust, offering the double-punch of texture and flavor that can carry any dish to another level.

Per tsp: 10 calories, 0 g fat, 1 g carbs

38. BEST MAYONNAISE

Kraft with Olive Oil Reduced Fat

Making mayo with olive oil instead of soybean oil displaces inferior omega-6 acids for heart-healthy monounsaturated fat.

Per Tbsp: 45 calories, 4 g fat, 2 g carbs

39. BEST BBQ SAUCE

Dinosaur Bar-B-Que Roasted Garlic Honey

It expertly balances the sweetness with subtle notes of smoke and tang.

Per 2 Tbsp: 25 calories, 0 g fat, 6 g carbs

40. BEST PASTA SAUCE

Muir Glen Organic Tomato Basil

Organic tomatoes are one of the few fruits to be scientifically proven more nutritious than their conventional counterparts. Stock up.

Per ½ cup: 60 calories, 1 g fat, 12 g carbs, 2 g fiber

41. BEST SALSA

Desert Pepper Roasted Tomato Chipotle Corn

This jar has far more flavor than your standard Old El Paso. The chipotle gives it some smokey spice, while the corn lends a hint of sweetness.

Per 2 Tbsp: 10 calories, 2 g carbs

42. BEST PREMADE GUACAMOLE
Wholly Guacamole

Unlike many of its competitors, Wholly makes its guac with real avocadoes.

Per 2 oz: 50 calories, 4 g fat, 2 g fiber, 190 mg sodium

43. BEST PEANUT BUTTER
Smucker's Natural Chunky

You'll find no added oils, sweeteners, or fillers in this jar—just peanuts and salt. Sure you have to stir it, but that's a small price to pay for real, unadulterated peanut butter.

Per 2 Tbsp: 200 calories, 16 g fat, 90 mg sodium

44. BEST DIP
Guiltless Gourmet Mild Black Bean Dip

Functions great as a dip, but it also works as a flavorful spread for wraps and burritos.

Per 2 Tbsp: 40 calories, 0 g fat, 2 g fiber, 125 mg sodium

45. BEST HUMMUS
Sabra Roasted Red Pepper Hummus

Hummus is the most underutilized spread in your refrigerator. Try on deli sandwiches or alongside a piece of grilled meat or fish.

Per 2 Tbsp: 70 calories, 6 g fat, 1 g fiber, 120 mg sodium

46. BEST SALAD DRESSING
Drew's All Natural Smoked Tomato

The blend of sweetness and smokiness makes this great for a hearty salad, but maybe even better as an impromptu marinade. Try both and decide for yourself.

Per Tbsp: 50 calories, 5 g fat, 69 mg sodium

47. BEST RANCH REPLACEMENT
Annie's Naturals Organic Buttermilk Dressing

Made with low-fat buttermilk and plenty of herbs and spices, this is a dead ringer for ranch, with nearly a third of the calories.

Per 2 Tbsp: 60 calories, 6 g fat, 230 mg sodium

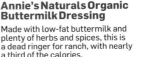

48. BEST EVERYDAY COOKING OIL
Newman's Own Organic Extra Virgin Olive Oil

A nicely balanced oil that's perfect for cooking or making homemade vinaigrettes.

Per Tbsp: 130 calories, 14 g fat

49. BEST COOKING BROTH
Swanson Certified Organic Free Range Chicken Broth

This has the best flavor of all the broths we tasted, and because it's organic, you'll have no trace antibiotics leaching into your family's food.

Per cup: 15 calories, 0.5 g fat, 550 mg sodium

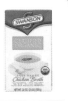

50. BEST SOY SAUCE
Kikkoman Less Sodium

Sodium is the Achilles' heal of soy sauce, but thankfully Kikkoman makes one that's reasonable. Combine it with brown sugar, chopped scallions, minced ginger, and minced garlic for a good all-purpose marinade.

Per Tbsp: 10 calories, 575 mg sodium

To find all our top picks, complete with customizable grocery list, go to
EATTHIS.COM.

Chapter

Breakfast
Satisfying morning meals to
supercharge your day

11 Instant Egg

1 Sauté an egg in olive oil. Slide on top of a bowl of hot spaghetti tossed with Parmesan, olive oil, and red pepper flakes.

2 Melt a pat of butter in a small nonstick pan. Add two beaten eggs and cook until a uniform layer begins to set in the pan. Grate plenty of real Parmesan into the center of the omelet, and, when fully set, fold the egg over the cheese and slide onto a plate. Eat for dinner with a salad and a glass of red wine.

3 Mix chopped-up hard-boiled eggs with mayonnaise, Dijon, capers, minced onion, and any fresh herbs you might have. Serve on a salad, in a pita, or sandwiched in a toasted English muffin.

4 *Denver scramble: Sauté chunks of ham, sliced mushrooms, onions, and bell pepper in a large nonstick sauté pan until the vegetables are soft and lightly browned. Add beaten eggs and scramble until the eggs are nearly set, then stir in a handful of sharp Cheddar.*

5 *Place a pizza of your choice in the oven and bake for 5 minutes. Slide out of the oven and crack an egg in the center of the dough, as if frying it. Return to the oven and bake until the white has just set but the yolk is still runny.*

6 Scramble eggs gently over low heat. Stir in pieces of broken tortillas, canned roasted chiles, and diced tomatoes. Season with salt, pepper, and a few shakes of hot sauce.

CHAPTER 2

Recipes

7 Roast or blanch asparagus spears until tender. Arrange four or five on a plate, top with sunny-side up eggs, and finish with a grating of Parmesan and salt and pepper.

Arrange a pile of frisée or arugula on plates. Top each with a poached egg, pieces of crumbled bacon, toasted walnuts, and a drizzle of olive oil and white wine or champagne vinegar.

9

10 Bring a pot of water to a vigorous boil. Carefully lower in eggs and cook for 5 minutes and 15 seconds. Remove to a bowl filled with ice water. Peel and serve each egg on top of a piece of toasted wheat bread. Tabasco is optional, but highly recommended.

8 Heat a tablespoon of butter in a nonstick pan over medium-low heat until brown and nutty, then add in beaten eggs. Slowly scramble until the eggs are soft and beginning to set, then fold in a few spoonfuls of ricotta cheese and fresh chopped chives. Serve on top of crusty bread.

Spoon some of your favorite jarred tomato sauce into ramekins or individual baking dishes. Crack an egg or two directly into the sauce, top with red pepper flakes, and bake at 400°F until the eggs whites just set, about 10 minutes.

11

Cook This!

Oatmeal with Peanut Butter and Banana

Oatmeal has a justified reputation as a healthy staple of the breakfast table, but that doesn't make this humble grain infallible. Problem is, plain oats are too boring to eat on a regular basis, and flavored oats carry a bevy of excess sugars and other ingredients that don't belong in your breakfast bowl. We solve both problems by using peanut butter and almonds to provide a rich base of healthy fats and bananas for natural sweetness and a shot of potassium. This is the kind of oatmeal you could—and should—eat 5 days a week.

You'll Need:

4½ cups water
2 cups rolled oats
Pinch of salt
2 bananas, sliced
2 Tbsp peanut butter
¼ cup chopped almonds
2 Tbsp agave syrup

How to Make It:

- In a medium saucepan, bring the water to a boil. Turn the heat down to low and add the oatmeal and salt. Cook, stirring occasionally, for about 5 minutes, until the oats are tender and have absorbed most of the liquid.
- Add the bananas, peanut butter, almonds, and agave syrup and stir to incorporate evenly. If the oatmeal is too thick, add a splash of milk.

Makes 4 servings / Cost per serving: $0.55

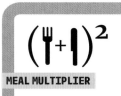

$$(\text{\textbf{¶}} + \text{\textbf{¶}})^2$$

MEAL MULTIPLIER

Peanut butter and banana may be our favorite oatmeal embellishment, but there are dozens of ways to trick out a plain bowl of boiled oats, including a few surprising ones (a hat tip to Mark Bittman, the first to introduce us to the idea of savory oatmeal).

- Diced apples (raw or sautéed in a bit of butter), toasted walnuts, and a pinch of cinnamon
- Sliced peaches, brown sugar, and chopped pecans (think peach cobbler)
- Soy sauce, scallions, and a fried egg (trust us—this makes a lot of sense)

320 calories
10 g fat
(1 g saturated)
17 g sugars

370 calories
6 g fat
(1 g saturated)
19 g sugars

Not That!

Au Bon Pain Large Apple Cinnamon Oatmeal
Price: $3.39

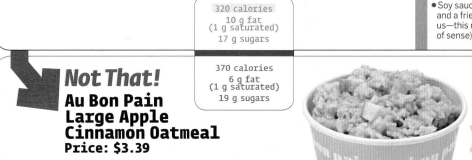

Save!
50 calories
and $2.84!

20

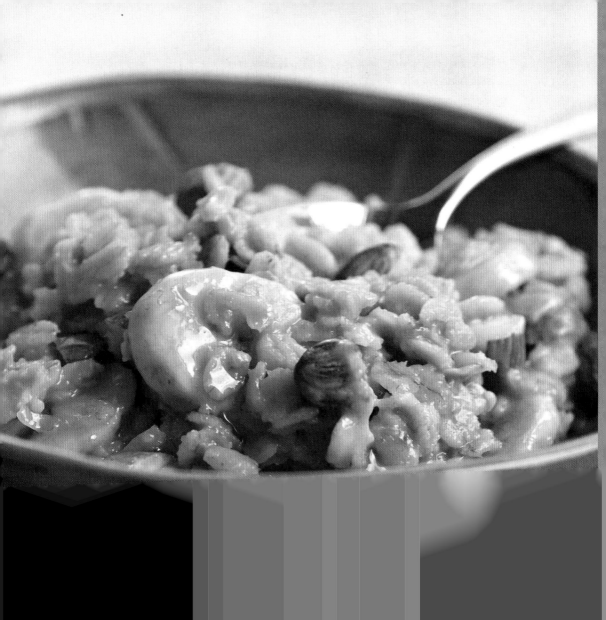

Egg Sandwich with Pastrami and Swiss

Is there anything more satisfying than a good breakfast sandwich? We think not, especially when we can chew comfortably knowing that we're starting our day in one of the best possible ways, which is to say, with a metabolism-jolting dose of protein and fiber. The combination of pastrami and Swiss has long been confined to the realm of the lunchtime deli counter, but we think it works beautifully with soft scrambled eggs—especially because pastrami trounces both sausage and bacon in the calorie department. Give it a try.

You'll Need:

- ½ Tbsp butter
- 4 oz lean pastrami (or turkey pastrami), cut into strips
- 6 eggs
- 2 Tbsp milk
- Salt and black pepper to taste
- 4 slices low-fat Swiss cheese
- 4 whole-wheat English muffins, lightly toasted

How to Make It:

- Melt the butter in a large nonstick skillet over medium heat. Add the pastrami and sauté for 2 to 3 minutes. Turn the heat down to low. Combine the eggs with the milk and a few pinches of salt and pepper. Whisk lightly, then add to the pan. Use a wooden spoon to constantly stir the eggs, scraping from the bottom as they set, as they'll continue to cook once removed from the stovetop.
- Place a slice of Swiss on the bottom of each English muffin. Divide the scrambled eggs among the muffins, top with the muffin tops, and serve.

Makes 4 servings / Cost per serving: $1.88

If pastrami is not your thing, this will work with any deli cut. Try roast beef, ham, or turkey.

325 calories
16 g fat
(6 g saturated)
860 mg sodium

770 calories
55 g fat
(18 g saturated)
2,310 mg sodium

Not That!
Hardee's Monster Biscuit
Price: $2.99

Save!
445 calories
and $1.11!

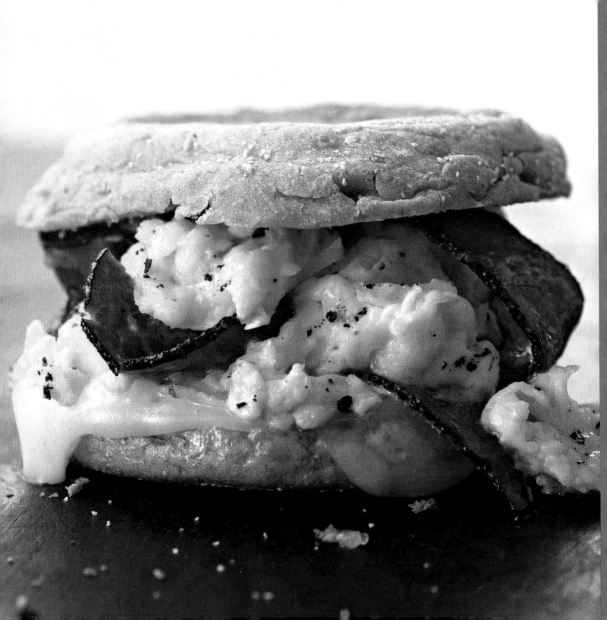

Cook This!

Breakfast Tacos with Bacon & Spinach

Americans have been taco crazy for decades, yet most of us have never thought of the tortilla as a breakfast food. Not the case in Austin, Texas, where 99-cent tacos stuffed with scrambled eggs, beans, and salsa mark the beginning of the day for many a local. Infectiously delicious, to be sure, but also a perfectly healthy start to your day, assuming you stick to corn tortillas, which have half the calories and twice the fiber of their flour counterparts.

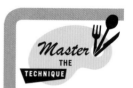

Tortilla treatment

Corn tortillas trounce their floury cousins in the nutrition department, but most people still have a problem making the jump to the more authentic taco base. The main issue? Texture. A cold corn tortilla is worthless, but a hot, toasty one is incomparable. If you have a gas stovetop, you can warm the tortillas directly over a low flame for 20 seconds a side. Or use a cast-iron skillet or nonstick sauté pan set over medium heat. Working with a few tortillas at a time, cook until the surface of each tortilla is lightly browned, about 30 seconds per side.

You'll Need:

- 4 strips bacon, chopped
- ½ onion, chopped
- 2 cups sliced mushrooms
- 1½ cups frozen spinach, thawed
- 6 eggs, beaten
- Salt and black pepper to taste
- 8 corn tortillas
- ½ cup shredded Monterey Jack cheese
- Pico de Gallo (see page 307) or bottled salsa

How to Make It:

- Cook the bacon in a large nonstick skillet over medium heat for 5 minutes, until the fat renders out and the bacon begins to crisp. Remove with a slotted spoon and reserve on a paper towel.
- Discard all but a thin film of the bacon grease from the pan. Add the onion and mushrooms and cook for about 3 minutes, until the onion is translucent. Add the spinach and continue cooking until the spinach is heated all the way through. (If any water has accumulated in the pan, carefully pour it out into the sink.)
- Add the eggs and use a wooden spoon to consistently scrape them from the bottom of the pan as they set. (The goal is to have light, fluffy eggs, and constant movement of the spoon will help you achieve that.) Season with salt and pepper.
- Heat the tortillas in a pan over medium heat. (Or, if short on time, wrap in a damp paper towel and microwave for 30 seconds.) Divide the cheese among the tortillas, top with the eggs, and spoon over as much salsa as you'd like.

Makes 4 servings /
Cost per serving: $1.52

360 calories
17 g fat
(6 g saturated)
450 mg sodium

610 calories
36 g fat
(14 g saturated)
1,390 mg sodium

Not That!
McDonald's McSkillet Burrito with Sausage
Price: $2.81

Save!
250 calories and $1.29!

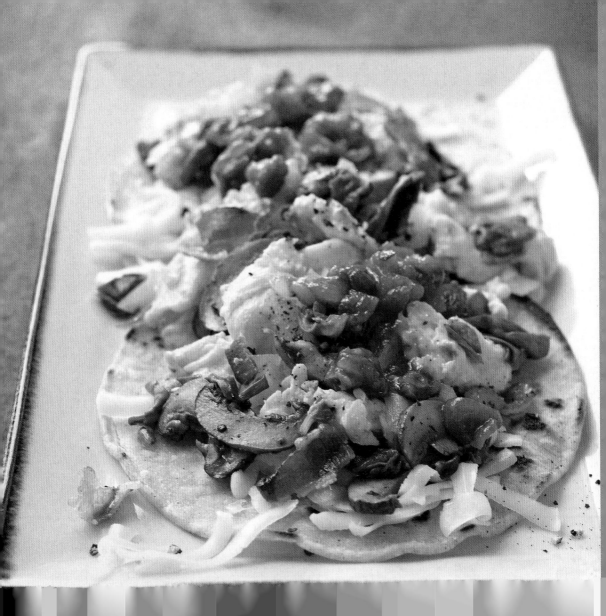

Cook This!
Oatmeal Pancakes with Cinnamon Apples

Banish the Bisquick! The ubiquitous dry mix is fine in a pinch, but if you could make healthier, more delicious pancakes by spending an extra 2 minutes at the mixing bowl, why wouldn't you? Oats and wheat flour give these pancakes a fiber and protein boost, helping stabilize your blood sugar levels as your body absorbs the rush of carbs that comes with a stack of flapjacks.

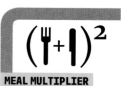

$$\left(\sf{f+l}\right)^2$$

MEAL MULTIPLIER

Supermarket maple syrup is either a) incredibly expensive or b) totally fake, awash in high-fructose corn syrup. Either way, you lose. Fret not, for all of these fruit toppings are not only better for you than normal syrup, they're also considerably more exciting. Combine in a small saucepan and simmer for 10 minutes:

- 2 cups frozen (or fresh) blueberries, 2 tablespoons sugar, and 1 tablespoon grated ginger
- 2 cups frozen strawberries, 1 tablespoon sugar, and 2 tablespoons balsamic vinegar
- 2 cups diced pineapple simmered in 1 cup lite coconut milk and 2 Tbsp shredded coconut

You'll Need:

1½ cups buttermilk

¾ cup instant rolled oats

¾ cup whole-wheat flour

2 Tbsp milk

1 Tbsp melted butter

1½ tsp baking powder

½ tsp baking soda

Pinch of cinnamon, plus ⅛ tsp for the apples

Pinch of nutmeg

1 Granny Smith apple, peeled, cored, and chopped

½ cup apple juice

2 Tbsp brown sugar

Butter or cooking spray

Confectioners' sugar

How to Make It:

- In a large mixing bowl, combine the buttermilk, oats, flour, milk, butter, baking powder, baking soda, pinch of cinnamon, and nutmeg. Stir to gently combine, then set aside to rest for a few minutes.
- Combine the apple, apple juice, brown sugar, and remaining ⅛ teaspoon cinnamon in a small saucepan and bring to a simmer. Cook until the apple has softened and the liquid has thickened.
- Preheat the oven to 200°F. Heat a large nonstick or cast-iron skillet over medium heat. Adding a bit of butter or cooking spray before each round, scoop ¼-cup portions of batter into the skillet and use a spatula to spread into thin, even circles. Cook until small bubbles form in the top of the batter, 2 to 3 minutes, then flip and cook for another 2 minutes. Keep pancakes warm in the oven while you finish cooking. Serve topped with the warm apples and a bit of confectioners' sugar, if you like.

*Makes 4 servings /
Cost per serving: $0.63*

260 calories
6 g fat
(2.5 g saturated)
19 g sugars

940 calories

Not That!
IHOP Harvest Grain 'N Nut Pancakes
with Cinnamon Apple Compote
Price: $7.99

Save!
680 calories and $7.36!

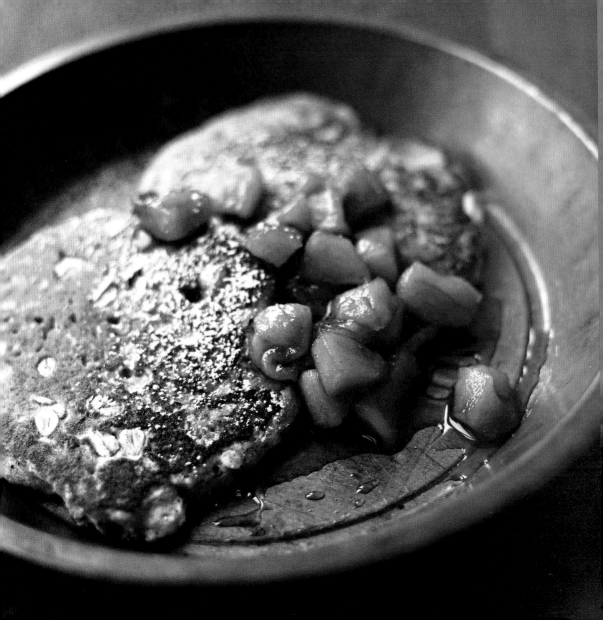

Cook This!

Yogurt with Pineapple, Kiwi, Mango, and Ginger Syrup

Don't be fooled: Flavored yogurt is only a small step away from ice cream. In fact, with some cups carrying up to 30 grams of sugar—as much as you'd find in two scoops of Breyer's All-Natural Vanilla—and it might actually be worse. You'll always be better off starting with plain yogurt, then flavoring it yourself. This refreshing concoction pairs tropical fruit with a spicy-sweet blast of ginger syrup.

You'll Need:

- 1 cup water
- ¼ cup sugar
- 1" piece peeled fresh ginger, sliced
- 24 oz Greek-style yogurt (four 6-oz containers)
- 2 kiwis, peeled and sliced
- 1 cup chopped pineapple
- 1 mango, peeled, pitted, and chopped
- ½ cup granola

How to Make It:

- Combine the water, sugar, and ginger in a small saucepan and bring to a boil. Simmer for 10 minutes. Let cool for at least 10 minutes. Discard the ginger pieces.
- Divide the yogurt among four bowls, top with the fruits and granola, then drizzle with the ginger syrup. For a more dramatic presentation, layer the yogurt, fruit, granola, and syrup in tall glasses, like parfaits.

Makes 4 servings / Cost per serving: $2.07

Fage, our favorite Greek yogurt, contains 7 grams of sugar per serving. The majority of the sugar in this recipe is naturally occurring sugar from the fruit.

The granola is added for texture, but use it sparingly: Those little clusters are dense with calories.

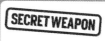
330 calories
4 g fat
(0.5 g saturated)
43 g sugars

640 calories
13 g fat
(4 g saturated)
72 g sugars

Not That!

Au Bon Pain Large Vanilla Yogurt
with Blueberries and Granola Topping
Price: $3.29

Save!
310 calories and $1.22!

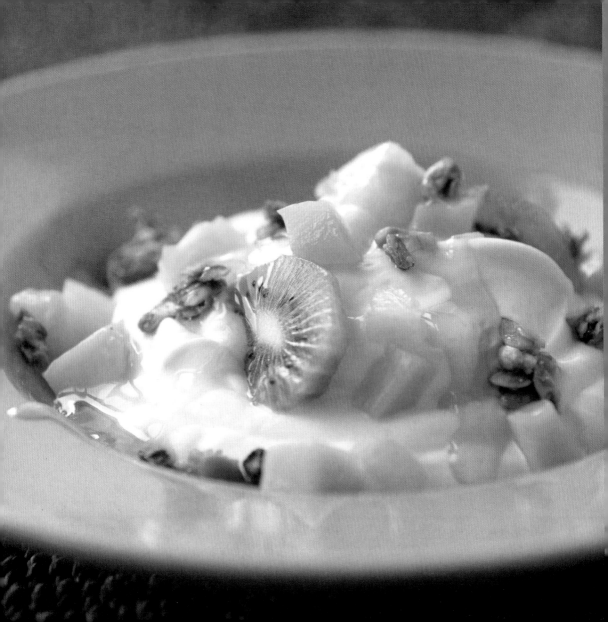

Frittata with Arugula and Pepper

At its core, a frittata is a crustless quiche that's both considerably easier to make and substantially healthier to eat. Make one at the beginning of the week, then slice off a wedge each morning for breakfast. You could even stuff a piece between a toasted English muffin for a gourmet breakfast sandwich.

You'll Need:

½ Tbsp olive oil

¼ cup bottled roasted red peppers, chopped

1 clove garlic, minced

4 cups baby arugula or baby spinach

4 thin slices prosciutto or other good ham, cut into strips

8 eggs, beaten

Salt and black pepper to taste

½ cup crumbled goat cheese •——— *Other cheeses can be used with awesome results. Try smoked gouda, ricotta, or feta. It's your world.*

How to Make It:

● Preheat the broiler. Heat the olive oil in a nonstick, 12" oven-safe skillet over medium-low heat. Add the roasted pepper and garlic and cook for about 1 minute, until the garlic is fragrant but not browned. Stir in the arugula and cook for another 2 minutes or so, until lightly wilted. Add the prosciutto, then pour the eggs over the top. Season the eggs with a good amount of salt and pepper, then dot with the crumbled goat cheese.

● Cook on the stovetop for 5 to 6 minutes, until most of the egg has set. Place the pan 6" under the broiler and cook for about 3 minutes, until the rest of the egg has fully set and the top of the frittata has begun to brown. Cool slightly, remove from the pan, and cut into wedges.

Makes 4 servings / Cost per serving: $2.09

$$(\Psi + \mathbf{I})^2$$

MEAL MULTIPLIER

Don't take the ingredients in this recipe too literally; rather, learn the basic technique, then play around with the filling based on what you like or what your refrigerator happens to be sheltering. Here are a few ideas to get the wheels turning:

● Sautéed chorizo, onions, and poblano peppers

● Leftover chicken or steak; pesto; and ricotta cheese

● Mushrooms, spinach, sundried tomatoes, and feta

325 calories
21 g fat
(6 g saturated)
480 mg sodium

673 calories
48 g fat
(26 g saturated)
1,140 mg sodium

Not That!

Così Quiche Lorraine
Price: $3.49

Save!
348 calories
and $1.40!

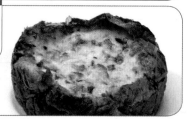

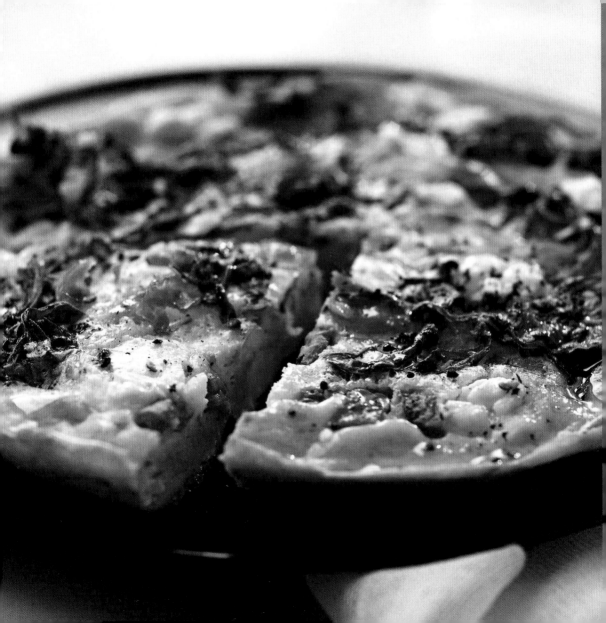

Black Bean Omelet

Why shell out your hard-earned dollars for an overpriced gut bomb when you can make something better, healthier, and cheaper at home in 10 minutes flat? That is the question that defines this book's mission, and nowhere is it more relevant than with omelets. Which would you prefer: an $11 spinach omelet with nearly 1,000 calories, or a $1.50 omelet filled with an oozing center of black beans and cheese, for 330 calories?

You'll Need:

- 1 can (14–16 oz) black beans, drained
- Juice of 1 lime
- ¼ tsp cumin
- Hot sauce
- 8 eggs
- Salt and black pepper to taste
- ½ cup feta cheese, plus more for serving
- Pico de Gallo (see page 307) or bottled salsa
- Sliced avocado (optional)

How to Make It:

- Pulse the black beans, lime juice, cumin, and a few shakes of hot sauce in a food processor until it has the consistency of refried beans, adding a bit of water to help if necessary.

- Coat a small nonstick pan with nonstick cooking spray or a bit of butter or olive oil and heat over medium heat. Crack two eggs into a bowl and beat with a bit of salt and pepper. Add the eggs to the pan, then use a spatula to stir and then lift the cooked egg on the bottom to allow raw egg to slide under. When the eggs have all but set, spoon a quarter of the black bean mixture and 2 tablespoons feta down the middle of the omelet. Use the spatula to fold over a third of the egg to cover the mixture in the center, then carefully slide the omelet onto a plate, using the spatula flip it over at the last second to form one fully rolled omelet.

- Repeat with the remaining ingredients to make four omelets. Garnish with pico de gallo, avocado slices if you like, and bit more crumbled feta.

Makes 4 servings /
Cost per serving: $1.47

330 calories
8 g fat
(6 g saturated)
480 mg sodium

980 calories

Perfect omelets

Cooking an omelet is like scrambling a batch of eggs, only you let it set in a single unified layer before adding your filling. Follow the steps below.

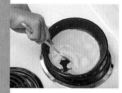

Step 1: *Let raw egg slide underneath the cooked egg*

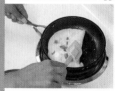

Step 2: *When egg is set, fold the ends over the filling*

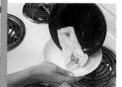

Step 3: *Slide the omelet out onto a warm plate*

Not That!
IHOP Spinach and Mushroom Omelette
Price: $10.99

Save!
650 calories and $9.52!

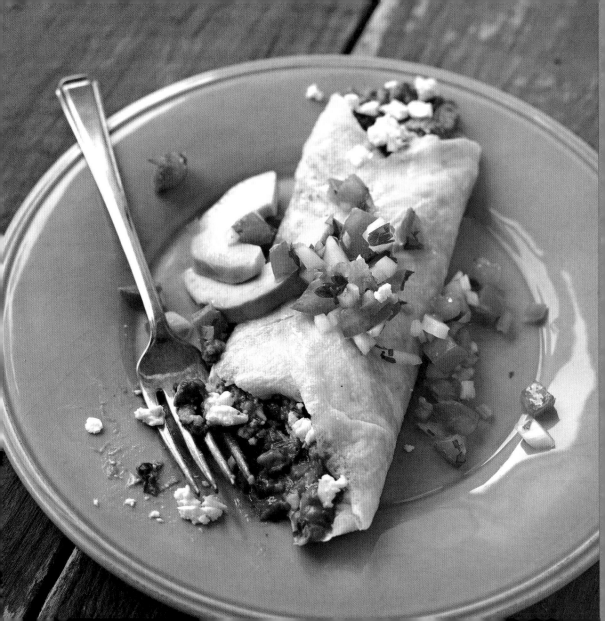

Cook This!

French Toast Stuffed with Strawberries

Odds are, if the word "stuffed" is in the menu description, the dish is dangerous. That's because restaurants choose to use "stuffed" as an excuse to sandwich extra quantities of the cheapest ingredients they have on hand—fat, sugar, salt—into an already-troubled creation. Case in point: IHOP's over-the-top French toast. Its stuffing technique takes a few pieces of bread and some fruit and turns them into a dish with more than half your day's caloric allotment. Done correctly, stuffing can actually be a nutritional boon: Here, it adds a dose of low-cal protein, fiber, and all the energy-boosting vitamins from fresh strawberries. Plus, it's simple enough to pull off on a weekday morning.

You'll Need:

- 1 cup low-fat ricotta or cottage cheese
- ½ cup skim milk
- 2 cups strawberries, sliced
- 2 Tbsp honey
- 2 Tbsp sliced or chopped almonds
- 1 Tbsp butter
- 2 eggs
- 1 cup milk
- ¼ tsp cinnamon
- 1 tsp vanilla extract
- 8 slices whole-wheat bread

Powdered sugar (optional)

How to Make It:

- Place the ricotta, milk, strawberries, honey, and almonds in a mixing bowl and stir gently to combine. Set aside.
- Heat the butter in a large cast-iron skillet or nonstick pan over medium heat. Beat the eggs with the milk, cinnamon, and vanilla in a shallow dish. Working one slice at a time, place the bread in the egg mixture, turning it over once to thoroughly coat, then add it directly to the hot pan. Repeat until the pan is full.
- Cook each slice for 2 to 3 minutes per side, until a golden brown crust is formed. Remove from the pan. Divide the strawberry mixture among four slices of toast, spreading to evenly coat. Top them each with another slice to make a sandwich, then slice on the diagonal to create two equal triangles. Serve with a shake of powdered sugar or a drizzle of pure maple syrup, if you prefer.

Makes 4 servings / Cost per serving: $2.11

370 calories
12 g fat
(4 g saturated)

1,180 calories

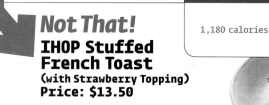

Not That!

IHOP Stuffed French Toast
(with Strawberry Topping)
Price: $13.50

Save!
810 calories and $11.39!

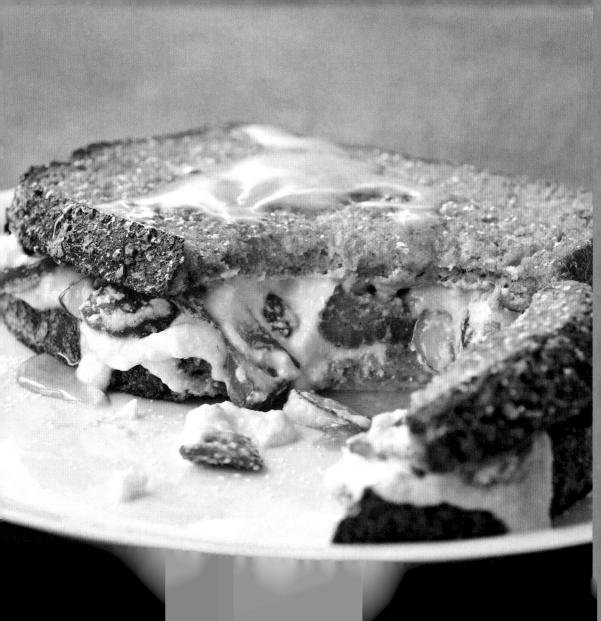

Breakfast Pizzas

In years of restaurant research, we've seen every kind of pizza imaginable—Mexican pizza, Thai chicken pizza, dessert pizza—but, shockingly enough, no breakfast pizza. Befuddling, given just how easy and tasty it can be. Start with the ultimate breakfast bread—the fiber-dense whole-wheat English muffin—as your base and salsa as your sauce, then add eggs, ham, and cheese for flavor, substance, and plenty of protein. Beats an 800-calorie breakfast sandwich any day.

You'll Need:

½ Tbsp butter

6 eggs, beaten

Salt and black pepper to taste

4 oz ham, cut into thin strips

4 whole-wheat or multigrain English muffins, split and lightly toasted

1 cup prepared salsa

1 cup shredded low-fat Jack or Cheddar

How to Make It:

● Preheat the broiler. Heat the butter in a large nonstick pan. When the butter is fully melted, season the eggs with salt and pepper, then add to the pan, along with the ham strips. Cook, using a wooden spoon or rubber spatula to keep stirring the eggs as they set. Remove the pan from the heat about 30 seconds before the eggs are fully done (they'll continue to cook in the pan and in the oven).

● Slather each English muffin half with a good spoonful of salsa. Divide the eggs among the English muffins, then top with the cheese. Place all the English muffins on a baking sheet and broil (6" from the heat is ideal) until the cheese is fully melted and browned around the edges.

Makes 8 pizzas, or 4 servings / Cost per serving: $1.96

Thomas Multi-Grain Light English Muffins are the best in the aisles, packing 8 grams of fiber and just 100 calories.

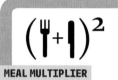

$$\left(\textbf{Y}+\textbf{I}\right)^2$$

MEAL MULTIPLIER

These individual pizzas have Mexican flavors at the base, but breakfast pizza can be interpreted in dozens of different ways. Here are a few other combinations (all include scrambled egg as part of the creation) that will get your day off to a rousing start:

● Pesto, mozzarella, and a few slices of tomato

● Marinara, provolone or fontina cheese, and shredded chicken

● Guacamole, Swiss, turkey, and tomato

350 calories
19 g fat
(8 g saturated)
900 mg sodium

780 calories
42 g fat
(16 g saturated)
2,580 mg sodium

Not That!

Denny's Moons Over My Hammy
Price: $7.99

Save!

430 calories and $6.03!

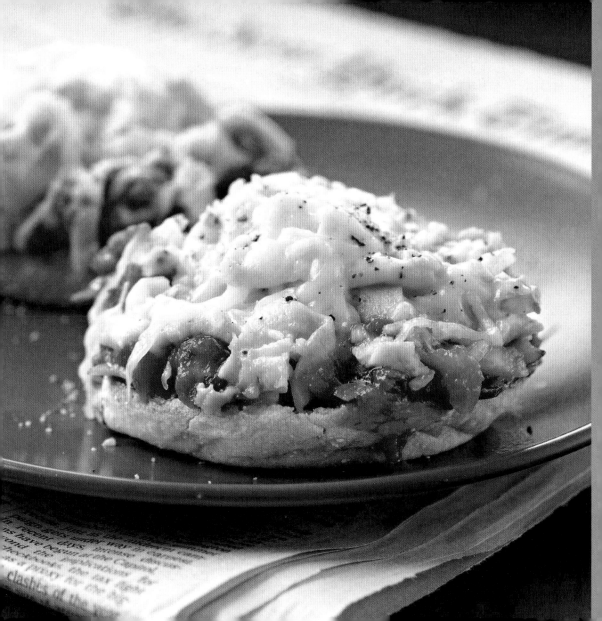

Cook This!

Baked Egg with Mushrooms and Spinach

Looking for some excitement in your weekday breakfast routine? Then ditch the cereal, drop the frozen waffles, and, for goodness sake, put down that bagel! Instead, pick up a ramekin and preheat the oven. The little ceramic vessels are perfect for housing eggs, meat, cheese, and vegetables and then tossing in the oven. What emerges 10 minutes later is a perfectly cooked egg—whites soft but firm, yolk gloriously runny—surrounded by a tasty and filling supporting cast. Use a larger ramekin if you'd prefer two eggs for breakfast. Either way, we suggest some whole-wheat toast soldiers to dip directly into the dish.

You'll Need:

- 1 **Tbsp olive oil**
- 1 **small onion, chopped**
- 2 **cups mushrooms, sliced**
- 4 **slices Canadian bacon or deli ham, cut into thin strips**
- ½ **(10 oz) bag frozen spinach, thawed**
- ½ **(7 oz) can roasted green chiles**
- **Salt and black pepper to taste**
- 4 **eggs**

How to Make It:

- Preheat the oven to 375°F. Heat the oil in a large skillet set over medium heat. Add the onion and cook for about 3 minutes, until translucent. Add the mushrooms and cook for about 5 minutes, until lightly browned. Stir in the bacon, spinach, and chiles and cook for a few minutes, until the spinach is heated through. If any water from the spinach accumulates in the pan, carefully drain. Season with salt and pepper.
- Divide the mixture among 4 6-ounce oven-safe ramekins that have been lightly greased with butter. Carefully crack an egg into each, making sure to keep the yolks intact. Place the ramekins in a baking dish and bake until the whites are just set but the yolks are still runny, about 10 minutes.

Makes 4 servings /
Cost per serving: $1.76

150 calories
9 g fat
(2.5 g saturated)
560 mg sodium

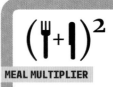

$$(\Upsilon + \rceil)^2$$

MEAL MULTIPLIER

Toss one of these in the oven when you wake up and it will be ready to eat when you get out of the shower. Keep it fresh and exciting by changing the supporting ingredients as often as possible (or just use it as an excuse to get rid of vegetables, deli meats, and cheeses sitting around in your fridge). Invent at will, but take these ideas for inspiration:

- Leftover chicken, salsa verde, and crumbled feta
- Chili, diced onions, and Cheddar
- Chopped fresh herbs (parsley, thyme, rosemary) and a splash of cream

Not That!

Panera Bread Spinach and Artichoke Egg Soufflé
Price: $3.59

540 calories
34 g fat
(19 g saturated,
0.5 g trans)
910 mg sodium

Save!
390 calories
and $1.83!

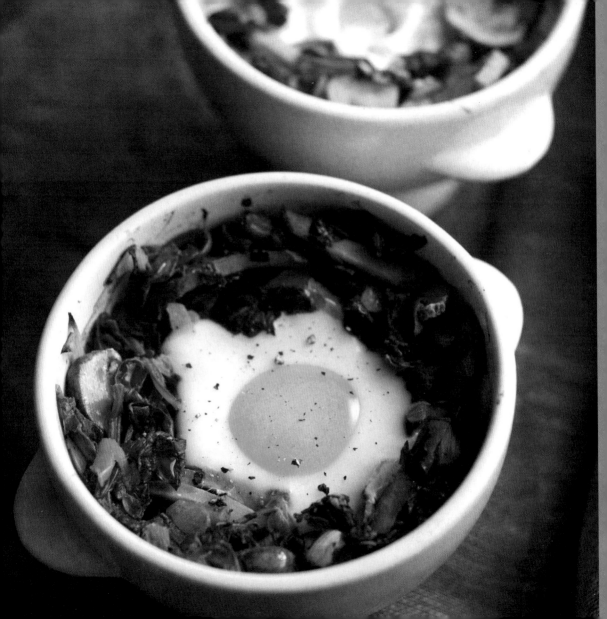

Breakfast Hash with Sweet Potato and Chicken Sausage

For years now, hash has carried a certain negative connotation, conjuring up images of either murky, over-salted slop eaten from a can or a group of peripatetic hippies on their first trip to Morocco. The former can be made from any combination of protein and vegetables; and by replacing the beef with lean chunks of chicken sausage and the greasy spuds with crispy sweet potato nuggets and bell pepper, you end up with a whole that is far greater than the sum of its parts. Served with a Bloody Mary chaser, this is exactly the kind of meal you want to soak up the excesses of a big night out.

You'll Need:

- 2 medium sweet potatoes, peeled and cut into ¼" cubes
- ½ Tbsp olive oil
- 2 links uncooked chicken sausage (chicken-apple works nicely)
- 1 medium yellow onion, chopped
- 1 red bell pepper, chopped
- ⅛ tsp cayenne pepper
- Salt and black pepper to taste
- 4 eggs, fried sunny-side up (see right)
- Tabasco sauce

How to Make It:

- Place the potatoes in a medium saucepan and cover with water. Bring to a boil and cook until fork tender, about 10 minutes. Drain.
- Heat the oil in a large cast-iron or nonstick skillet over medium heat. Cut open the sausage casing and squeeze the meat directly into the pan, discarding the casing. Sauté for 4 to 5 minutes, until the meat is cooked through. Transfer to a plate.
- In the same pan, add the reserved sweet potatoes, the onion, and red pepper. Cook until the potatoes and vegetables are browned, about 7 minutes. Return the sausage to the pan, season with the cayenne and salt and pepper, and stir to mix.
- Divide the hash among four plates or bowls. Top each serving with a fried egg and Tabasco.

Makes 4 servings /
Cost per serving: $1.50

230 calories
11 g fat
(4.5 g saturated)
290 mg sodium

Master THE TECHNIQUE

Perfect fried eggs

Impatience is the easiest way to ensure a tough, underwhelming egg. Heat a nonstick skillet over medium-low heat and add just enough butter or olive oil to lightly coat the pan. Crack the eggs directly into the pan and let them sit, undisturbed, until the whites fully coagulate, but the yolks are still wobbly, about 5 minutes. Season with salt and pepper.

Not That!
Bob Evans Pot Roast Hash
Price: $7.49

681 calories
45 g fat
(14 g saturated)
1,205 mg sodium

Save!
451 calories
and $5.99!

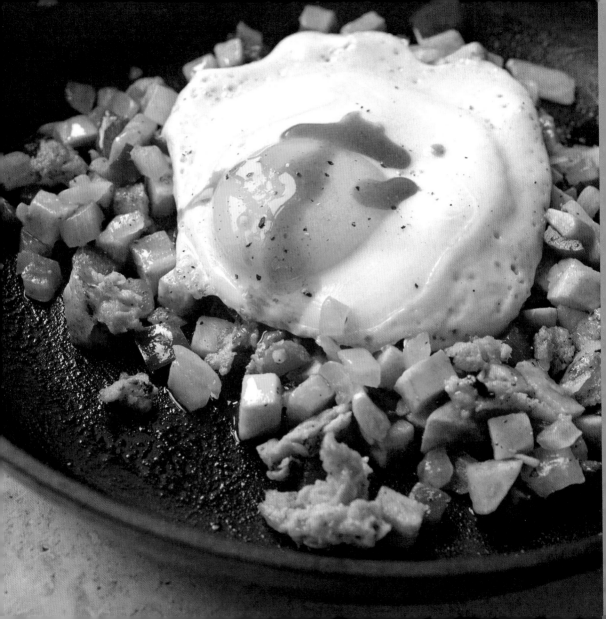

Cook This!

Smoked Salmon Sandwich

This is a New York classic, minus the bagel. All the great flavors that make this such a satisfying breakfast are still here—the richness of smoked salmon, the bite of onion and capers, the sweetness of tomato—but by ditching the oversize bagel in favor of whole-wheat toast, you save about 200 calories and trade a ton of refined carbs for a boost of fiber. The end result is a sandwich you can feel good about eating every day of the week, and given that it takes about as much time to make as it does to pour a bowl of cereal, why not?

You'll Need:

- ¼ cup whipped cream cheese
- 8 slices whole-wheat or 9-grain bread, toasted
- 2 Tbsp capers, rinsed and chopped
- ½ red onion, thinly sliced
- 2 cups mixed baby greens
- 1 large tomato, sliced
- Salt and black pepper to taste
- 8 oz smoked salmon

How to Make It:

- Spread 1 tablespoon of the cream cheese on each of four slices of toast. Top each with capers, onion, greens, and a slice or two of tomato. Lightly salt the tomato, then add as much pepper as you'd like (this sandwich cries out for a lot of it). Finish by draping a few slices of smoked salmon over the tomatoes and topping with the remaining slices of toasted bread.

Makes 4 sandwiches / Cost per serving: $3.17

Not only is whipped cream cheese easier to spread, it's also less calorie-dense than the stuff that comes in a block.

280 calories
10 g fat
(3 g saturated)
460 mg sodium

530 calories
19 g fat
(7.5 g saturated)
820 mg sodium

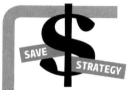

SAVE $ STRATEGY

As much as we love smoked salmon—not just for its full-throttle flavor and silky texture, but also for its concentration of omega-3 fatty acids—it's not cheap. Granted, it takes only a few slices to make an excellent sandwich, but if you want a more affordable way to make this a part of your breakfast repertoire, try subbing in smoked turkey, ham, or even canned tuna. The nutritional info won't change much and it will still be twice as satisfying as any breakfast sandwich you can score from a drive-thru window.

Not That!

Dunkin' Donuts Multigrain Bagel
with Reduced Fat Smoked Salmon Cream Cheese
Price: $2.43

Save!
250 calories
9 grams of fat!

42

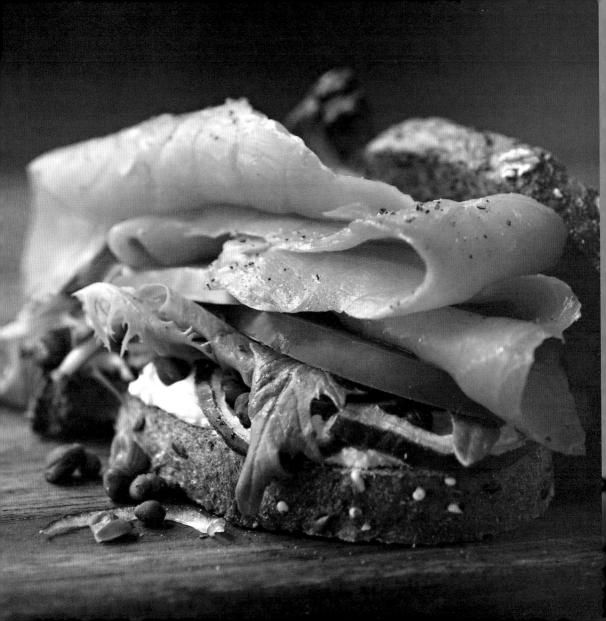

Cook This!
Tortilla Española

Anyone who has ever spent time in Spain will recognize this recipe as the humble national staple found on nearly every bar counter from Barcelona to Malaga, a tender omelet layered with potatoes and sweet onions. The simplicity of the ingredient list belies the depth, nuance, and soul-satisfying deliciousness a properly cooked tortilla is capable of achieving. A true Spaniard would cook the potatoes and onions in a liter of olive oil and would never use the broiler to finish the cooking, but we've cut back the fat and employed the oven to make this addictive dish easier on you, and your waistline.

You'll Need:

- 3 medium Yukon Gold potatoes (about 1 ½ pounds), diced into ⅓" cubes
- 2 Tbsp olive oil
- 1 large yellow onion, diced
- 1 tsp salt
- 8 eggs, beaten

How to Make It:

- Fill a large cast-iron skillet or 12" sauté pan with water. Add the potatoes and bring to a boil. Cook for about 10 minutes, until the potatoes have softened but aren't completely tender. Drain.
- Preheat the broiler. Return the potatoes to the same pan, along with the olive oil and onion, and cook over medium-low heat, stirring occasionally, for about 5 minutes, until the onions begin to brown and the potatoes are cooked through. Season with the salt.
- Add the eggs to the pan, cover, and cook for about 10 minutes, until most of the egg is set. Uncover and finish by placing the pan 6" under the broiler for 3 to 4 minutes to brown the top of the tortilla. Let the tortilla rest for a few minutes. When ready to eat, slip from the pan and cut into wedges.

Makes 6 servings / Cost per serving: $1.06

Omelets should be the first restaurant food you give up, given how no food comes with a higher caloric markup.

255 calories
10 g fat
(2.5 g saturated)
480 mg sodium

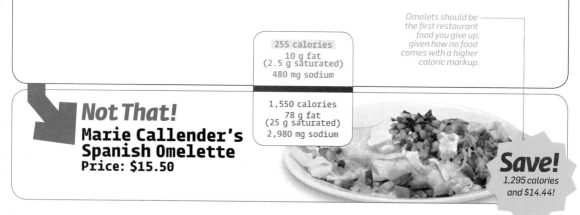

Not That!
Marie Callender's Spanish Omelette
Price: $15.50

1,550 calories
78 g fat
(25 g saturated)
2,980 mg sodium

Save!
1,295 calories and $14.44!

44

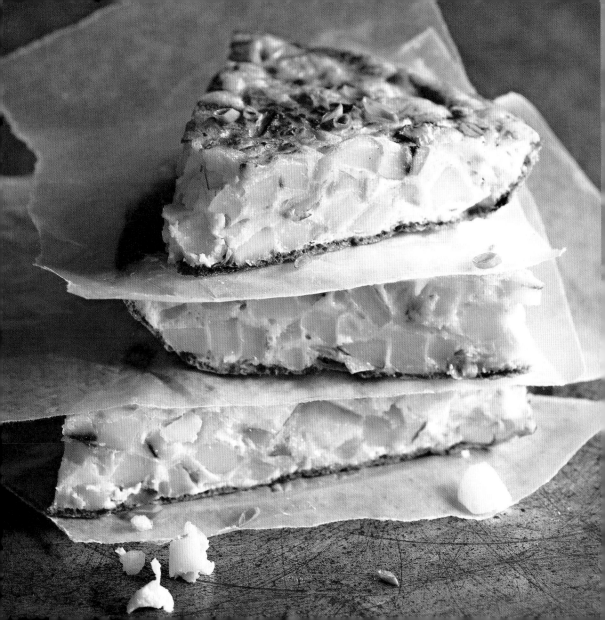

Banana Bread

Most banana bread recipes call for twice the amount of butter used here, but to keep the loaf moist and rich and tasting intensely of its namesake fruit, we cut the butter and added an extra banana and Greek-style yogurt. This is no breakfast of champions, but it's a healthier alternative to other banana breads or, even worse, a banana, bran, or blueberry muffin (hard to believe, but they truly are bad for you). A slice of this will treat you well at breakfast. Better yet, make it for dessert. Toast it up and serve with a bit of whipped cream.

You'll Need:

- 4 very ripe bananas, peeled and mashed (about 2 cups)
- ½ cup Greek-style yogurt
- 4 Tbsp butter, melted
- 2 large eggs
- 1 tsp vanilla
- 2 cups flour
- ¾ cup sugar
- ½ cup toasted walnuts, coarsely chopped
- 1 tsp baking soda
- 1 tsp baking powder
- ½ tsp ground cinnamon
- ½ tsp salt

How to Make It:

- Preheat the oven to 350°F. Butter a 9" x 5" x 3" loaf pan.
- Combine the bananas, yogurt, butter, eggs, and vanilla in a large mixing bowl, stirring to blend. In a separate bowl, mix together the flour, sugar, walnuts, baking soda, baking powder, cinnamon, and salt. Gently fold the dry ingredients into the wet banana mixture and stir until fully incorporated.
- Scrape the batter into the prepared pan. Bake on a low oven rack for about 50 minutes, until a toothpick inserted into the center of the bread comes out clean. Let cool for 5 minutes in the pan. Eat warm or at room temperature.

Makes 4 servings / Cost per serving: $0.96

$$(\Psi + \mathbf{I})^2$$

MEAL MULTIPLIER

Banana bread can be tricked out in a variety of different ways, some making it healthier and more suitable for breakfast, others bringing a level of decadence that edges it into the dessert realm. Stir in any of the following add-ons just before pouring the batter into the pan:

- 1 cup blueberries, fresh or frozen
- ¼ cup shredded coconut
- 1 cup semisweet chocolate chips
- 2 tablespoons smooth peanut butter

350 calories
12 g fat
(4.5 g saturated)
27 g sugars

490 calories
19 g fat
(2.5 g saturated)
46 g sugars

Not That!
Starbucks Banana Nut Loaf
Price: $2.16

Save!
140 calories and $1.20!

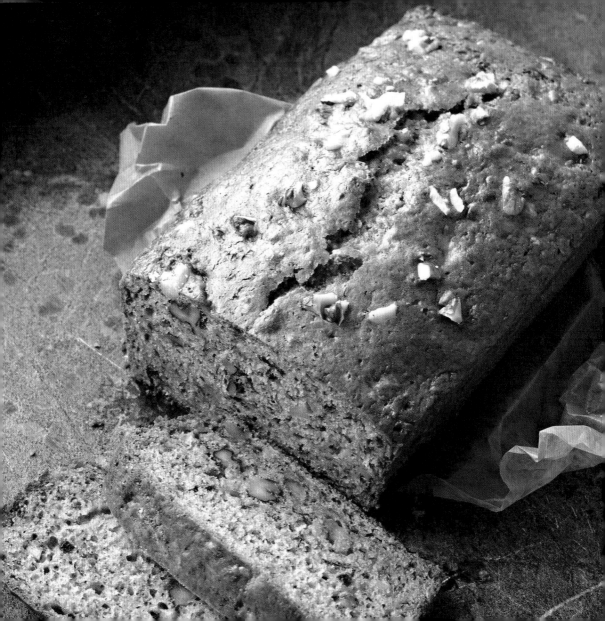

Chapter

Appetizers & Small Bites
The perfect start to any meal

Cook This!
Ultimate Guacamole

Nobody should be without a solid guacamole recipe. Sure, it's a healthy, incredibly delicious condiment that makes almost anything it touches taste better, but there's an even more compelling reason to commit this recipe to memory: It's because having an awesome guac recipe is one of the easiest ways to impress others. Master it and you become the "guac guy" or "guac girl," that person who needs to be at the party on Saturday and who needs to bring along the best guacamole ever. We hope this recipe helps you achieve such a vaunted status.

You'll Need:

- ¼ cup chopped cilantro
- 2 cloves garlic, minced

Salt to taste

- 2 ripe avocados, pitted and peeled
- ¼ cup minced onion
- 2 Tbsp minced jalapeño pepper

Juice of 1 lemon

- 2 oz tortilla chips

How to Make It:

● Combine the cilantro and garlic on a cutting board and use the back of a chef's knife to work them into a fine paste; a pinch of coarse salt helps this process. (If you own a mortar and pestle, there's never been a better time to use it.) Transfer the paste to a bowl and add the avocado. Use a fork to smash the avocado into a mostly smooth—but still slightly chunky—puree. Stir in the onion, jalapeño, lemon juice, and salt. Serve with tortilla chips or warm corn tortillas.

Makes 4 servings / Cost per serving: $0.93

Always buy Hass, or California, avocados—the ones with the dark pebbly skin. They have a higher healthy fat content and creamier taste and texture.

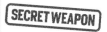

SECRET WEAPON

Mortar and pestle

The mortar and pestle is a critical tool for unlocking the flavors behind many of the world's most thrilling culinary creations, from pesto from Italy to curries from Thailand to salsa and guacamole from Mexico. By pounding ingredients like herbs and spices, garlic cloves, and chiles, you release their essential oils, infusing dishes with an intense flavor that is impossible to achieve with a knife or a food processor. While ceramic mortars are good-looking, look for a volcanic or granite base with a slightly rough exterior; it's abrasion you're looking for to unlock those essential oils, and this tool does it the best.

190 calories
15 g fat
(1.5 g saturated)
440 mg sodium

1,340 calories
83 g fat
(8 g saturated,
2.5 g trans)
950 mg sodium

Not That!
Baja Fresh Chips and Guacamole
Price: $3.49

Save!
1,150 calories
and $2.56!

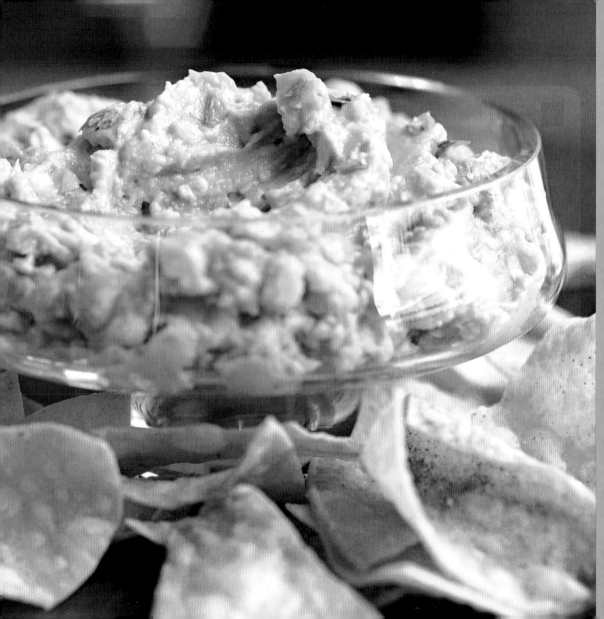

Cook This!

Hummus

Hummus earned a reputation in the United States a few decades back as hippie food, the provenance of people with knotted dreadlocks and rainbow bumper stickers. But its ubiquity in the refrigerator section of the average market these days shows that it has endeared itself to quite a few Johnny and Sally Punchclocks, and that's a great thing. The store-bought stuff is fine, but it can't touch the hummus you can make in your food processor with a few flicks of the wrist.

You'll Need:

- 3 whole-wheat pitas, cut into wedges
- 1 can (14–16 oz) garbanzo beans (aka chickpeas), drained
- 2 Tbsp tahini
- Juice of 1 lemon
- 2 cloves garlic, minced
- ½ tsp cumin
- ½ tsp salt
- 2 Tbsp olive oil

How to Make It:

- Preheat the oven to 400°F. Place the pita wedges on a baking sheet and bake for 10 minutes, until hot and lightly crisped.
- Combine the beans, tahini, lemon juice, garlic, cumin, and salt in a food processor and puree. With the motor running, drizzle in the olive oil until the hummus has a thick, creamy consistency. If the mixture is still too thick, add a bit of water to thin it out. Serve with the toasted pita wedges. Keeps in the refrigerator for up to a week.

Makes 6 servings / Cost per serving: $0.74

Tahini is a paste made from ground sesame seeds. Thanks to hummus's popularity, it's easy to find these days, but if you can't, try 1 tablespoon of smooth peanut butter for the 2 tablespoons of tahini here.

$$(\Psi + I)^2$$

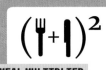

MEAL MULTIPLIER

Hummus is dying to be embellished. The best part about making it from scratch at home (besides the money you'll save) is that you can punch it up however you like. Try these additions:

- 5 or 6 whole roasted garlic cloves
- ½ cup bottled roasted red peppers
- 2 teaspoons canned chipotle pepper
- ¼ cup sundried tomatoes, minced
- ¼ cup chopped black olives
- Fresh herbs: basil, rosemary, thyme, or parsley

210 calories
9 g fat
(2 g saturated)
460 mg sodium

861 calories
4 g saturated fat
1,562 mg sodium

Not That!

California Pizza Kitchen Tuscan Hummus
with Traditional Pita
Price: $6.49

Save!

651 calories and $5.75!

52

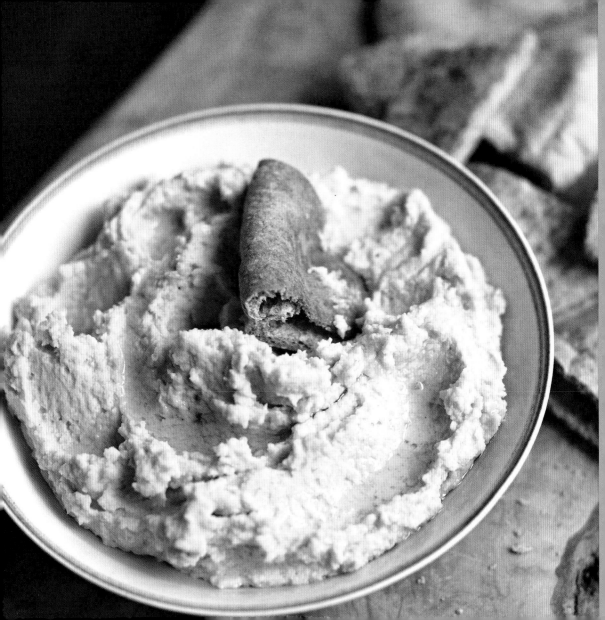

Cook This!
Cheese Fries

When we released our first list of the 20 Worst Foods in America back in 2007, Outback's Aussie Cheese Fries occupied the top slot, packing an outrageous 2,900 calories and 182 grams of fat. While the steakhouse has managed to trim those numbers ever so slightly, the prospect of eating fried potatoes covered in cheese at a restaurant is as dangerous as ever. This easy home version keeps the calories low by baking the potatoes until crisp, applying just the right amount of cheese, and using a few hunks of crumbled bacon and a handful of pickled jalapeños to give the impression of decadence without the four-digit damage.

You'll Need:

- 2 large russet potatoes, peeled and cut into ¼" fries
- 1 Tbsp olive oil
- 1 tsp chili powder
- ¼ tsp smoked paprika (optional)

Salt and black pepper to taste

- 1 cup shredded Pepper Jack cheese
- 4 slices bacon, cooked and crumbled
- 5 scallions, chopped

Pickled Jalapeños (see page 307)

How to Make It:

- Preheat the oven to 425°F. Toss the potatoes with the olive oil, chili powder, smoked paprika (if using), and salt and pepper. Spread out on a rimmed baking sheet and bake for about 20 minutes, until deep brown and crispy on the outside. Top with the cheese, bacon, and scallions, and return to the oven. Bake until the cheese is fully melted and beginning to brown. Garnish with pickled jalapeños.

Makes 4 servings / Cost per serving: $1.21

The cut of the fry is critical. Slice off the lengths of the potato to create flat surfaces, then cut the potato into 1/4-inch planks. Stack the planks and cut into 1/4-inch fries.

300 calories
13 g fat
(5 g saturated)
310 mg sodium

2,136 calories
151 g fat
(72 g saturated)
2,344 mg sodium

Not That!
Outback Aussie Cheese Fries
Price: $7.95

Save!
1,836 calories and $6.74!

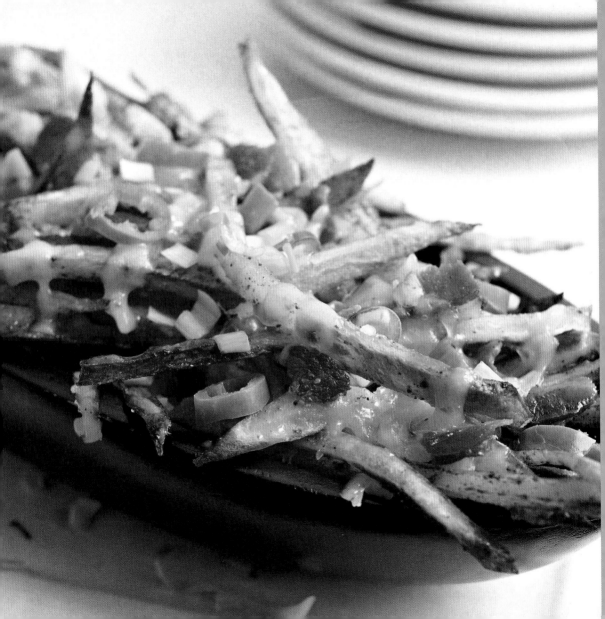

Cook This!
Shrimp Cocktail

If there's a better way to start a meal, we haven't found it. Shrimp derives about 80 percent of its calories from protein, making it one of the leanest sources of the belly-filling, metabolism-revving macronutrient. Problem is, eating shrimp cocktail outside of the house is a recipe for sodium overload, as restaurants tend to turn cocktail sauce into a saline solution. We cut back on the salt by making a fiery homemade cocktail sauce and improve matters with the shrimp by skipping the precooked store-bought kind (most of which are pretty disappointing) in favor of quickly oven-roasting fresh crustaceans tossed in Old Bay. The only thing this recipe is missing is a frosty beer.

You'll Need:

- 1 lb raw shrimp, peeled and deveined (see right)
- 1 Tbsp olive oil
- ½ tsp Old Bay seasoning (optional)
- Salt and black pepper to taste
- ½ cup ketchup
- Juice of ½ lemon
- 1 Tbsp prepared horseradish
- 1 tsp sriracha or other hot sauce

How to Make It:

- Preheat the oven to 400°F. On a baking sheet, toss the shrimp with the olive oil, Old Bay (if using), and salt and pepper. Bake for about 5 minutes, until the shrimp are pink and just firm.
- While the shrimp cook, combine the ketchup, lemon juice, horseradish, and sriracha. Taste and adjust the spice level to your preference. Serve with the shrimp.

Makes 4 servings / Cost per serving: $2.83

Save!
460 calories and $5.66!

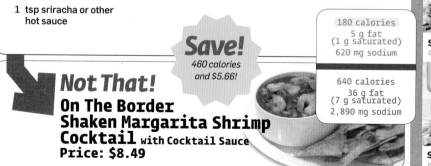

```
180 calories
5 g fat
(1 g saturated)
620 mg sodium
```

```
640 calories
36 g fat
(7 g saturated)
2,890 mg sodium
```

Not That!
On The Border Shaken Margarita Shrimp Cocktail with Cocktail Sauce
Price: $8.49

STEP-BY-STEP

Deveining shrimp

The vein running down the back of the shrimp is actually its digestive tract, so removing it is a pretty good idea before cooking. Luckily, it's also super simple.

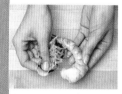

Step 1: *Peel off the shrimp shell and legs*

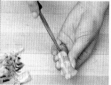

Step 2: *Make an incision down the back of the shrimp*

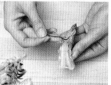

Step 3: *Remove the vein with a knife or your hands*

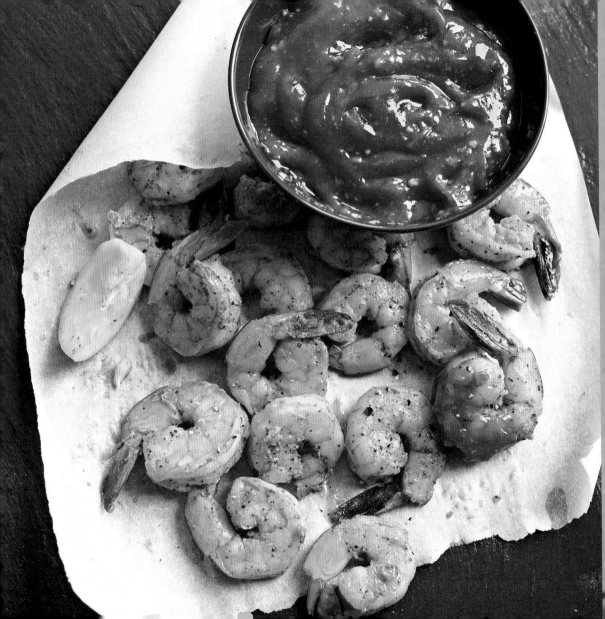

Beijing Wings

Even if you're a lifelong wing junkie, it's unlikely that you've ever had one that wasn't a) deep fried and b) slathered in hot sauce and melted butter. There are two fundamental flaws in this unshakeable two-pronged approach. First, chicken wings have plenty of natural fat, so cooking them in boiling oil is like committing a fat-on-fat crime. As for the Buffalo treatment, hot sauce and butter are great, but wings scream out for other bold treatments. We soak these wings in an Asian marinade, then roast them at high temperature in the oven (though a grill would be nice, too) to crisp them up. Once you go Beijing, you'll have a hard time finding your way back to Buffalo.

You'll Need:

- ½ cup low-sodium soy sauce
- ¼ cup brown sugar
- 4 cloves garlic, minced
- 1 Tbsp grated fresh ginger
- 2 lbs chicken wings
- 2 Tbsp butter
- 1 Tbsp sriracha
- Juice of ½ lime
- Sesame seeds and chopped scallions (optional)

How to Make It:

- Combine the soy sauce, half the brown sugar, the garlic, and ginger in a sealable plastic bag. Add the wings, mix to coat, and seal the bag. Marinate in the refrigerator for at least 1 hour or up to 8.

- Preheat the oven to 450°F. Remove the wings from the marinade and lay out on a baking sheet lined with lightly oiled aluminum foil (for easier cleanup), making sure they're evenly spaced. Roast for about 15 minutes, until the meat firms up and is cooked through and the skin begins to caramelize and crisp up.

- Heat the butter, sriracha, lime juice, and remaining brown sugar in a large nonstick skillet. When the butter has melted, add the wings and sauté for 2 to 3 minutes, until the sauce clings lightly to the chicken. Garnish with the sesame seeds and scallions (if you like).

Makes 4 servings / Cost per serving: $1.94

290 calories
10 g fat
(4.5 g saturated)
890 mg sodium

1,377 calories
100 g fat
(31 g saturated)
3,819 mg sodium

Not That!
Outback Kookaburra Wings
Price: $7.95

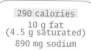

Save!
1,087 calories and $6.01!

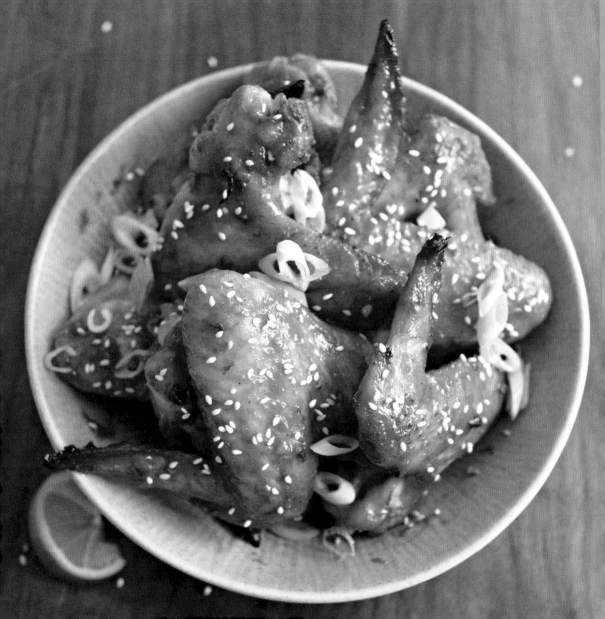

Cook This!
Chipotle Shrimp Quesadilla

The key to a world-class quesadilla is careful crisping of the tortilla exterior. Restaurants make up for their sloppy cooking by adding more cheese and oil to the equation, which is why we've never, in years of analyzing nutritional information, found a restaurant quesadilla with fewer than 900 calories and 50 grams of fat. This quesadilla is plenty cheesy, but the abundance of spicy shrimp and caramelized vegetables teamed with the shattering crust of the tortilla means we can cut fat without sacrificing flavor.

You'll Need:

- 8 oz medium shrimp, peeled and deveined
- ½ cup orange juice
- 1 Tbsp canned chipotle pepper
- 2 cloves garlic, minced
- ½ Tbsp canola oil
- 1 medium onion, sliced
- 1 red or yellow bell pepper, sliced

Salt and black pepper to taste

- 4 large whole-wheat tortillas
- 2 cups shredded Monterey Jack cheese

Salsa

Guacamole (see page 50), optional

How to Make It:

- Combine the shrimp with the orange juice, chipotle, and garlic. Marinate for 15 minutes.
- Heat the oil in a large cast-iron skillet or sauté pan over medium-high heat. When the oil is lightly smoking, add the onion and pepper and cook for about 10 minutes, until lightly charred on the outside. Push the vegetables to the perimeter of the pan and add the the shrimp to the center. Sauté until cooked through, about 10 minutes. Season with salt and pepper to taste. Remove from the heat.
- Coat a separate nonstick pan with cooking spray, oil, or butter and heat over medium-low heat. Place one tortilla in the bottom, sprinkle with half of the cheese, then top with half of the shrimp mixture and a second tortilla. Cook for about 5 minutes, until the bottom is very crisp, then flip and cook for another 2 to 3 minutes. Cut the quesadillas into wedges and serve with salsa and a bit of guacamole, if you like.

Makes 4 servings /
Cost per serving: $3.45

Master THE TECHNIQUE

Crisp Quesadillas

Cooking quesadillas, one side at a time, in a cast-iron or non-stick skillet is the best, but by no means is it the only, method. Have a big batch? Fire up the grill and place them directly on the well-oiled grates for a few minutes a side. Or pop them in a 450°F oven for 12 minutes, flipping them once midway through.

340 calories
15 g fat
(8 g saturated)
750 mg sodium

1,465 calories
89 g fat
3,528 mg sodium

Not That!
Ruby Tuesday Buffalo Shrimp Quesadilla
Price: $11.99

Save!
1,125 calories and $8.54!

60

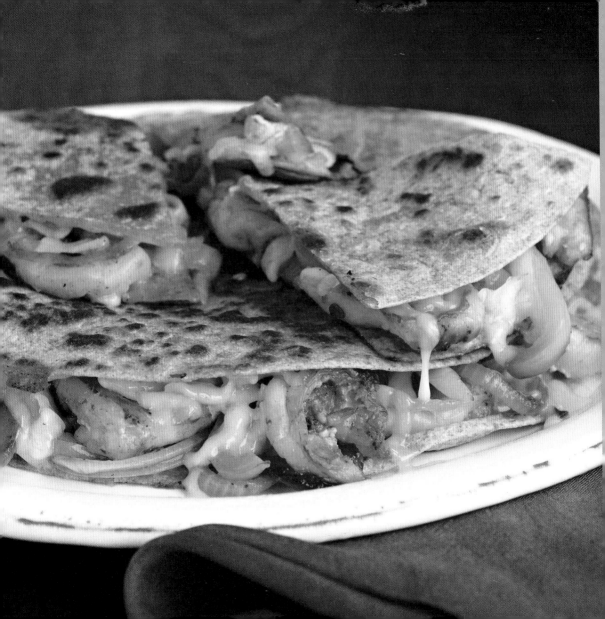

Cook This!

Mussels with Garlic and White Wine

The only shellfish most cooks bother messing with at home is shrimp, which is a shame, because clams, oysters, and especially mussels are begging for an invite to your dinner table. Packed with protein, omega-3s, and a cache of energy-boosting B vitamins, they make an ideal way to start a meal. Or add a salad and call it dinner. Build a flavor base with onions, garlic, and other aromatics, then add the mussels and enough liquid to create some steam. Cover and cook until they pop open, about 5 minutes or so. And make sure you have plenty of crusty bread for dunking in the sumptuous broth at the bottom of the bowl.

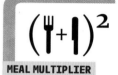

$$(\text{\textipa{Y}}+\text{I})^2$$

MEAL MULTIPLIER

Mussels are a blank protein canvas, ready to be embellished endlessly with bold international flavors. Follow the same basic technique highlighted here, but for the wine, tomatoes, and parsley, trade in one of these combinations:

- Light coconut milk, red curry paste, and chopped fresh cilantro or scallions
- Diced bacon, caramelized onion, Dijon, and chicken stock
- Canned tomato puree, chopped olives, red pepper flakes, and red wine

You'll Need:

- 1 Tbsp butter
- 1 small red onion, thinly sliced
- 4 cloves garlic, minced
- 1 large tomato, chopped
- Salt to taste
- 1 cup white wine
- 1 tsp saffron (optional)
- 2 lbs mussels, scrubbed and debearded
- Chopped fresh parsley for garnish

How to Make It:

- Heat the butter in a large stockpot over medium heat. Add the onion and garlic and cook for 5 minutes, until the onion is translucent. Add the tomato and cook for 2 to 3 minutes, until softened. Season with a pinch of salt.
- Pour in the wine and add the saffron (if using), then dump in the mussels. Cover and cook until the mussels have opened, about 5 minutes (discard any that don't open). Season again with a few pinches of salt and top with parsley. Serve the mussels straight from the pot, or in individual bowls, with hunks of bread to sop up the juices at the bottom.

Makes 6 appetizer servings (or 4 meal servings)/
Cost per serving: $2.66

260 calories
7 g fat
(2 g saturated)
510 mg sodium

960 calories

Not That!

Carrabba's Small Cozze in Bianco
Price: $8

Save!
*700 calories
and $5.34!*

62

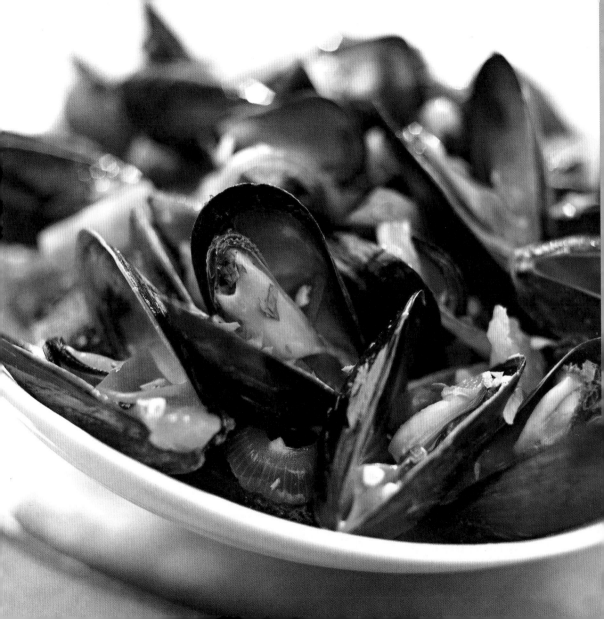

Stuffed Jalapeños

Matt's first cooking job had him stuffing jalapeños in a steamy North Carolina kitchen at the tender age of 14. Between the mountains of cheese, the thick blankets of batter, and the inevitable pile of oil-soaked peppers that emerged from the deep fryer, it was an eye-opening introduction to the excesses of the restaurant world. Those specific excesses are still on full display in most family-style restaurants and sports bars across America, but we found a way to harness the heat of jalapeños and the creaminess of cheese without shackling you with a full day's worth of calories.

You'll Need:

- **4 oz fresh Mexican-style chorizo, casings removed**
- **1 cup cremini or button mushrooms, diced**
- **½ onion, minced**
- **½ cup shredded Monterey Jack cheese**
- **½ cup whipped cream cheese**
- **Salt and black pepper to taste**
- **12 jalapeño peppers**

How to Make It:

- Preheat the oven to 400°F.
- Cook the chorizo in a skillet over medium heat, using a wooden spoon to break up any clumps that form. Once cooked through, remove the meat and drain off all but a thin layer of fat. Add the mushrooms and onion to the pan and cook for about 3 minutes, until the onion is translucent and the mushrooms are lightly browned. Stir back in the chorizo.
- In a mixing bowl, combine the chorizo mixture, cheese, cream cheese, and a good pinch of salt and pepper.
- Halve the jalapeños vertically. Use a paring knife to cut and scrape out as much of the white membranes and seeds in each pepper as possible (this is where the real heat of the pepper comes from; be sure to wash your hands carefully after).
- Stuff each pepper half with a spoonful of the cheese-chorizo mixture. Line up the stuffed peppers on a baking sheet. Bake for about 15 minutes, until the peppers soften and the cheese browns and bubbles.

Makes 4 servings / Cost per serving: $1.59

250 calories
19 g fat
(9 g saturated)
620 mg sodium

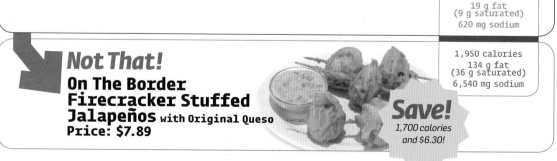

1,950 calories
134 g fat
(36 g saturated)
6,540 mg sodium

Not That!
On The Border Firecracker Stuffed Jalapeños with Original Queso
Price: $7.89

Save!
1,700 calories and $6.30!

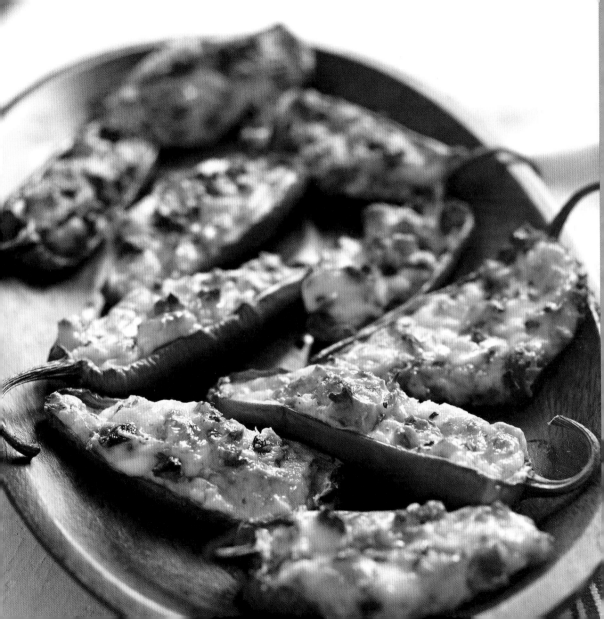

Mozzarella Spiedini

We're not sure what type of diabolical mind dreamed up the idea of deep-frying cheese, but if you've made it this far in the book, we probably don't need to explain why it's a bad thing for your waistline and overall well-being. Rather than chase fried mozz down its dubious rabbit hole, we decided to reinvent the concept entirely. By grilling cheese, bread, and tomatoes together, you've essentially re-engineered the whole fried mozzarella package on skewers (*spiedini* in Italian): gooey melted cheese and crunchy bits of bread, plus a burst of tomato to finish it off.

You'll Need:

- 8 **rosemary branches**
- 16 **cherry tomatoes**
- ½ **baguette, crust removed, cut into ¾" cubes**
- 6 oz **fresh mozzarella, cut into ½" cubes**
- 1 Tbsp **olive oil, plus more for drizzling**
- **Salt and black pepper to taste**

How to Make It:

- Preheat a grill. Strip the rosemary branches of enough of their leaves to make room for the tomatoes, bread, and cheese. Chop the leaves and reserve.
- Alternating between each, thread the tomatoes, bread cubes, and mozzarella cubes onto the rosemary skewers (cutting the tip of the branch into a sharp point makes this easier). Drizzle with the olive oil and season with salt and pepper.
- Place the skewers on a cooler part of the grill and cook for 7 to 10 minutes, until the bread toasts and the cheese begins to melt. (This can happen very quickly if the grill is too hot. Either way, it's important to turn the skewers throughout so that all sides are exposed to the heat.) Serve with another drizzle of olive oil and garnish with the reserved rosemary leaves.

Makes 4 servings / Cost per serving: $2.24

If you can't find sturdy rosemary branches, soak normal wooden skewers in water for 20 minutes.

160 calories
10 g fat
(4 g saturated)
270 mg sodium

770 calories

Not That!
T.G.I. Friday's Fried Mozzarella
Price: $7.89

Save!
610 calories and $5.65!

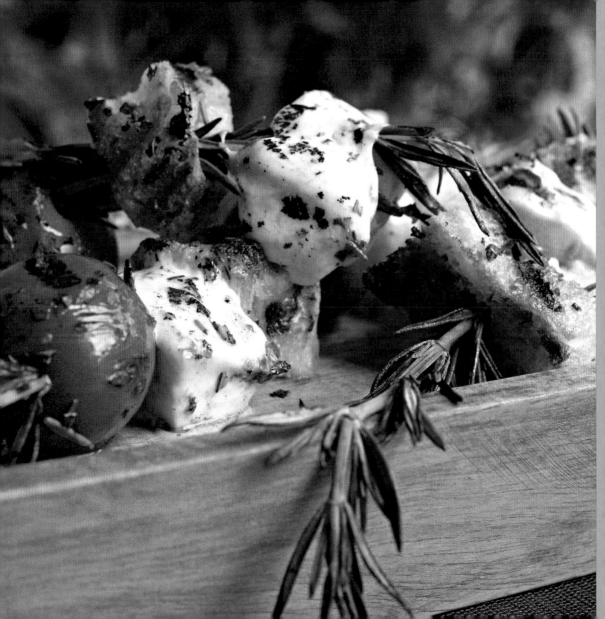

Cook This!
Coconut Shrimp

Shrimp may be among the world's leanest sources of protein, but when entombed in a deep-fried coconut cocoon, all bets are off. We free the crustaceans from the fry job, but not from the crunchy coconut coating that makes this dish a mainstay on so many American restaurant menus. Naturally, this works great as an appetizer, but with sides of cumin-spiked black beans and roasted asparagus, these crunchy crustaceans also make for a pretty sound meal.

You'll Need:

- 1 cup panko bread crumbs
- ½ cup shredded sweetened coconut
- 1 tsp salt
- ½ tsp black pepper
- ½ cup flour
- 2 eggs, beaten
- 12 oz large shrimp, peeled and deveined

Sweet Asian chili sauce for dipping •———

Look for sweet Asian chili sauce in the international section of your supermarket or an Asian specialty grocery. The balance of heat and sweet make this a must-have condiment.

How to Make It:

- Preheat the oven to 450°F. Combine the panko, coconut, salt, and pepper on a plate. Place the flour on a separate plate and the egg in a shallow bowl. Working with a few at a time, coat the shrimp with flour, then egg, then finally with the bread crumb mixture, rolling the shrimp around so they are fully covered.
- Place the breaded shrimp on a nonstick baking sheet and bake for 10 minutes, until the shrimp are firm and cooked through and the coating is nicely browned and crispy. Serve with chili sauce for dipping.

Makes 4 servings / Cost per serving: $2.89

Save!
780 calories
and $11.10!

200 calories
6 g fat
(4 g saturated)
690 mg sodium

980 calories
55 g fat
(12 g saturated)
1,950 mg sodium

Not That!
Red Lobster Parrot Isle Jumbo Coconut Shrimp
Price: $13.99

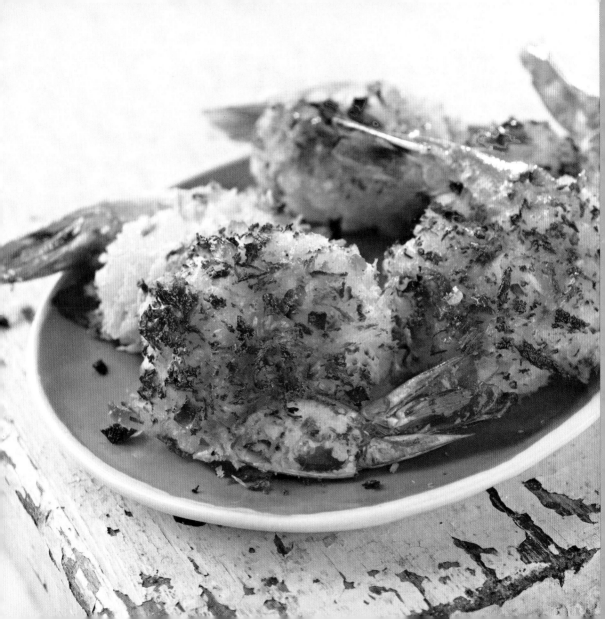

Cook This!
Queso Fundido

Crocks of melted cheese are burbling in corporate kitchens across America, and admittedly, it's difficult to resist their fatty allure. Despite our considerable calorie-cutting capabilities here at CTNT HQ, making a dish of pure melted cheese relatively healthy was a serious challenge. In this case, we took inspiration from industrious Mexican cooks, who stretch a bit of cheese into a larger dish by bolstering it with vegetables: tomatoes, mushrooms, onions, chiles. In a miraculous turn of events, queso fundido is not just better for you, it's a lot more satisfying to eat. Just make sure you serve this one right away; once it cools, it loses its full potential. If you have a fondue pot, now is the time to use it.

You'll Need:

6 **corn tortillas, cut into triangles**

1 ½ **Tbsp canola oil**

1 **small onion, minced**

2 **cloves garlic, minced**

2 **cups mushrooms, diced**

1 **cup diced tomato**

Salt and black pepper to taste

1 **can (4 oz) green chiles**

1 ½ **cups shredded Pepper Jack cheese**

How to Make It:

● Preheat the oven to 425°F. Toss the tortillas with 1 tablespoon of the oil and arrange on a large baking sheet. Bake until lightly brown and crispy, about 10 minutes.

● Heat the remaining ½ tablespoon oil in a large cast-iron skillet or sauté pan over medium heat. Add the onion and garlic and cook for 2 to 3 minutes, until the onion is translucent. Add the mushrooms and tomato and cook for 2 to 3 minutes, until softened. Season with salt and pepper. Turn the heat down to low and add the chiles and cheese, stirring constantly so the cheese melts uniformly. When the cheese has fully melted and starts to bubble, immediately remove from the heat and serve, using the tortilla chips to scoop directly from the pan.

Makes 4 servings / Cost per serving: $1.46

Homemade chips, as superior as they are to the bagged stuff, aren't essential here. Snyder's of Hanover Multigrain chips are the best in show, with 130 calories and 3 grams of fiber per serving.

340 calories
21 g fat
(10 g saturated)
470 mg sodium

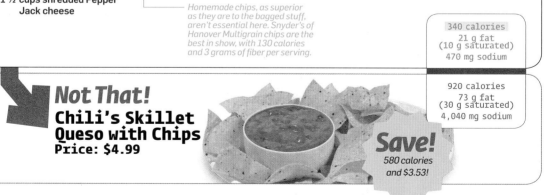

920 calories
73 g fat
(30 g saturated)
4,040 mg sodium

Not That!
Chili's Skillet Queso with Chips
Price: $4.99

Save!
580 calories and $3.53!

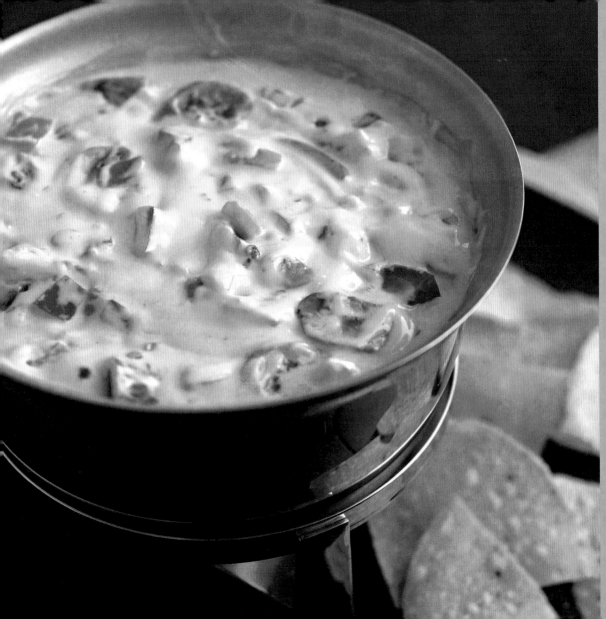

Cook This!
Summer Roll with Shrimp and Mango

Not to be confused with the deep-fried spring roll, the summer roll is a prime example of how a few healthy, relatively boring ingredients can be carefully coerced into something much greater than the sum of their parts. The combination of shrimp, sweet mango, and crunchy strips of red pepper makes for seriously good eating, but once you master the simple wrapping technique, feel free to fiddle with the filling.

You'll Need:

- 1 Tbsp chunky peanut butter
- 1 Tbsp sugar
- ½ Tbsp fish sauce
- ½ Tbsp rice wine vinegar, plus more for the noodles
- 2 oz vermicelli or thin rice noodles (capellini or angel hair pasta also works)
- 8 sheets of rice paper
- ½ lb cooked medium shrimp, each sliced in half
- ½ red bell pepper, thinly sliced
- 1 mango, peeled, pitted, and cut into thin strips
- 4 scallion greens, cut into thin strips
- ¼ cup cilantro or mint leaves

How to Make It:

- Combine the peanut butter, sugar, fish sauce, and vinegar with 1 tablespoon warm water. Stir to thoroughly combine. Set the peanut sauce aside.
- Cook the noodles according to package instructions. Drain and toss with a few shakes of vinegar to keep them from sticking.
- Dip a sheet of rice paper in a bowl of warm water for a few seconds, until just soft and bendable. Lay the paper on a cutting board. Leaving a ½" space at each end of the wrapper, top with noodles, 3 or 4 shrimp halves, bell pepper, mango, scallion, and a few whole cilantro leaves. Fold the ends of the rice paper toward the center, then roll tight like a burrito. Repeat with the remaining 7 wrappers. Serve with the peanut sauce.

Makes 4 servings / Cost per serving: $3.02

Save!
363 calories and $5.47!

270 calories
3.5 g fat
(0 g saturated)
390 mg sodium

633 calories
2 g saturated fat
3,693 mg sodium

Not That!
California Pizza Kitchen Singapore Shrimp Rolls
Price: $8.49

Rice paper rolls

Rice paper is delicate, so work with one piece at a time and soak in water just long enough so that it's soft and foldable. Then follow these steps:

Step 1: *Arrange ingredients in the center of the wrapper*

Step 2: *Carefully fold the ends over the filling*

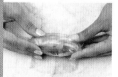

Step 3: *Gently roll into a tight, compact burrito*

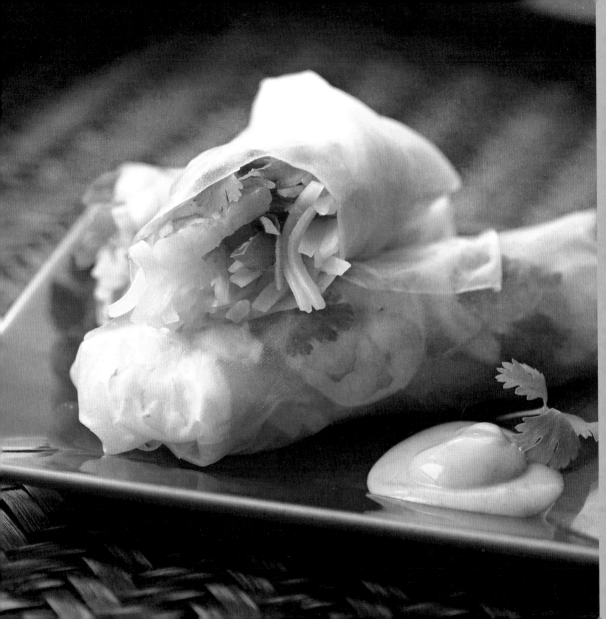

Cook This!
Steak Nachos

The beloved nacho, in all its gooey glory, has won over the hearts of women, children, and beer-swilling, face-painting sports fans alike. Too bad the average plate of restaurant nachos packs more than 1,500 calories. This recipe uses a spicy cheese sauce (which actually saves calories), a healthy amount of salsa, and plenty of fixings to deliver a high-flavor, low-calorie plate of goodness.

You'll Need:

- 8 oz skirt or flank steak
- 1 tsp chili powder
- Salt and black pepper to taste
- 1 Tbsp butter
- 1 Tbsp flour
- ¾ cup low-sodium chicken stock
- 1½ cups shredded reduced-fat Jack cheese
- ½ cup bottled salsa verde
- 4 oz tortilla chips
- ½ (14–16 oz) can pinto beans
- 1 jalapeño pepper, thinly sliced
- 1 red onion, diced
- 2 Roma tomatoes, diced
- Chopped fresh cilantro or scallions (optional)

How to Make It:

- Preheat a grill, grill pan, or cast-iron skillet. Season the steak with the chili powder, salt, and pepper and grill for 3 to 4 minutes per side, until medium-rare. Let the steak rest.

- Preheat the oven to 400°F. Heat the butter in a medium saucepan over medium heat. Stir in the flour and cook for a minute, then slowly whisk in the stock. Simmer for a few minutes, then stir in the cheese and salsa and continue stirring until the cheese is fully melted.

- Chop the steak into small pieces. Arrange the chips in a single layer on a large cookie sheet or baking pan. Top evenly with the beans and steak, then drizzle on three-quarters of the cheese sauce. Top with the jalapeño and onion. Bake for about 15 minutes, until the cheese is fully melted. Top with the remaining cheese sauce, tomatoes, and cilantro if using.

Makes 4 servings /
Cost per serving: $2.73

360 calories
14 g fat
(6 g saturated)
610 mg sodium

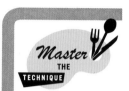

Master THE TECHNIQUE

Nacho architecture

Don't you hate how your nachos arrive fully covered in greasy add-ons, only to find the toppings all but disappear as you work through the layers? The secret to a great nacho is balance. Put too much on and that little chip grows soggy and overburdened. Add too little and they're not really nachos, are they? To hit the sweet spot, spread a single layer of chips (the bigger, the better) on a baking sheet. Start with beans, followed by cheese, meats, and vegetables. Save all cold toppings (guac, salsa, etc.) for after the nachos emerge from the oven.

Not That!
Baja Fresh Charbroiled Steak Nachos
Price: $7.89

2,120 calories
118 g fat
(44 g saturated, 4.5 g trans)
2,990 mg sodium

Save!
1,760 calories and $5.16!

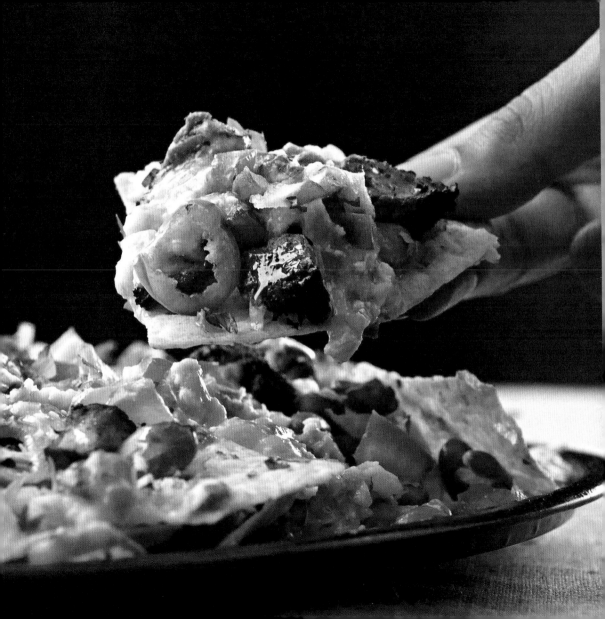

Smoky Deviled Eggs

Have we mentioned our affinity for the egg? Beyond being a near-perfect nutritional substance (ignore what antiquated nutritionists tell you about cholesterol—nearly all current research shows that eggs have no effect on overall cholesterol), no food is so versatile: It is capable of being fried, poached, baked, boiled, scrambled, and emulsified. And, of course, deviled. It might not be the healthiest way to eat an egg (that honor would go to boiling or poaching), but in terms of snacks and finger food, it's hard to beat this Southern specialty.

You'll Need:

8 eggs

¼ cup olive oil mayonnaise

½ Tbsp Dijon mustard

2 tsp canned chipotle pepper

Salt and black pepper to taste

Paprika (preferably the smoked Spanish-style paprika called pimentón) •

2 strips bacon, cooked and finely crumbled

How to Make It:

● Bring a pot or large saucepan of water to a full boil. Carefully lower the eggs into the water and cook for 8 minutes. Drain and immediately place in a bowl of ice water. When the eggs have cooled, peel them while still in the water (the water helps the shell slide off).

● Cut the eggs in half and scoop out the yolks. Combine the yolks with the mayo, mustard, chipotle, and a good pinch of salt and pepper. Stir to combine thoroughly. Scoop the mixture into a sealable plastic bag, pushing it all the way into one corner. Cut a small hole in the corner. Squeeze to pipe the yolk mixture back into the whites. Top each with a sprinkle of paprika and a bit of crumbled bacon.

Makes 4 servings / Cost per serving: $0.70

Spanish-style paprika adds more than just a visual pop: It brings a smoky note to the eggs that reinforces the smoke from the bacon and the chipotle.

220 calories
17 g fat
(4 g saturated)
370 mg sodium

Save!
1,090 calories
and $7.29!

Not That!
T.G.I. Friday's Loaded Potato Skins (half order)
Price: $7.99

1,310 calories

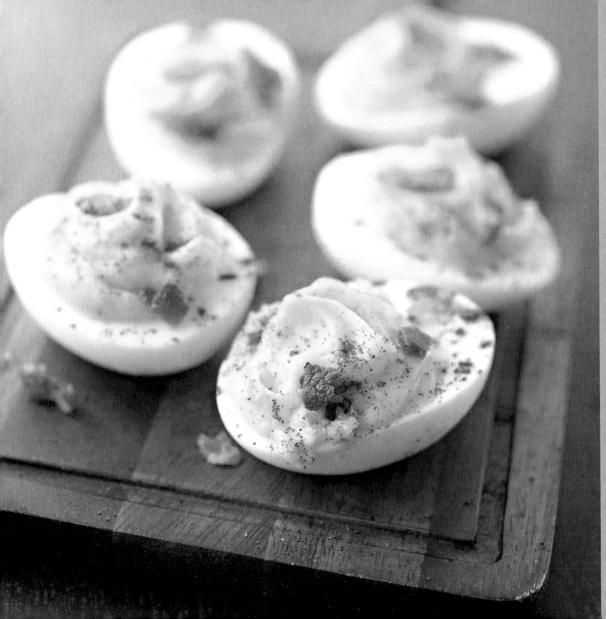

Cook This!
Stuffed Dates

Sometimes it's truly astounding just how little effort it takes to make food taste great; this recipe, as much as any, proves that point. Sweet, salty, smoky, creamy: In a single bite, these tiny packages take you through the highest peaks of flavor country. Show up at a party or a potluck with these little gems and suddenly you—and your dates—will be inundated with invites to swanky soirees all across town.

You'll Need:

- 8 **Medjool dates**
- 8 **almonds**
- ¼ **cup crumbled blue cheese**
- 4 **strips bacon, cut in half**
- **Black pepper to taste**

How to Make It:

- Preheat the oven to 425°F. Using a sharp paring knife, make a slit across the length of a date so that the pocket in the fruit is exposed. Remove the small pit inside the date and replace with an almond. Spoon about ½ tablespoon of blue cheese into the pocket, so that it's tightly stuffed but not overflowing with cheese. Place the date at the bottom of a bacon strip half and roll up as tightly as possible. Secure with a toothpick. Repeat with the remaining 7 dates.
- Place the dates on a nonstick baking sheet and bake for about 20 minutes, until the bacon has rendered and is brown and crispy. Top each with a bit of black pepper and serve.

Makes 4 servings / Cost per serving: $1.76

Some people are turned off by the funk of blue cheese, but it's nicely tempered here by the sweetness of the fruit and the smoke of the bacon. Still don't love it? Goat cheese and feta are good substitutes.

Save!
973 calories and $7.24

```
220 calories
7 g fat
(3 g saturated)
300 mg sodium
```

```
1,193 calories
63 g fat
(26 g saturated)
1,609 mg sodium
```

Not That!
Houlihan's Jumbo Stuffed Shrooms
Price: $9

STEP-BY-STEP

Stuffing dates

Stuffing dates isn't rocket science, as this recipe will teach you. Just be sure to wrap the bacon extra tight, and to only use just enough to cover the date once.

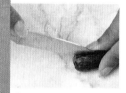

Step 1: *Make a cut across the fruit; scoop out seed*

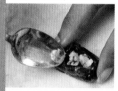

Step 2: *Stuff with almond and a spoonful of cheese*

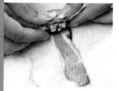

Step 3: *Wrap very tightly with a single layer of bacon*

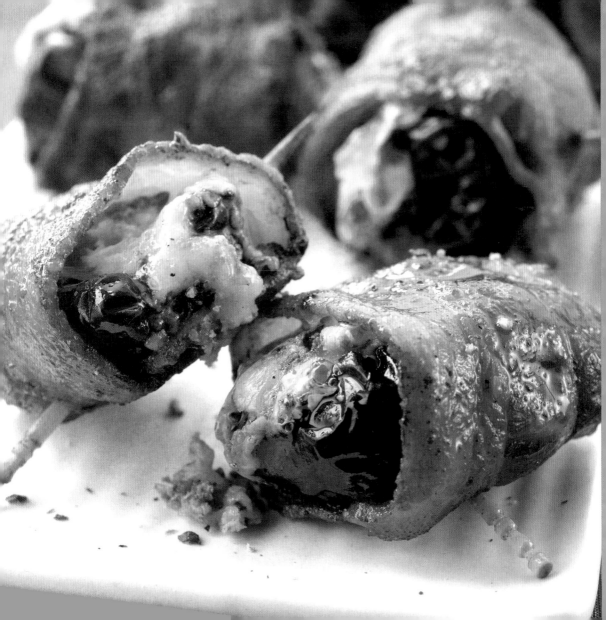

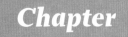
Chapter

4

Soups & Salads
Never has food this healthy
tasted so good

The Salad Matrix

Few foods differ more dramatically on the nutrition front than a heavy, overloaded chain restaurant salad and one made quickly but carefully at home. Save your hard-earned cash and conserve your precious calories by following the blueprints before you. Whether you want a simple side salad to serve before the main event or a filling, palate-pleasing entrée-size bowl to squash your ravenous hunger, we have you covered.

Four Super Salads

For a seriously satisfying salad, pick a lettuce or a mix of lettuces, then choose at least one item from the remaining four rows. And remember, you can never have too much produce in a salad.

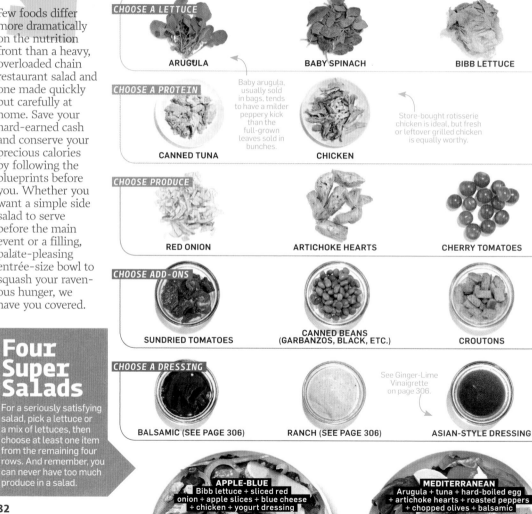

CHOOSE A LETTUCE

ARUGULA   BABY SPINACH   BIBB LETTUCE

Baby arugula, usually sold in bags, tends to have a milder peppery kick than the full-grown leaves sold in bunches.

CHOOSE A PROTEIN

CANNED TUNA   CHICKEN

Store-bought rotisserie chicken is ideal, but fresh or leftover grilled chicken is equally worthy.

CHOOSE PRODUCE

RED ONION   ARTICHOKE HEARTS   CHERRY TOMATOES

CHOOSE ADD-ONS

SUNDRIED TOMATOES   CANNED BEANS (GARBANZOS, BLACK, ETC.)   CROUTONS

CHOOSE A DRESSING

BALSAMIC (SEE PAGE 306)   RANCH (SEE PAGE 306)   ASIAN-STYLE DRESSING

See Ginger-Lime Vinaigrette on page 306.

APPLE-BLUE
Bibb lettuce + sliced red onion + apple slices + blue cheese + chicken + yogurt dressing

MEDITERRANEAN
Arugula + tuna + hard-boiled egg + artichoke hearts + roasted peppers + chopped olives + balsamic

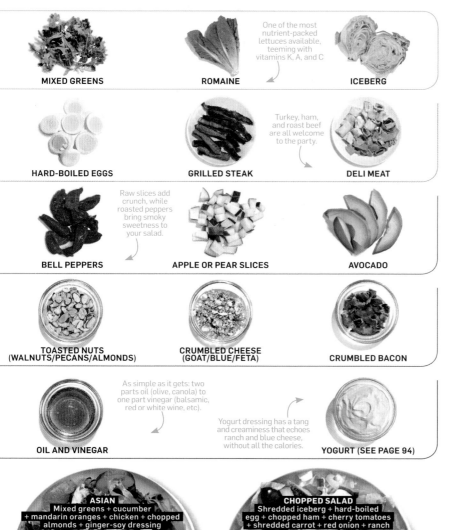

CHAPTER 4

MIXED GREENS

ROMAINE

One of the most nutrient-packed lettuces available, teeming with vitamins K, A, and C

ICEBERG

HARD-BOILED EGGS

GRILLED STEAK

Turkey, ham, and roast beef are all welcome to the party.

DELI MEAT

Raw slices add crunch, while roasted peppers bring smoky sweetness to your salad.

BELL PEPPERS

APPLE OR PEAR SLICES

AVOCADO

TOASTED NUTS (WALNUTS/PECANS/ALMONDS)

CRUMBLED CHEESE (GOAT/BLUE/FETA)

CRUMBLED BACON

As simple as it gets: two parts oil (olive, canola) to one part vinegar (balsamic, red or white wine, etc).

Yogurt dressing has a tang and creaminess that echoes ranch and blue cheese, without all the calories.

OIL AND VINEGAR

YOGURT (SEE PAGE 94)

ASIAN
Mixed greens + cucumber + mandarin oranges + chicken + chopped almonds + ginger-soy dressing

CHOPPED SALAD
Shredded iceberg + hard-boiled egg + chopped ham + cherry tomatoes + shredded carrot + red onion + ranch

Rules of the Salad

Rule 1
Keep it clean. Lettuce needs to be thoroughly washed and dried; any water that remains on the leaves will prevent the dressing from adhering to the salad. Invest in a salad spinner today.

Rule 2
Match your toppings to your lettuce. Sturdier leaves like iceberg and romaine are fit to hold bulkier ingredients and thicker dressings, while delicate lettuces like arugula and baby spinach tend to be best suited for vinaigrettes and lighter toppings.

Rule 3
Think balance, both in terms of nutrition and flavor. For a salad to be filling, it needs protein (chicken, eggs, deli meat) and fiber (beans, avocado). To maximize flavor, pair sweet (tomatoes, apples) with sharp (onion, olives) and savory (meat, cheese). Plus, a salad needs crunch; nuts and raw bell pepper are your best bets.

Rule 4
Don't drown your leaves. Add dressing, 1 tablespoon at a time, in a large mixing bowl, tossing to distribute evenly.

Baked Potato Soup

In its normal restaurant iteration, this is the only soup that can compete with brocco-li-Cheddar soup or clam chowder in terms of sheer caloric impact. Most versions you'll find start with a base of heavy cream, making for a bowl that can easily pack 400 calories or more. We slice the calories dramatically by switching to chicken stock as the foundation, then adding a splash of half-and-half. The creamy potato flavor still shines through, and the bacon, cheese, and Tabasco give it the indulgent taste of a fully loaded spud. Add a bowl of mixed greens tossed with olive oil and balsamic and you've got dinner.

You'll Need:

- 3 strips bacon, sliced
- 4 scallions, whites and greens separated, chopped
- 2 cloves garlic, minced
- 1 Tbsp flour
- 8 cups low-sodium chicken stock (or a mix of stock and water)
- 2 medium russet potatoes, baked (leftover potatoes work great here)
- ½ cup half-and-half
- Salt and black pepper to taste
- Shredded Cheddar
- Tabasco sauce to taste

How to Make It:

- Heat a large soup pot over medium heat. Add the bacon and cook for about 5 minutes, until crispy. Remove with a slotted spoon and reserve.
- Discard all but a thin film of the bacon fat. Add the scallion whites and garlic to the pot and cook for a minute or two, until fragrant and the scallions are translucent. Add the flour and stir to coat the ingredients. Pour in the stock, whisking to help prevent any lumps from forming.
- Remove the peel from one of the potatoes, chop, and add to the pot. Use a potato masher to smash the potato into the broth. (For a smoother, more uniform soup, you can puree the soup in a blender.) Cube the other potato, leaving the peel on, and add to the soup, along with the half-and-half. Season with salt and pepper. Turn the heat all the way down and simmer for 5 to 10 minutes.
- When ready to serve, ladle into bowls and garnish with the bacon, scallion greens, a bit of cheese, and a few shakes of Tabasco.

Makes 4 servings / Cost per serving: $1.69

220 calories
9 g fat
(4 g saturated)
650 mg sodium

420 calories
30 g fat
(14 g saturated)
1,230 mg sodium

Not That!
Applebee's Baked Potato Soup
(bowl)
Price: $4.76

Save!
200 calories
and $3.07!

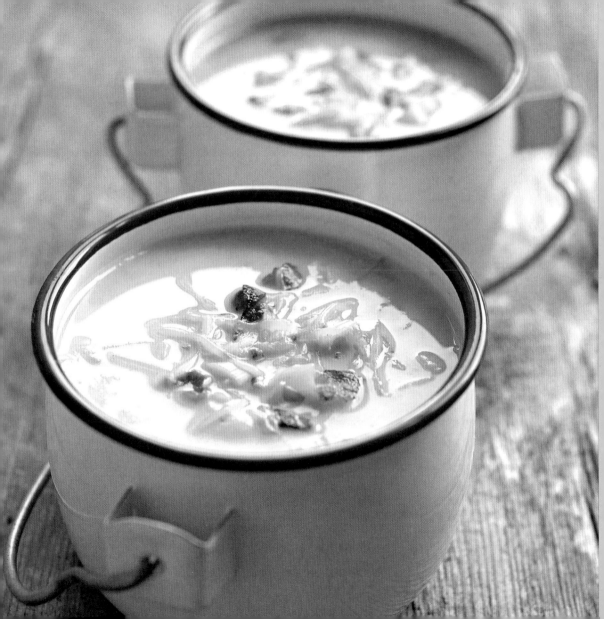

Cook This!
Minestrone with Pesto

Nearly 9 out of 10 Americans don't consume enough fruits and vegetables on a daily basis. This hodgepodge soup will go a long way in making sure you're not one of them. Vary the specific vegetables depending on what's in your fridge and what looks good in the market, but be sure to finish with a spoonful of jarred pesto, which helps tie the whole bowl together.

$$\left(\text{Y} + \text{I} \right)^2$$

MEAL MULTIPLIER

You'll Need:

- 1 Tbsp olive oil
- 1 medium onion, chopped
- 2 cloves garlic, minced
- 8 oz Yukon gold or red potatoes, cubed
- 2 medium carrots, peeled and chopped
- 1 medium zucchini, chopped
- 8 oz green beans, ends trimmed, halved
- Salt and black pepper to taste

- 1 can (14 oz) diced tomatoes
- 8 cups low-sodium chicken stock (or a mixture of stock and water)
- ½ tsp dried thyme
- ½ (14–16 oz) can white beans (aka cannellini), drained
- Pesto
- Parmesan for grating

How to Make It:

- Heat the olive oil in a large pot over medium heat. Add the onion and garlic and cook until the onion is translucent, about 3 minutes. Stir in the potatoes, carrots, zucchini, and green beans. Season with a bit of salt and cook, stirring, for 3 to 4 minutes to release the vegetables' aromas. Add the tomatoes, stock, and thyme and turn the heat down to low. Season with salt (if still needed) and pepper to taste. Simmer for at least 15 minutes, and up to 45.

- Before serving, stir in the white beans and heat through. Serve with a dollop of pesto and bit of grated Parmesan.

Makes 4 servings /
Cost per serving: $2.15

The best part about minestrone is that the same basic technique can be applied to nearly any combination of vegetables. Change up this recipe depending on the season, keeping the onion, garlic, potatoes, pesto, tomatoes, and stock intact but adding one of these timely teams:

- Fall: Cubed butternut squash and halved Brussels sprouts
- Winter: Chopped Swiss chard, shredded cabbage, and chopped celery
- Spring: Start with cauliflower, then add asparagus and green peas or fava beans in the final minutes before serving

200 calories
5 g fat
(1.5 g saturated)
490 mg sodium

280 calories

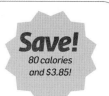

Not That!
Carrabba's
Minestrone (bowl)
Price: $6.00

Save!
80 calories and $3.85!

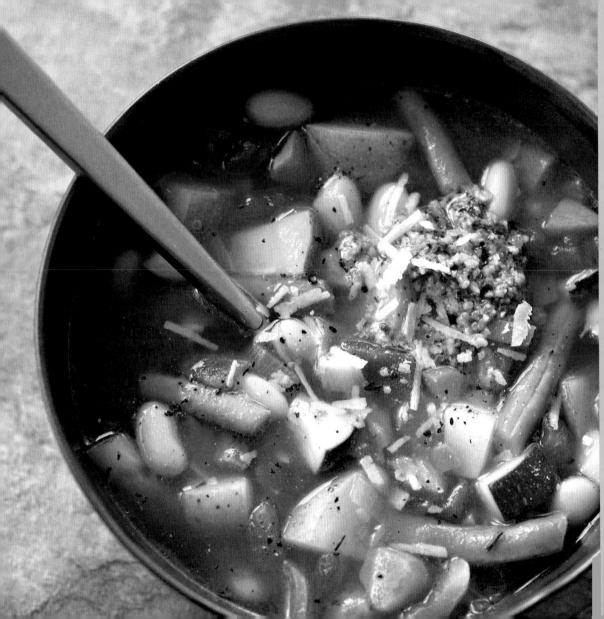

Cook This!
Broccoli-Cheddar Soup

Traditionally, broccoli-Cheddar soup is about the cheese, the broccoli playing second fiddle to a bowl of glorified fondue. We turn the tables on tradition, giving broccoli its proper due and using only a handful of sharp Cheddar to give this soup a rich, creamy texture and beer—preferably a full-flavored ale like Bass—to give it body and soul. Just 8 ounces is needed, which leaves you 4 to sip on while the soup simmers away.

You'll Need:

- 1 Tbsp butter
- 1 yellow onion, diced
- 1 large carrot, diced
- 1 head broccoli, cut into florets and stem thinly sliced
- 2 cloves garlic, chopped
- 1 Tbsp flour
- 1 cup low-sodium chicken stock
- 1 cup beer
- 2 cups milk
- 1 cup shredded sharp Cheddar cheese

Salt and black pepper to taste

Tabasco sauce to taste

- 4 Parmesan crisps •

How to Make It:

- ● Heat the butter in a large pot over medium heat. Add the onion, carrot, broccoli, and garlic and cook for about 5 minutes, until the vegetables soften. Stir in the flour and cook until it evenly coats all of the vegetables. Add the stock and beer, stirring vigorously to keep the flour from clumping. Simmer for a few minutes, then pour the mixture (working in batches, if need be) into a blender and puree until mostly smooth (a bit of texture can be nice here). You can also use a hand blender to puree the soup in the pot.
- ● Return the soup to the pot and bring to a simmer over low heat. Stir in the milk and cheese. After the cheese has fully melted into the soup, season with salt and pepper and a few good shakes of Tabasco. Serve each bowl of soup with a Parmesan crisp floating in the middle.

Makes 4 servings / Cost per serving: $2.21

Make crisps by topping thin slices of baguette with Parmesan and baking in the oven until golden brown, about 12 minutes.

290 calories
17 g fat
(9 g saturated)
580 mg sodium

Not That!
Uno Chicago Grill
Broccoli
& Cheddar Soup
Price: $5.29

Save!
160 calories and $3.08!

450 calories
34.5 g total fat
(19.5 g saturated)
2,175 mg sodium

88

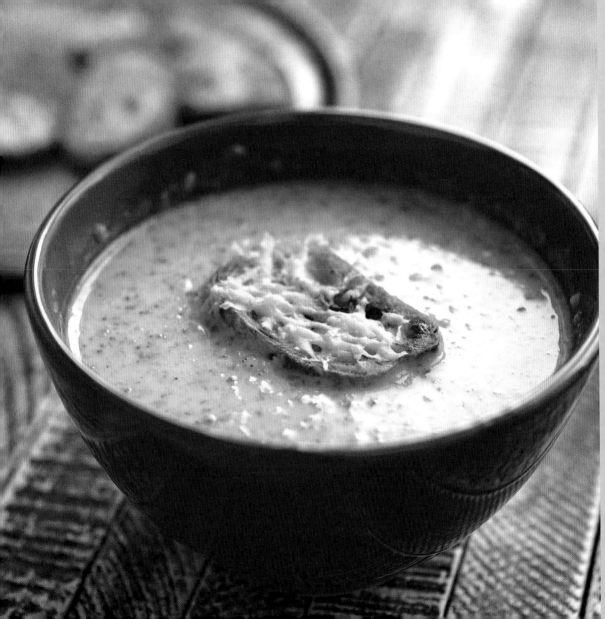

Gazpacho

Ever feel the urge to cool off on a sweltering summer day with a bowl of hot tomato soup? Apparently the Spaniards didn't, either, which is why they created gazpacho to fend off the oppressive heat of August in Andalusia. Beyond beating the heat, gazpacho is also best in August and September because tomatoes are at their peak in late summer when they're sweet and ripe and cheap. Gazpacho is a garden in a bowl, which means it's better for you than plain, one-dimensional tomato soup.

You'll Need:

- 2 cups chopped tomatoes
- 1 red or green bell pepper, chopped
- 1 medium red onion, diced
- 1 cup diced English cucumber
- 1½ cups low-sodium V8 or other tomato juice
- Juice of 1 lemon
- 2 Tbsp olive oil, plus more for serving
- 1 Tbsp white or red wine vinegar
- 2 cloves garlic, chopped
- 1 tsp salt

How to Make It:

- Combine the tomatoes, bell pepper, onion, and cucumber in a large mixing bowl and mix well. Transfer one-fourth of the mixture to a small bowl, cover, and refrigerate. Add the tomato juice, lemon juice, olive oil, vinegar, garlic, and salt to the vegetables in the large bowl and mix to combine. If you have the time, it's best at this point to allow the ingredients to mingle in the fridge for an hour or two—or even overnight. (If not, simply proceed with the recipe.)

- Working in batches if necessary, add the tomato juice mixture to a blender and puree, stopping just short of creating a smooth soup (a bit of texture here is nice). If you didn't refrigerate before, place the gazpacho in the fridge for 20 or 30 minutes to cool down.

- When ready to serve, divide the gazpacho among 4 or 6 bowls. Chop the reserved vegetables on a cutting board until you have a rough salsa. Garnish each bowl with a bit of the reserved vegetables and a drizzle of olive oil.

Makes 4 to 6 servings / Cost per serving: $1.54

English cucumbers are great because there is no need to peel or seed them. If you use more common hothouse cucumbers, be sure to remove both.

120 calories
7 g fat
(1 g saturated)
650 mg sodium

Not That!
Au Bon Pain Old Fashioned Tomato Soup (large)
Price: $4.59

270 calories
10 g fat
(4 g saturated)
1,540 mg sodium

Save!
150 calories
and $3.05!

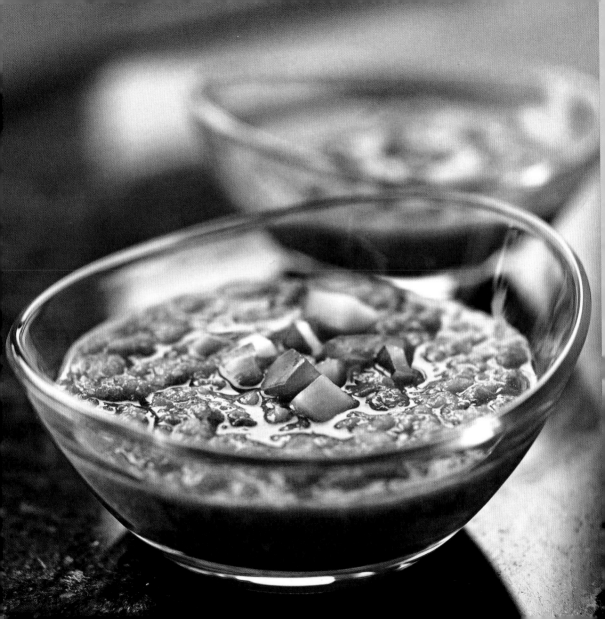

Cook This!
Asian Beef Noodle Soup

When it comes to soups that serve as meals, no one can touch the Asian cuisines. From the thick, heady ramens of Japan to the funky, darkly satisfying beef noodle soups of China, to the spice-suffused bowls of pho from Vietnam, the entire continent seems to have mastered the art of transforming a few scraps of meat and vegetables into a magical eating experience. The slow-cooker soup here takes a cue from all three, combining a rich ginger- and soy-spiked broth with chunks of fork-tender beef, a tangle of springy noodles, and—for a fresh, high note to pair with the dark, brooding ones—a pile of fresh bok choy. This is no appetizer soup; this is a full-on meal.

You'll Need:

- ½ Tbsp peanut or canola oil
- 1½ pounds chuck roast, cut into ½" chunks
- Salt and black pepper to taste
- 4 cups low-sodium beef stock
- 6 cups water
- ¼ cup low-sodium soy sauce
- 2 medium onions, roughly chopped
- 4 cloves garlic, peeled
- 1" piece peeled fresh ginger, sliced into thin coins
- 4 whole star anise pods
- 12 oz Japanese udon noodles, rice noodles, or fettuccine
- 1 head bok choy, leaves chopped into 1" pieces, stems thinly sliced
- Sriracha, hoisin, cilantro leaves, and/or fresh basil leaves for serving

How to Make It:

- Heat the oil in large pot over high heat. Season the beef all over with salt and pepper. Working in batches if necessary, sear the beef on all sides for 3 to 4 minutes, until browned. Transfer to a slow cooker and add the stock, water, soy sauce, onions, garlic, ginger, and star anise. Cook on low for 6 hours, until the beef is very tender. (Or, simmer everything in the pot over a very low flame for 2 to 3 hours.)
- When the beef is nearly ready, prepare the noodles according to package instructions. Add the bok choy to the soup and simmer for about 10 minutes, until tender. Season to taste with salt (if it needs any) and plenty of black pepper. Divide the noodles among 8 large bowls. Ladle the broth, along with a generous amount of beef and bok choy, into each bowl. Top with any of the garnishes you like.

Makes 8 servings /
Cost per serving: $2.44

More than calories, you'll save nearly 2 days' worth of sodium by making this soup.

350 calories
8 g fat
(2 g saturated)
550 mg sodium

Not That!
P.F. Chang's Hot and Sour Soup (bowl)
Price: $5.95

400 calories
15 g fat
(5 g saturated)
5,000 mg sodium

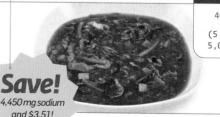

Save!
4,450 mg sodium
and $3.51!

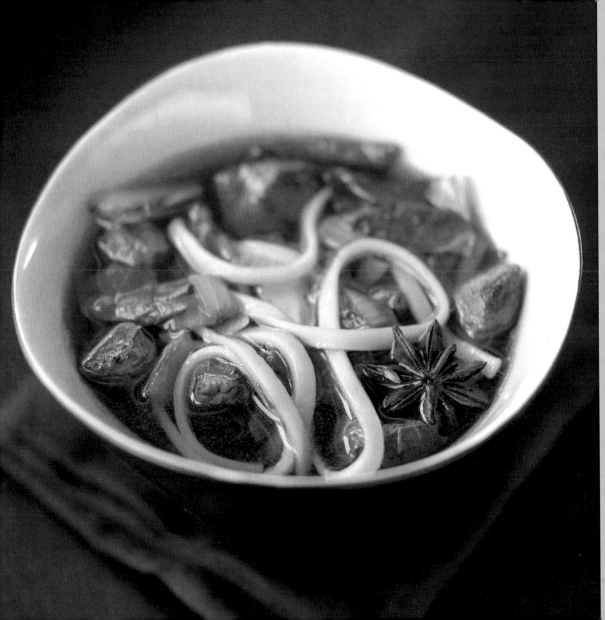

Cook This!

Turkey BLT Salad

Bacon, lettuce, and tomato may be the finest combination ever introduced to sliced bread (sorry, PB&J . . . but you are a close second), but that doesn't mean you need a sandwich to make this cozy relationship work. By turning the bread into crunchy croutons and the lettuce into the base of a salad, you minimize the refined carbs and maximize the healthiest part of the equation. Toss in a handful of cubed deli turkey to boost the protein and suddenly you have a salad with substance and style to tuck into.

You'll Need:

- 2 slices whole-wheat bread, cut into cubes
- ½ Tbsp olive oil
- 4 strips bacon, cooked and crumbled
- 1 large tomato, chopped
- ½ English cucumber, chopped
- 8 oz roast turkey from the deli, cut into cubes
- 1 large head romaine lettuce, chopped
- Low-fat ranch dressing (we like Bolthouse Farms) or Homemade Ranch (see page 306)

How to Make It:

- Preheat the oven to 400°F. Toss the bread cubes with the olive oil, place on a baking sheet, and bake for about 10 minutes, until golden brown and crispy. Combine the croutons with the bacon, tomato, cucumber, turkey, and romaine in a large salad bowl. Toss with just enough dressing to lightly coat the leaves. Divide among four plates.

Makes 4 servings /
Cost per serving: $1.81

Rather than slice it thinly, have the deli sell you one large slab of turkey, or use the Herb-Roasted Turkey on page 228.

230 calories
11 g fat
(2 g saturated)
910 mg sodium

SECRET WEAPON

Yogurt-Based Dressings

Most creamy dressings start with mayonnaise or egg and oil (i.e., mayonnaise) as their base. But Greek yogurt, with its creamy texture and pronounced tang, makes a perfect low-cal substitute. Combine 1 cup yogurt with the juice of a lemon and 2 tablespoons olive oil. That's your base. Now you can add garlic, fresh herbs, a drizzle of honey—anything you'd like to tack on for flavor.

Not That!

Quiznos Classic Cobb Regular Chopped Salad
Price: $5.99

780 calories
56 g fat
(18 g saturated)
1,790 mg sodium

Save!
550 calories
and $4.18!

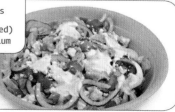

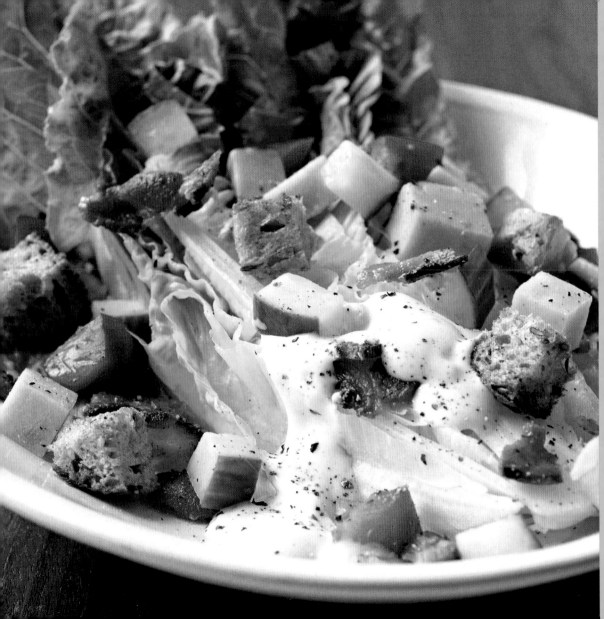

Cook This!
Grilled Mexican Steak Salad

We've long lamented the Mexican-style restaurant salad, in all of its greasy, overwrought, hypercaloric absurdity. Whether from the drive-thru or at a sit-down establishment, no salad is likely to be worse for you than the one with "fiesta" or "olé" or "Southwest" in the title. That's too bad, because the flavors that define the cuisine of our neighbors to the south should form the perfect base for an intensely satisfying, relatively healthy lunch or dinner. We've reengineered the standard, underachieving Mexican salad to be just that.

You'll Need:

- 3 corn tortillas, cut into thin strips
- 4 small Roma tomatoes, chopped
- 1 red onion, diced
- 1 jalapeño pepper, minced
- ½ cup chopped fresh cilantro
- Juice of 1 lime
- 8 oz flank steak
- Salt and black pepper to taste
- ½ Tbsp red wine vinegar
- 1 tsp canned chipotle pepper
- ½ Tbsp honey
- 2 Tbsp olive oil
- 1 head romaine lettuce, chopped
- ½ can (14–16 oz) black beans, drained
- 1 avocado, pitted, peeled, and thinly sliced

How to Make It:

- Preheat the oven to 400°F. Place the tortilla strips on a baking sheet and bake for 8 to 10 minutes, until lightly brown and crispy. Set aside.
- In a mixing bowl, combine the tomatoes, onion, jalapeño, cilantro, and half the lime juice. Set the salsa aside.
- Preheat a grill or grill pan. Season the steak with salt and pepper. Once the grill or pan is fully heated, toss on the steak. Cook for 4 to 5 minutes per side, depending on thickness, until firm but yielding. Let the steak rest for 5 minutes before slicing it thinly against the grain of the meat.
- Combine the remaining lime juice with the vinegar, chipotle, and honey. Slowly drizzle in the olive oil, whisking to combine. Toss the lettuce with enough vinaigrette to lightly coat, then divide among 4 plates. Top each serving with slices of steak, black beans, avocado, a heaping spoonful of salsa, and a few tortilla strips.

Makes 4 servings / Cost per serving: $3.17

340 calories
18 g fat
(4 g saturated)
460 mg sodium

1,800 calories

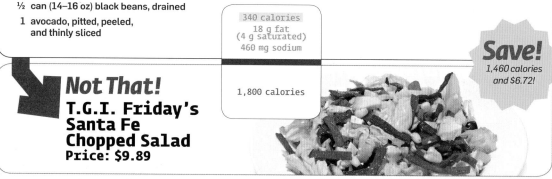

Not That!
T.G.I. Friday's Santa Fe Chopped Salad
Price: $9.89

Save!
1,460 calories
and $6.72!

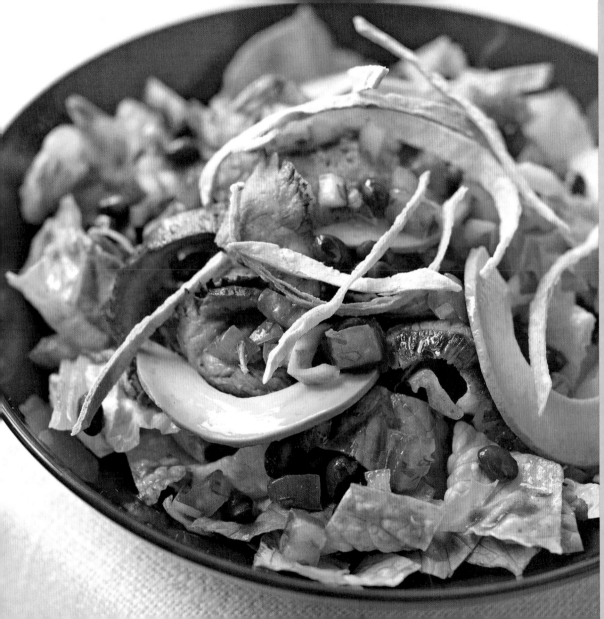

Avocado-Crab Salad

Crab doesn't come out much in the kitchen, but when it does, the idea is to do as little to it as possible. Otherwise, why spend the money on such a delicate ingredient? With the exception of a few salty Marylanders, nobody knows crabs better than the cooks of Southeast Asia, so we follow their light-handed lead here. Cucumber and onion for crunch, chiles for heat, and a bit of fish or soy sauce for a slick of savory salt. An avocado half makes the perfect vessel for this salad, its rich, creamy texture boosting the sweetness of the crab.

You'll Need:

- 1 can (8 oz) crabmeat, preferably jumbo lump, drained
- ½ cup diced seeded and peeled cucumber
- ¼ cup minced red onion
- ¼ cup chopped cilantro
- 1 jalapeño pepper (preferably red), minced
- 1 Tbsp fish sauce (in a pinch, soy sauce will do)
- 1 Tbsp sugar
- Juice of 1 lime
- Salt
- 4 small Hass avocados, halved and pitted
- 1 lime, quartered

How to Make It:

- Combine the crab, cucumber, onion, cilantro, jalapeño, fish sauce, sugar, and lime juice in a mixing bowl. Stir gently to combine, being careful not to break up the bigger lumps of crab. Lightly salt the flesh of the avocados, then divide the crab mixture among the 8 halves, spooning it directly into the bowls created by removing the pits. Serve with the lime quarters.

Makes 4 servings /
Cost per serving: $3.55

Jumbo lump gives you the largest, sweetest hunks of crab, but it also comes with the steepest price tag. Backfin crab is a more affordable variety made from broken-up lumps.

SAVE $ STRATEGY

Don't feel like springing for expensive crabmeat? Luckily, there are half a dozen different ways to make this recipe, all of them delicious, some of them incredibly cheap. The most obvious swap is also the cheapest: a can of tuna, drained. Or try cooked shrimp, chopped into bite-size pieces. If it's meat you seek, a pile of leftover chicken, diced, is the best way to go. And for vegetarians, a few hard-boiled eggs can stand in as the protein foundation.

355 calories
25 g fat
(4 g saturated)
550 mg sodium

1,182 calories
61 fat
(9 g saturated)
1,719 mg sodium

Not That!
Houlihan's Fire Grilled BBQ Salmon Salad
Price: $14.95

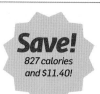

Save!
827 calories and $11.40!

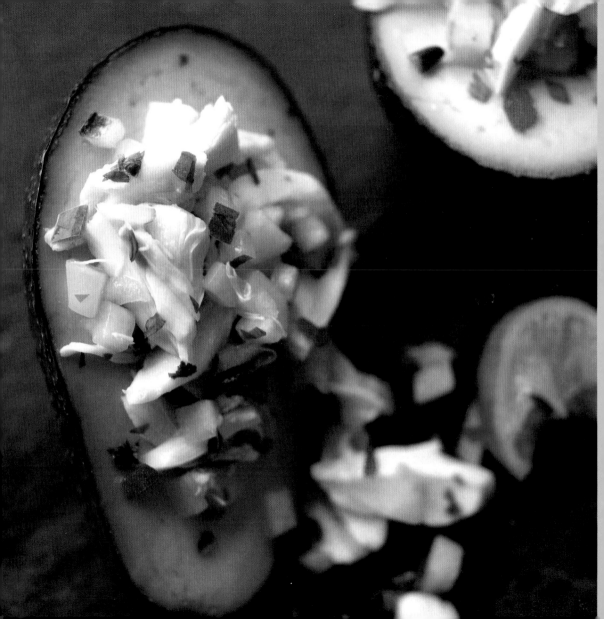

Fig & Prosciutto Salad

Fruit and meat make a pretty good team, especially in salads, since a huge helping of lettuce becomes immensely more attractive when interspersed with bursts of sweet and savory goodness. Most major restaurants take a stab at it, but they often end up with something like Red Robin's 800-calorie Apple Harvest Chicken debacle. This version—with a quarter of the calories—pairs strips of salty, intense prosciutto with juicy, ripe figs. Add the tang of fresh goat cheese and the subtle, earthy crunch of toasted pine nuts and this makes for one inspired salad.

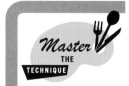

Master THE TECHNIQUE

Mason-jar vinaigrettes

Considering how easy it is to make vinaigrette at home, there's no reason to buy bottled dressing at all, especially since most bottles are awash in salt and high-fructose corn syrup. A bowl and a whisk work just fine, but a clean mason jar is even better. Add your base flavorings—Dijon, minced garlic, shallot, herbs—then a vinegar and oil of choice (no more than 2 parts oil to 1 part vinegar). Season with salt and pepper and shake like crazy for 20 seconds. Done. Store any leftovers in the fridge for up to a week.

You'll Need:

- 12 **cups baby arugula**
- 8 **figs (preferably Mission)**
- 6 **slices prosciutto, cut into thin strips**
- ¼ **cup pine nuts, toasted**
- ½ **cup crumbled fresh goat cheese**
- **Salt and black pepper to taste**
- **Balsamic Vinaigrette (see page 306)**

How to Make It:

- Combine the arugula, figs, prosciutto, pine nuts, and goat cheese in a large salad bowl, along with a few pinches of salt and plenty of black pepper. Pour in just enough vinaigrette to cling lightly to the lettuce and toss gently. Divide among 4 plates.

Makes 4 servings / Cost per serving: $3.73

Can't find figs at the local market? Sliced ripe peaches or strawberries make an excellent substitute.

The best way to toast nuts is to spread them on a baking sheet and bake in a 375°F oven for about 10 minutes. A few minutes in a pan set over medium-low heat will also do the trick.

230 calories
12 g fat
(3.5 g saturated)
690 mg sodium

Not That!
Red Robin Apple Harvest Chicken Salad
Price: $10.49

812 calories
44 g total fat
1,769 mg sodium

Save!
582 calories and $6.76!

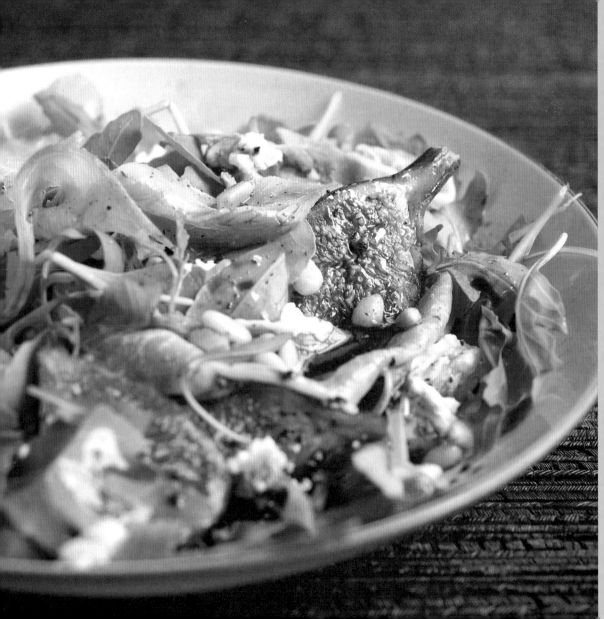

Cook This!
Greek Salad

When it comes to good eating, the Greeks have it right. Though the idea of the Mediterranean diet has echoes throughout Spain, Italy, and southern France, it's really the Greek culinary ethos that forms the backbone of this fabled eating approach. Healthy fats, lots of vegetables, lean protein—all are cornerstones of their diet, and all are captured in this simple and satisfying chopped salad. Incidentally, ask a Greek and he'll tell you: It's not a diet, it's a lifestyle. Amen to that.

You'll Need:

- 2 cups shredded or chopped cooked chicken
- 1 large cucumber, peeled, seeded, and chopped
- 1 red bell pepper, chopped
- 4 Roma tomatoes, chopped
- 1 red onion, chopped
- ½ (14–16 oz) can garbanzo beans, drained
- ¾ cup crumbled feta
- 2 Tbsp red wine vinegar
- 1 tsp dried oregano
- Salt and black pepper to taste
- ¼ cup olive oil

How to Make It:

● Combine the chicken, cucumber, bell pepper, tomato, onion, beans, and feta in a large salad bowl. In a separate bowl, combine the vinegar and oregano with a few generous pinches of salt and pepper. Slowly drizzle in the olive oil, whisking to combine. Toss the dressing with the salad. You can serve now, but it's best to let this one sit in the fridge for 30 minutes or so, which gives all the ingredients a chance to get friendly.

Makes 4 servings / Cost per serving: $2.35

This salad would be just as good made with canned tuna, chopped hard boiled egg, or no main protein at all.

360 calories
22 g fat
(7 g saturated)
580 mg sodium

517 calories
47 g fat
(10 g saturated)
1,480 mg sodium

Not That!
Così
Greek Salad
Price: $7.79

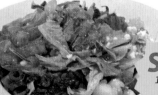

Save!
157 calories
and $5.44!

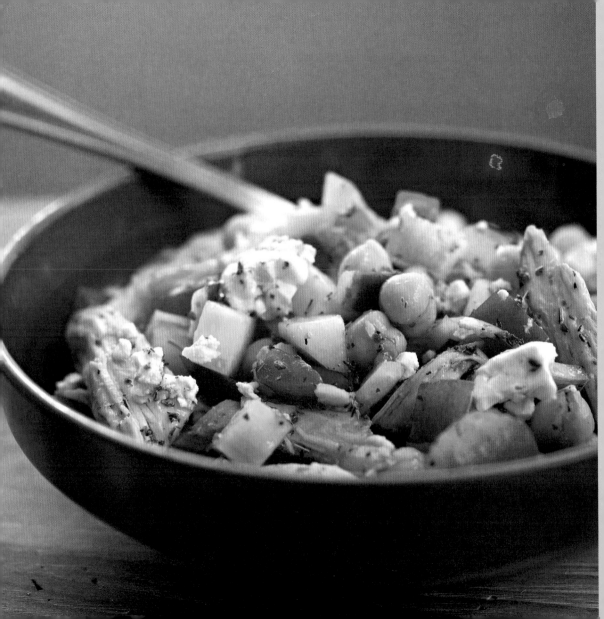

Grilled Ratatouille Salad

Pixar embedded the Provençal vegetable dish in the brains of kids and adults alike with their 2007 animated smash hit, *Ratatouille*. Whatever it takes—even a prodigiously gifted anthropomorphic rat—to get people thinking about eating more vegetables works for us. This is by no means a traditional ratatouille; it merely takes inspiration from the variety of vegetables that make up the ancient peasant dish from France. Nor does this recipe require every vegetable listed below, nor should it be confined to these ingredients. Don't have squash? No problem. Love tomatoes? Toss them directly onto the grill. That's the whole point of cooking: You—not some oily-faced teenager and his over-achieving rat—are in control.

You'll Need:

- 1 large red onion, cut into ¼"-thick slices
- 1 red bell pepper, quartered, stems and seeds removed
- 1 medium eggplant, cut into ¼"-thick planks
- 1 large portobello mushroom cap, cut into ¼"-thick slices
- 1 large zucchini, cut into ¼"-thick planks
- 2 medium yellow squash, cut into ¼"-thick planks

- 12–16 asparagus stalks, woody ends removed
- 4 Tbsp olive oil
- Salt and black pepper to taste
- 1 Tbsp prepared pesto
- 2 Tbsp red wine vinegar
- 2 Tbsp pine nuts, toasted
- ¼ cup grated Parmesan

How to Make It:

- Preheat a grill. Toss the vegetables with 2 tablespoons olive oil and generously season with salt and pepper. Grill the vegetables until cooked through and lightly charred, removing each individually when it has reached this stage. Some vegetables (like the onion and pepper) will take longer than others (like the asparagus and squash).
- Combine the pesto and vinegar in a small bowl, then slowly drizzle in the remaining 2 tablespoons olive oil. Cut the red pepper into thin slices, then toss all of the vegetables with the vinaigrette, pine nuts, and Parmesan.

Makes 4 servings / Cost per serving: $3.84

270 calories
19 g fat
(2.5 g saturated)
385 mg sodium

810 calories
8 g saturated fat
2,104 mg sodium

Save!

540 calories and $10.15!

California Pizza Kitchen Grilled Vegetable Salad
Price: $13.99

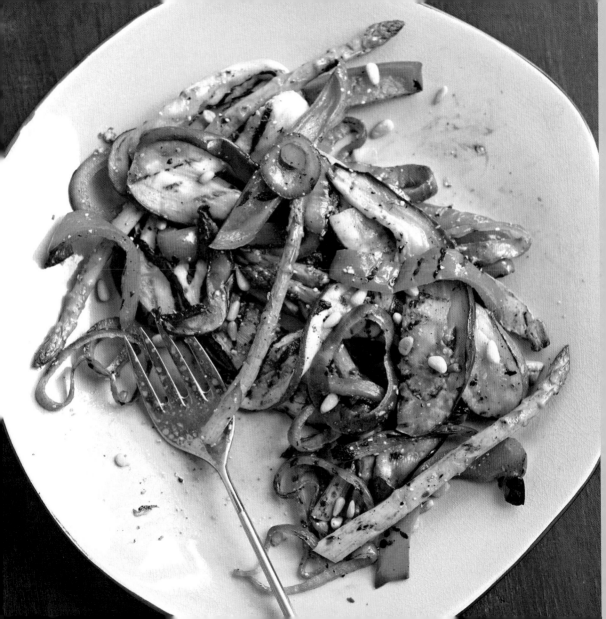

Chapter

Sandwiches & Burgers

Heroic handheld meals to satisfy any appetite

Cook This!
The Sandwich Matrix

Sandwich making at its finest is an exalted craft, one capable of packing a delicately balanced, well-proportioned, and even healthy array of meat, vegetables, and condiments into a handheld vessel. Too bad what we get from most places are poorly conceived subs long on calories and short on flavor. Enough! Use the grid to form myriad specimens that will restore the sandwich to its rightful place as one of the world's greatest forms of food.

Four Super Sand-wiches

Choose the right bread and the right condiments and a tasty 350-calorie sandwich is well within reach. Make sure your next sandwich stacks up.

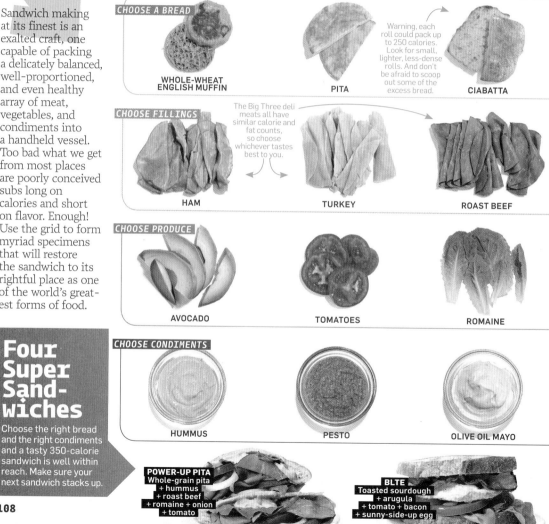

CHOOSE A BREAD

WHOLE-WHEAT ENGLISH MUFFIN

PITA

Warning, each roll could pack up to 250 calories. Look for small, lighter, less-dense rolls. And don't be afraid to scoop out some of the excess bread.

CIABATTA

CHOOSE FILLINGS

The Big Three deli meats all have similar calorie and fat counts, so choose whichever tastes best to you.

HAM

TURKEY

ROAST BEEF

CHOOSE PRODUCE

AVOCADO

TOMATOES

ROMAINE

CHOOSE CONDIMENTS

HUMMUS

PESTO

OLIVE OIL MAYO

POWER-UP PITA
Whole-grain pita
+ hummus
+ roast beef
+ romaine + onion
+ tomato

BLTE
Toasted sourdough
+ arugula
+ tomato + bacon
+ sunny-side-up egg

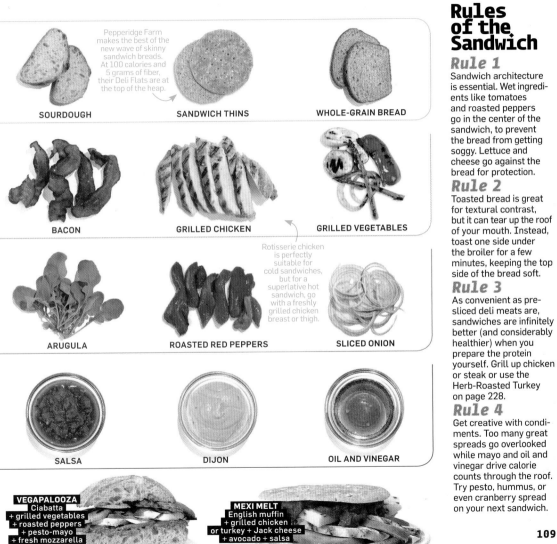

Rules of the Sandwich

Rule 1

Sandwich architecture is essential. Wet ingredients like tomatoes and roasted peppers go in the center of the sandwich, to prevent the bread from getting soggy. Lettuce and cheese go against the bread for protection.

Rule 2

Toasted bread is great for textural contrast, but it can tear up the roof of your mouth. Instead, toast one side under the broiler for a few minutes, keeping the top side of the bread soft.

Rule 3

As convenient as pre-sliced deli meats are, sandwiches are infinitely better (and considerably healthier) when you prepare the protein yourself. Grill up chicken or steak or use the Herb-Roasted Turkey on page 228.

Rule 4

Get creative with condiments. Too many great spreads go overlooked while mayo and oil and vinegar drive calorie counts through the roof. Try pesto, hummus, or even cranberry spread on your next sandwich.

Pepperidge Farm makes the best of the new wave of skinny sandwich breads. At 100 calories and 5 grams of fiber, their Deli Flats are at the top of the heap.

SOURDOUGH

SANDWICH THINS

WHOLE-GRAIN BREAD

BACON

GRILLED CHICKEN

GRILLED VEGETABLES

Rotisserie chicken is perfectly suitable for cold sandwiches, but for a superlative hot sandwich, go with a freshly grilled chicken breast or thigh.

ARUGULA

ROASTED RED PEPPERS

SLICED ONION

SALSA

DIJON

OIL AND VINEGAR

VEGAPALOOZA
Ciabatta
+ grilled vegetables
+ roasted peppers
+ pesto-mayo
+ fresh mozzarella

MEXI MELT
English muffin
+ grilled chicken
or turkey + Jack cheese
+ avocado + salsa

12 Ways to a Better

1

Combine ground lamb with salt, pepper, and fresh or dried rosemary. Sandwich on toasted buns with garlic- and olive oil-spiked yogurt, arugula, and roasted red peppers.

3

Rub portobello caps with olive oil, salt, and pepper, and grill until soft and lightly charred.

4

Brush a turkey or beef burger with your favorite barbecue sauce a minute or two before it finishes cooking. Top with sharp cheddar and caramelized or grilled onions (and bacon, if you really want to indulge).

5

Breakfast burger: Mix ground turkey with chunks of apple, some maple syrup, and a pinch of cinnamon. Grill or cook patties in a skillet, then place on a toasted English muffin and crown with a fried egg.

2

Combine a can of black beans with half a chopped onion, a few spoonfuls of salsa, a quarter cup of bread crumbs, the juice of one lime, and salt and pepper to taste. Whirl through a food processor. Form into patties, grill or broil, and serve on buns topped with more salsa.

6

Top a grilled beef burger with Swiss, a slice or two of ham, pickle slices, and a good bit of Dijon. Cook the entire burger in a cast-iron skillet, turning once, using a heavy pan to compress the burger, as if making a crispy panini.

Burger

Fiesta burger: Grill beef or chicken patties for 4 minutes on one side, flip, and top with a scoop of canned roasted chilies and a slice of Jack cheese. Dress with salsa and guacamole.

8

11
Mix ground turkey with minced shallot, fresh thyme, and Dijon. Grill or broil patties, adding a slice of brie just before they finish cooking. Place on toasted English muffins with baby mixed greens, Dijon, and thinly sliced apple.

7
Grill patties made with lean pork or chicken and glaze with bottled teriyaki sauce as they cook. Grill slices of onion and pineapple at the same time. Combine the burgers with the onion, pineapple, sliced jalapeño, and more teriyaki on toasted buns.

9
Remove a pound of chicken or turkey sausage from their casings and form into patties. Grill or broil—topping each with a slice of provolone after you flip—until cooked all the way through. Top with sautéed onions and peppers.

12
Form patties using lean ground sirloin. Make a deep indentation with your thumb into each and stuff with a tablespoon of blue or goat cheese, then fold the meat over to completely cover the cheese.

10
Black and blue: Rub bison or beef patties with blackening spices. Cook in a cast-iron skillet, and top with crumbled blue cheese and sautéed mushrooms.

Cook This!
Buffalo Chicken & Blue Cheese Sandwich

Given the rate of wing consumption in this country, clearly hot sauce-slathered chicken and blue cheese is a winning combination for American palates. Problem is, most take-out wings deliver more fat than flavor, and now chains such as Chili's and Ruby Tuesday are using the high-calorie combo to fatten up their sandwiches, too. We stay true to the flavors people love—basting the chicken in hot sauce butter after grilling, topping with a yogurt-based blue cheese sauce—but manage to do what no one else out there has done yet: make Buffalo chicken into a healthy meal. Try the same technique with grilled shrimp—with or without the bread.

You'll Need:

- ¼ cup crumbled blue cheese
- ½ cup Greek-style yogurt
- Juice of half a lemon
- Salt and pepper to taste
- 4 chicken breasts (6 oz each)
- ½ Tbsp chili powder
- 1 red onion, sliced
- 3 Tbsp favorite hot sauce (Frank's Red Hot works best here)
- 2 Tbsp butter, melted in the microwave for 20 seconds
- 4 large romaine lettuce leaves
- 4 sesame buns, toasted

How to Make It:

- Preheat a grill or grill pan. While it's heating, combine the blue cheese, yogurt, and lemon juice, plus a pinch of salt and pepper. Stir to combine, and set aside.
- Season the chicken breasts with salt, pepper, and the chili powder. Add the chicken to the hot grill and cook for 4 to 5 minutes the first side, then flip. Add the onions to the perimeter of the grill (if using a grill pan, you'll need to wait until you remove the chicken to grill the onions). Cook the chicken until firm and springy to the touch, another 4 to 5 minutes. Remove, along with the grilled onions.
- Combine the hot sauce and butter and brush all over the chicken after removing from the grill. Place one large leaf of romaine on the base of each bun. Top with a chicken breast, the blue cheese sauce, grilled onions, and then the top half of the bun.

Makes 4 servings / Cost per serving: $3.81

387 calories
15 g fat
(5 g saturated)
912 mg sodium

1,560 calories
86 g fat
(14 g saturated)
4,010 mg sodium

Not That!
Chili's Buffalo Chicken Ranch Sandwich
Price: $8.79

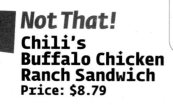

Save!
1,173 calories
and $4.98!

112

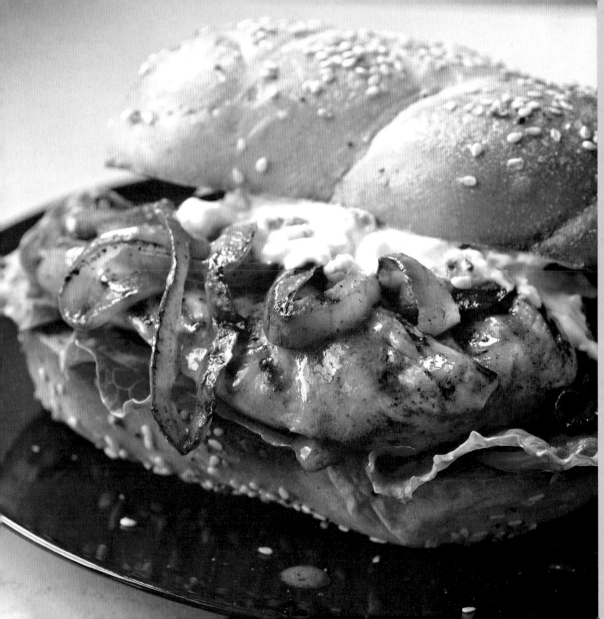

Turkey Burger Mediterranean Style

Thought you were doing yourself a favor by ordering the turkey burger? Think again. Whether scored from a big chain restaurant or a local dive, odds are you just ordered one of the worst items on the menu. Dark turkey packs as much fat and calories as most ground beef. Add to that the inevitable flurry of high-calorie condiments and you have a recipe for disaster. Here, we complement truly lean turkey with a barrage of big flavors—punchy olives, sweet red peppers, a layer of tangy feta cheese—that do little to compromise the overall nutritional picture. For once, you'll have a turkey burger you can eat with impunity.

You'll Need:

1 lb lean ground turkey

Salt and pepper to taste

½ tsp dried thyme

½ cup feta or fresh goat cheese

2 cups arugula

4 English muffins, split and lightly toasted

½ cup roasted red peppers

¼ cup olives, chopped

How to Make It:

- Preheat a grill or grill pan. Season turkey with a few big pinches of salt and pepper, plus the dried thyme. Form the meat into four patties, being careful not to overwork the meat (which will cause the proteins to bind, making for a tough burger). Use your thumb to make a small impression in the middle of each patty (as they cook, the middle will swell up; this simple step makes for a more evenly cooked burger).
- Cook over medium-high heat for 4 to 5 minutes on the first side, until lightly charred. Flip and immediately add the cheese to each patty. Cook for another 4 to 5 minutes, until the burgers feel firm and springy to the touch. Remove from the grill.
- Lay the arugula on the bottom of four English muffin halves. Top with the burger, then crown the burger with peppers, olives, and the other half of the English muffin.

Makes 4 servings /
Cost per serving: $2.89

317 calories
8 g fat
(3 g saturated)
710 mg sodium

Not That!
Ruby Tuesday Bella Turkey Burger
Price: $8.99

1,126 calories
69 g fat
2,760 mg sodium

Save!
809 calories and $6.10!

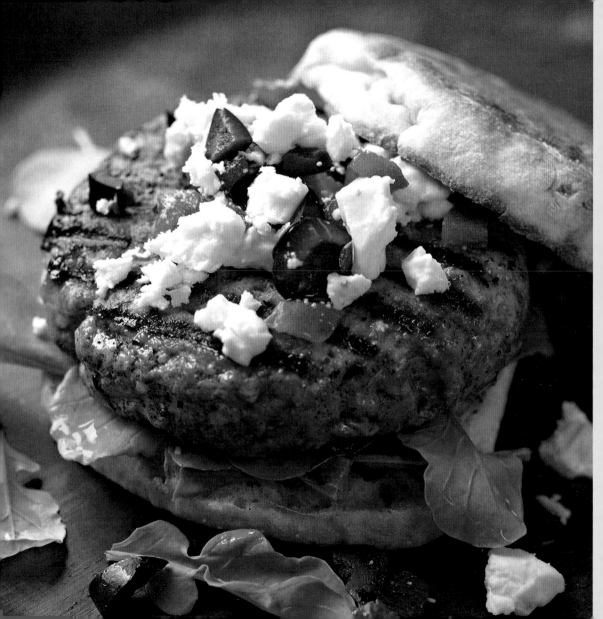

Italian Panini
with Provolone, Peppers, and Arugula

Philadelphians are justly proud of their robust sandwich culture. Sure, there's the epo-ny-mous cheesesteak, but there's also the roast pork, the scrapple and egg, and, of course, the inimitable Italian hoagie. Typically, this last sandwich contains three or four different cuts of Italian-style meats, plus provolone, some roughage, and oil and vinegar, all tucked into a massive squishy hoagie roll. Damage? About 1,000 calories. The chains that imitate this sandwich inflict similar damage upon their customers. Our version takes the same classic flavors of the Italian sandwich, but turns it into a crispy, melted panini. We promise you won't miss the bulky bread, the mound of meat, or the excess 600 calories.

You'll Need:

- 8 slices sourdough bread
- 4 slices provolone
- ½ red onion, very thinly sliced
- ½ cup roasted red pepper
- 4 cups arugula
- 8 slices reduced-fat spicy salami
- 8 oz sliced ham
- 1 Tbsp olive oil

How to Make It:

- Lay four slices of bread on a cutting board. Cover each with a provolone slice, then top with onion, peppers, and arugula. Layer the salami and ham over the arugula and top with the remaining four slices of bread.
- Heat half the oil in a grill pan or large cast-iron skillet over medium-low heat (naturally, if you're fortunate enough to have a panini press, use that). Add the sandwiches, being careful not to crowd, and use something to weigh them down (if cooking individually, a teakettle partly filled with water works nicely; if cooking together, a few cans in a large pasta pot will do the trick). Cook for 3 to 4 minutes, until the bottoms have toasted nicely and the cheese has begun to melt. Remove the weight, flip, reapply the weight, and cook for another 3 to 4 minutes. Cut the sandwiches on the diagonal and serve with a small salad or soup.

Makes 4 sandwiches /
Cost per serving: $2.33

$$(\Psi + I)^2$$

MEAL MULTIPLIER

Another two panini you should try immediately:

- Layer thinly sliced chicken on the bottom of the sandwich, cover in marinara, then top with grated mozzarella and fresh basil leaves
- Make a Cubano: Layer leftover pork with a slice of ham, plus Swiss, pickles, and a good swipe of Dijon mustard

350 calories
12 g fat
(4 g saturated)
1,010 mg sodium

1,040 calories
45 g fat
(17 g saturated,
1 g trans)
3,090 mg sodium

Not That!
Panera Bread Italian Combo on Ciabatta
Price: $7.19

Save!
690 calories
and $4.86!

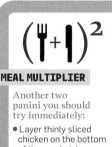

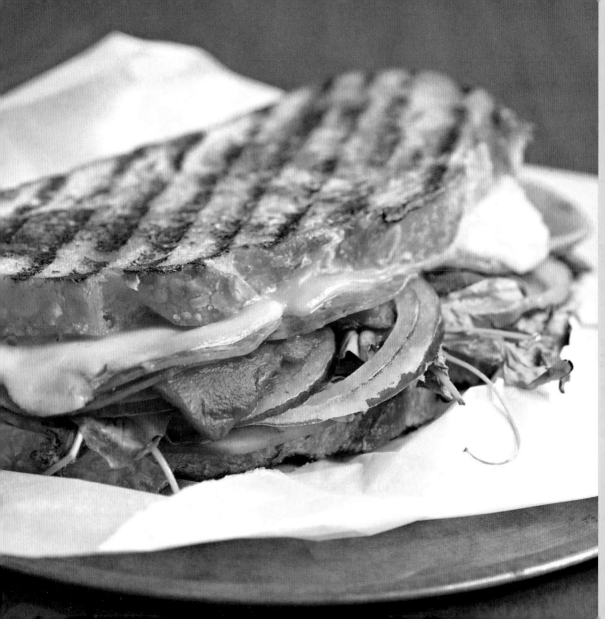

Sausage Sandwich with Peppers

Whether it's fennel-laced Italian links smothered in onions or plump bratwurst grilled before kickoff, few foods satisfy as deeply as sausages cooked over an open flame. Unfortunately, ounce for ounce, few foods are also as caloric. Pork sausage can contain up to 30 percent fat, meaning a single link of bratwurst on its own can pack 400 calories. Switching to a lean chicken or turkey sausage will bring that number to fewer than 150 calories, and a tangle of sautéed onions and peppers, a bit of melted cheese, and a slick of spicy mustard will ensure that you won't miss the pig.

You'll Need:

- 1 Tbsp olive oil
- 1 red bell pepper, sliced
- 1 yellow bell pepper, sliced
- 1 yellow onion, sliced

Salt and black pepper to taste

- ½ Tbsp red wine vinegar
- 4 links uncooked chicken or turkey sausage
- 4 hot dog buns (preferably potato buns)
- 4 slices provolone
Spicy mustard to taste

Provolone makes the most sense here from a flavor standpoint, but you'll cut calories by switching to Swiss or mozzarella.

How to Make It:

- Preheat a grill or grill pan.
- Heat the oil in a large skillet. Add the red and yellow peppers and the onion and cook, stirring occasionally, for about 10 minutes, until lightly blistered and soft. Remove from the heat, season with salt and pepper, and add the vinegar. Reserve.
- Grill the sausages for about 12 minutes, until lightly charred and cooked all the way through. This can also be done in a pan, over medium-low heat. Heat the rolls on the grill until warm and toasted, if you like. Lay a slice of cheese in each roll, drizzle with mustard, then top with a sausage. Divide the peppers and onions among the four sandwiches.

Makes 4 sandwiches / Cost per serving: $2.56

370 calories
20 g fat
(9 g saturated)
650 mg sodium

900 calories
49 g fat
(23 g saturated)
2,240 mg sodium

Not That!

Domino's Italian Sausage & Peppers Sandwich
Price: $5.59

Save!
530 calories and $3.03!

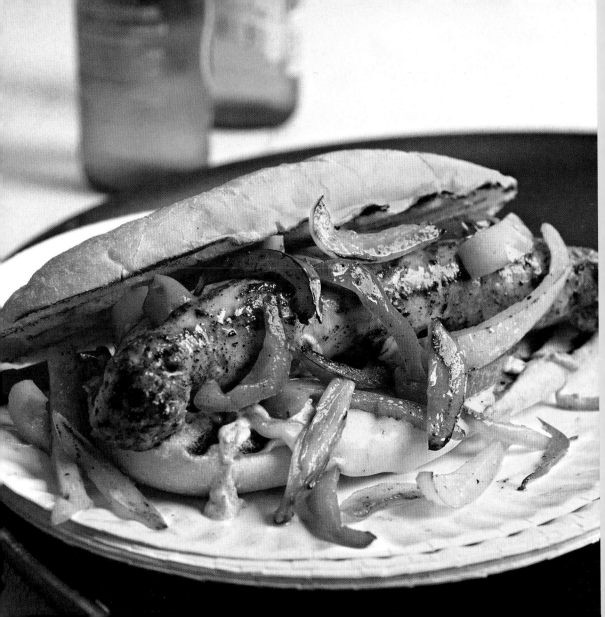

Jalapeño Cheeseburger

Americans have always been hamburger crazy, but never more so than now, as celebrity chefs like Bobby Flay rush to open burger outlets and mega chains continue to expand their menus of tricked-out patties. Applebee's new Realburgers from Across America menu fails to showcase a single burger with fewer than 1,000 calories. With a few simple tweaks (lean sirloin, olive oil mayonnaise), we've taken their Southwestern behemoth, improved its flavor, and cut its calories dramatically.

You'll Need:

- 2 Tbsp ketchup
- 2 Tbsp relish
- 1 Tbsp olive oil mayonnaise
- Salt and black pepper
- 1 lb ground sirloin
- 1 cup shredded Pepper Jack cheese
- 1 cup Caramelized Onions (see page 305)
- ¼ cup Pickled Jalapeños (see page 307)
- 4 potato buns, split

How to Make It:

- Combine the ketchup, relish, and mayo in a mixing bowl. Season with a pinch of salt and pepper and set aside.

- Preheat a grill, grill pan, or cast-iron skillet. Combine the ground sirloin with ½ teaspoon salt and ½ teaspoon pepper and mix gently. Without overworking the meat, form into four patties until the beef just comes together.

- When the grill or skillet is hot (if using a skillet, add a touch of oil), add the patties. Cook on the first side for 5 to 6 minutes, until a nice crust develops. Flip and immediately top with the cheese. Cook for another 2 to 3 minutes, until the cheese is melted and the burgers are firm but still yielding to the touch. Remove the burgers. While the grill or pan is hot, toast the buns.

- Slather the bottom buns with the reserved spread, then top each with a burger, caramelized onions, and pickled jalapeños. Crown with the bun tops and serve.

Makes 4 burgers /
Cost per serving: $2.41

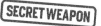
SECRET WEAPON

Potato buns

If you like burgers as much as we do, it's important to find the right bun for the base of your next master-piece. We love potato buns, not just because their squishy, compact size holds a 4-ounce patty perfectly, but because they tend to deliver a good dose of fiber for a light caloric toll. Take our favorite burger vessel, Martin's Potato Rolls. For 130 calories you get 3 grams of fiber and 6 grams of protein. Compare that with whole-wheat buns, many of which pack 150 or more calories and offer 2 or fewer grams of fiber, and you'll see why we love the humble spud rolls so much.

360 calories
14 g fat
(6 g saturated)
840 mg sodium

1,110 calories
70 g fat
(24 g saturated,
3 g trans)
2,100 mg sodium

Not That!

Applebee's Southwest Jalapeño Burger
Price: $9.99

Save!
750 calories and $7.58!

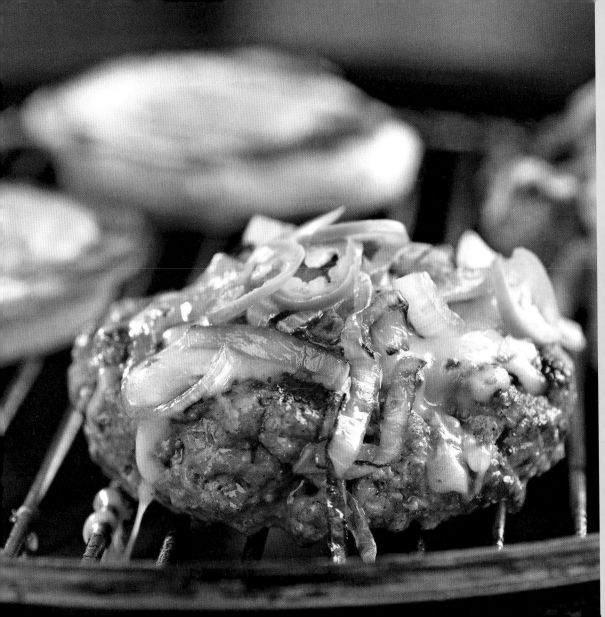

Cook This!
Grilled Cheese with Sautéed Mushrooms

To most people, grilled cheese means a few Kraft Singles sandwiched between slices of Wonder Bread. As comforting as it may be, the standard take offers only a glimpse of grilled cheese's full potential. A better grilled cheese needs substance, something to turn it from a high-calorie snack into a low-calorie meal, hence the mushrooms and the pile of caramelized onions here. Mushrooms and Swiss are close buddies, so out goes the processed American. And few breads offer less than high fructose corn syrup—laden white bread, so rye stands in as the better—and tastier—alternative. This all goes to show you that food, no matter how sacred, is meant to be played with.

You'll Need:

- ½ Tbsp olive oil
- 2 cups cremini mushrooms, sliced
- Salt and black pepper to taste
- 8 slices rye bread
- 2 cups shredded Swiss cheese
- 1 cup Caramelized Onions (see page 305)
- ½ Tbsp fresh thyme leaves (optional)
- 2 Tbsp softened butter

How to Make It:

- Heat the olive oil in a skillet over medium heat. Add the mushrooms and cook for about 6 minutes, until nicely caramelized. Season with salt and pepper.
- Lay out four slices of the rye bread on a cutting board. Top with half the Swiss, then the onions and mushrooms. Add the thyme (if using) and the remaining cheese. Top with the remaining slices of rye. Spread the softened butter on both sides of the sandwiches.
- Heat a large cast-iron or nonstick skillet over medium-low heat. Add the sandwiches, working in batches if you must, and cook for 5 to 6 minutes per side, until fully toasted and golden brown.

*Makes 4 sandwiches /
Cost per serving: $2.39*

$$(\text{\ding{}} + \text{\ding{}})^2$$

MEAL MULTIPLIER

Once you've successfully broken free from the shackles of standard grilled cheese, you'll be hungry to explore more genre-bending options. Here are a few of our favorites:

- Cream cheese, pickled jalapeños, grated Swiss, and crushed corn chips
- Goat cheese, sliced fig, and prosciutto
- Brie, pear, and turkey

340 calories
12 g fat
(6 g saturated)
570 mg sodium

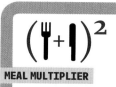

1,049 calories
31 g saturated fat
1,714 mg sodium

Not That!
Cheesecake Factory Grilled Cheese
Price: $8.73

Save!
*709 calories
and $6.34!*

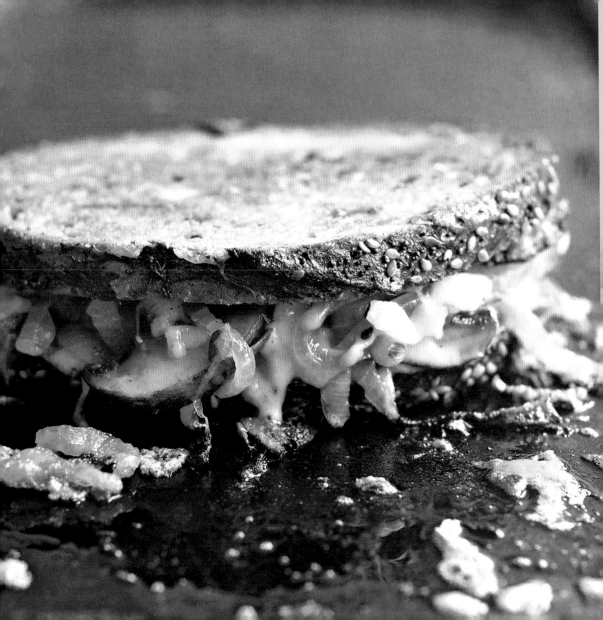

Turkey Reuben

For anyone who has spent time eating in New York, Reubens invariably conjure up the image of an oversize deli sandwich stacked so high with peppery beef you'd need an unhingeable snake jaw just to get your teeth around it—and a generous belt for waistline adjustment in the postprandial aftermath. We've taken the indulgent essence of the Jewish deli staple and distilled it to a sandwich with substance and soul, but without half a day's calories and a day and a half's worth of saturated fat (which is exactly what Applebee's, and nearly every other major establishment, offers with their version).

You'll Need:

- ¼ cup ketchup
- ¼ cup olive oil mayonnaise
- 2 Tbsp relish
- Few dashes Tabasco sauce
- Black pepper to taste
- 1 lb turkey pastrami (or, failing that, regular turkey)
- 4 slices low-fat Swiss cheese
- 8 slices rye bread, toasted
- 1 cup bottled sauerkraut

How to Make It:

- Combine the ketchup, mayo, relish, and Tabasco in a bowl and mix. Season with a bit of black pepper. Set the dressing aside.
- Divide the pastrami into four portions, pile on plates, and top each with a slice of cheese. Microwave briefly, about 30 seconds each, to melt the cheese.
- Layout four slices of the rye bread on a cutting board. Top each with sauerkraut and then pastrami and cheese. Drizzle with the dressing. Top with the remaining slices of bread.

Makes 4 sandwiches / Cost per serving: $2.94

You can always skip this step and buy a bottle of Russian or Thousand Island dressing, but it's never as good as the homemade stuff.

365 calories
14 g fat
(4 g saturated)
1,120 mg sodium

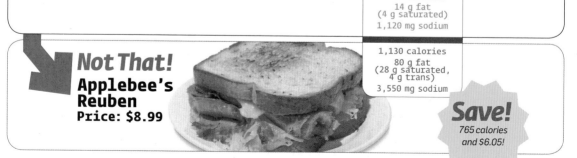

Not That!
Applebee's Reuben
Price: $8.99

1,130 calories
80 g fat
(28 g saturated,
4 g trans)
3,550 mg sodium

Save!
765 calories
and $6.05!

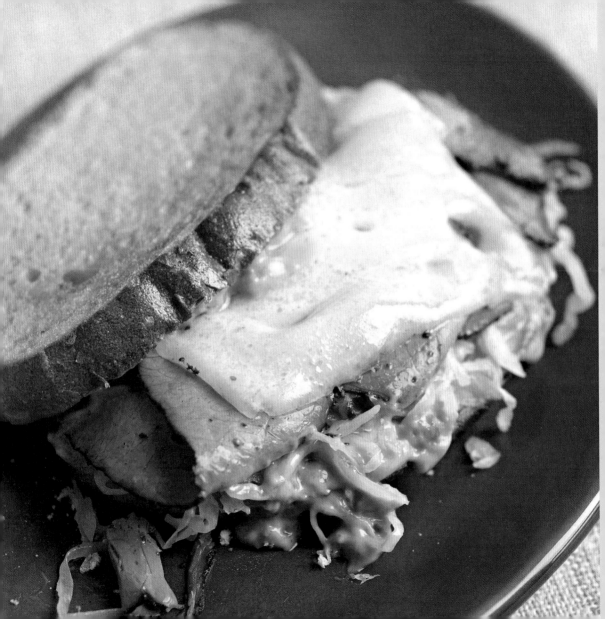

Chicken Burger with Sundried Tomato Aioli

Alternative burgers nearly always lead you astray in the restaurant world. Chicken burgers, turkey burgers, even veggie burgers tend to be every bit as unhealthy as their beefy brethren. Why bother? We've taken back the chicken burger, using a lean grind of meat and a hugely flavorful (but surprisingly low-calorie) spiked mayo to deliver on the promise of a truly healthy burger.

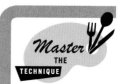

Master THE **TECHNIQUE**

Improvising aioli

Aioli is traditionally a garlic and olive oil mayonnaise made in France and Spain, and the combination of these two ingredients makes for a much healthier spread than your average jar of Hellmann's. You can do a quick approximation by mincing a clove or two of garlic, then using the back of your knife—along with a pinch of salt for abrasion—to grind the garlic into a paste. Add it to olive oil–based mayonnaise (made by Kraft and Hellmann's), along with any other flavor boosters. Some of our favorites: roasted red pepper, sriracha, chipotle, and balsamic vinegar.

You'll Need:

- 2 Tbsp olive oil mayonnaise
- 2 Tbsp chopped sundried tomatoes
- Juice of ½ lemon
- 2 cloves garlic, finely minced
- 1 tsp chopped fresh rosemary
- Salt and black pepper
- 1 lb lean ground chicken
- 4 whole-wheat or potato buns (or even English muffins), split
- 2 cups arugula, baby spinach, or mixed greens

How to Make It:

- In a mixing bowl, combine the mayonnaise, sundried tomatoes, lemon juice, garlic, and rosemary. Season with a pinch of salt and black pepper. Set the aioli aside.
- Preheat a grill, grill pan, or cast-iron skillet. Combine the ground chicken with ½ teaspoon salt and ½ teaspoon black pepper and mix gently. Without overworking the meat, form into four patties until the chicken just comes together.
- When the grill or skillet is hot (if using a skillet, add a touch of oil), add the burgers. Cook on the first side for 5 to 6 minutes, until a nice crust develops. Flip and cook for another 3 to 4 minutes, until the burgers are firm but ever so slightly yielding to the touch and cooked through. Remove the burgers. While the grill or pan is hot, toast the buns.
- Layer the bottom buns with the arugula, top each with a burger, then slather the aioli over the top of each. Crown with the bun tops and serve.

Makes 4 burgers /
Cost per serving: $1.80

330 calories
14 g fat
(3 g saturated)
730 mg sodium

Not That!
Whisky River BBQ Chicken Burger
Price: $9.59

965 calories
52 g fat
1842 mg sodium

Save!
635 calories
and $7.79!

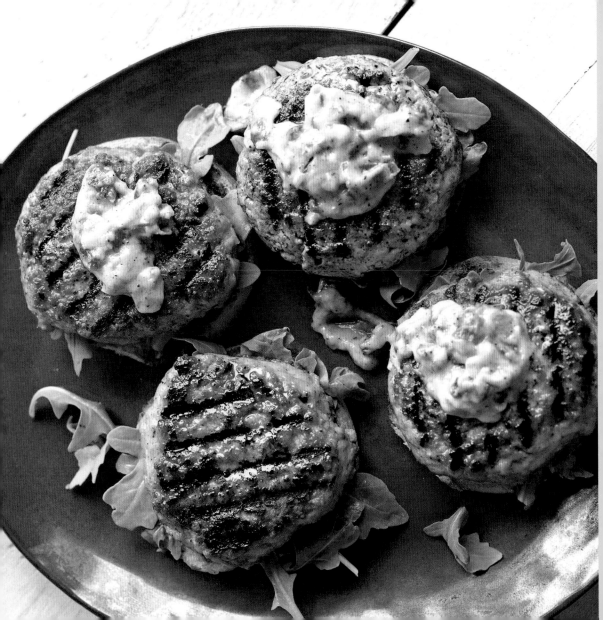

Grilled Vegetable Wrap

Can it be? A truly healthy wrap? We've been watching on the sidelines in shock and dismay as one person after the next is tricked into believing that a wrap is some sort of magical weight loss bullet. Unfortunately, sandwich shops and sit-down spots alike take advantage of the reputation to cram Frisbee-size tortillas with cheese, bacon, ranch, and any other high-calorie ingredients they can find. Even with a dusting of goat cheese and a spread of balsamic mayo, this wrap earns its healthy stripes by virtue of its low calorie counts and generous vegetable filling.

You'll Need:

- 12 asparagus spears, woody ends removed
- 2 portobello mushroom caps
- 1 red bell pepper, halved, seeds and stem removed
- 1 Tbsp olive oil
- Salt and black pepper to taste
- 2 Tbsp olive oil mayonnaise
- 1 Tbsp balsamic vinegar
- 1 clove garlic, minced
- 4 large spinach or whole-wheat tortillas or wraps
- 2 cups arugula, baby spinach, or mixed baby greens
- ¾ cup crumbled goat or feta cheese

How to Make It:

- Preheat a grill. Toss the asparagus, mushrooms, and bell pepper with the olive oil, plus a few pinches of salt and pepper. Place on the hottest part of the grill and cook, turning occasionally, until lightly charred and tender. The asparagus should take the least amount of time (about 5 minutes) and the peppers the most (about 10). Alternatively, you can roast the vegetables in a 450°F oven for 10 to 12 minutes. Slice the mushroom caps into thin strips. If possible, peel off the charred skin of the pepper and then slice.

- Combine the mayonnaise, vinegar, and garlic and stir to combine thoroughly. Heat the tortillas on the grill or in the microwave for 30 seconds. Spread the balsamic mayo down the middle of each tortilla, then top with the greens and cheese. Divide the grilled vegetables among the tortillas, then roll up tightly and slice each wrap in half.

Makes 4 wraps /
Cost per serving: $3.15

240 calories
13 g fat
(3.5 g saturated)
450 mg sodium

610 calories
29 g fat
(7 g saturated)
1,770 mg sodium

Not That!
Au Bon Pain Mediterranean Wrap
Price: $5.99

Save!
370 calories
and $2.84!

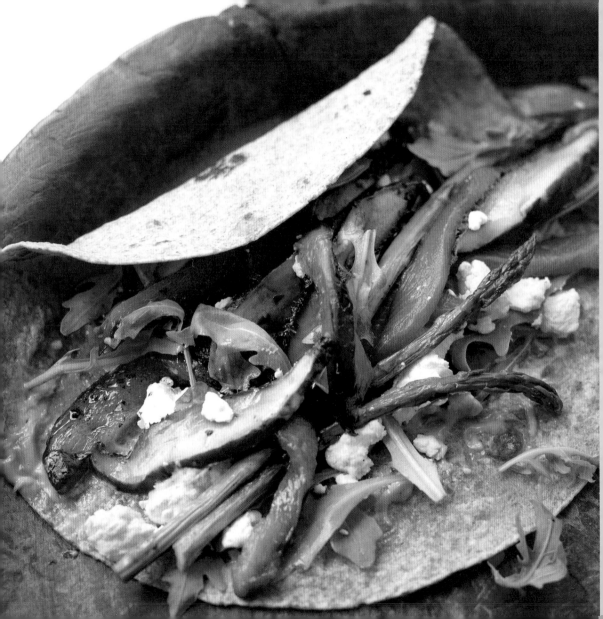

Cook This!
Asian Tuna Burgers with Wasabi Mayo

A firm, meaty fish like tuna is prime picking for the burger treatment. All it takes is a quick pulse in the food processor, or even just a bit of fine chopping. Either way, make sure the fish is very cold, which keep the proteins from binding into tough lumps. The resulting ground tuna is ready to be formed into patties and dressed up in dozens of different ways. If tuna isn't your fish of choice, salmon works every bit as well.

You'll Need:

- 1 lb fresh tuna
- 4 scallions, minced
- 1 tsp minced fresh ginger
- 1 Tbsp low-sodium soy sauce
- 1 tsp toasted sesame oil
- Canola oil, for grilling
- 2 Tbsp olive oil mayonnaise
- ½ Tbsp prepared wasabi (from powder or in premade paste)
- 4 whole-wheat sesame buns, split and lightly toasted
- 1 cup sliced cucumber, lightly salted
- 2 cups mixed baby greens

How to Make It:

- Chop the tuna into ½" cubes, then place in the freezer for 10 minutes to firm up (this will make grinding easier). Working in batches if necessary, pulse the tuna in a food processor to the consistency of ground beef. (Be sure not to overdo it; you only want to pulse it enough so that you can form patties.) Transfer to a mixing bowl and mix in the scallions, ginger, soy sauce, and sesame oil. Form into four equal patties. Place in the fridge for at least 10 minutes before grilling to firm up.

- Preheat a well-oiled grill or grill pan. When hot, add the patties and cook for 2 to 3 minutes a side, until browned on the outside, but still medium rare in the center. Flip and handle carefully, as these burgers are more delicate than beef burgers.

- Mix the mayo with the wasabi, then spread evenly onto the bun tops. Line the bottoms with cucumber and greens, top with the burgers, then crown with the bun tops.

Makes 4 burgers /
Cost per serving: $3.82

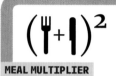

MEAL MULTIPLIER

Like any beef or turkey burger, these tuna patties are prime picks for an array of flourishes and accoutrements. Change up the burger with one of these treatments:

- Mix the tuna with Dijon and herbs (instead of the Asian seasonings), then top with slices of grilled tomato and tapenade
- Brush the Asian patties with teriyaki sauce and top with pickled jalapeños and rings of grilled pineapple
- Brush the Asian patties with hoisin and top with mayonnaise spiked with lime juice and sriracha

330 calories
11 g fat
(2 g saturated)
460 mg sodium

750 calories
47 g fat
(9 g saturated)
1,130 mg sodium

Not That!
Panera Bread Tuna Salad on Honey Wheat Sandwich
Price: $5.59

Save!
420 calories and $1.77!

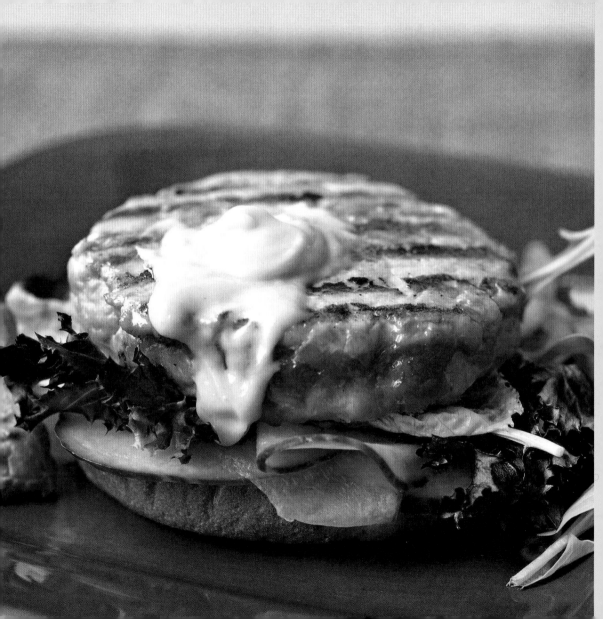

Steak Sandwich Open-Face on Garlic Toast

As nice as it is to pick up a meat- and vegetable-stuffed roll with both hands and chomp down on it, there's something especially alluring about the knife-and-fork approach that goes with the open-face sandwich. The brilliance of it is that the cutlery implies a certain heft and decadence—that this sandwich is too loaded to handle by hand—when in fact, you just saved yourself 100 empty calories by ditching half of the bread. To make matters even better, we rub the base with cut garlic cloves, giving you the impression that you're eating a cheesesteak on top of a big hunk of garlic bread.

You'll Need:

- 2 ciabatta rolls, split or 4 6-inch baguette halves
- 2 cloves garlic, peeled and cut in half
- ½ Tbsp olive oil
- 1 medium onion, sliced
- 1 lb sirloin, sliced into thin pieces
- Salt and black pepper to taste
- ¼ cup A.1. Steak Sauce
- 1 large tomato, cut into 4 thick slices
- 4 slices low-fat Swiss or provolone cheese

How to Make It:

- Preheat the oven to 450°F. Place the bread on a baking sheet and bake on an upper rack for about 5 minutes, until lightly toasted. Rub with the garlic cloves.
- Heat the oil in a large sauté pan over medium heat. Add the onion and cook for about 3 minutes, until translucent. Add the sirloin pieces and cook for about 7 minutes, until both the beef and onions are browned and the meat is cooked through. Season with salt and pepper, then stir in the A.1. Remove from the heat.
- Place a slice of tomato on top of each ciabatta half. Top with the beef mixture and then the cheese. Bake for 5 to 7 minutes, until the cheese is fully melted.

Makes 4 sandwiches / Cost per serving: $2.59

$$(\Psi + I)^2$$

MEAL MULTIPLIER

Other sandwich concepts that take well to the open-face approach:

- Ham, Swiss, and sliced tomato, slathered in honey mustard
- Grilled Ratatouille Salad (see page 104) topped with fresh goat cheese
- Herb-Roasted Turkey Breast (see page 228), stuffing, and turkey gravy or cranberry sauce

365 calories
16 g fat
(6 g saturated)
510 mg sodium

763 calories
20 g fat
(6 g saturated)
3,333 mg sodium

Not That!
Outback Roasted Filet Sandwich
Price: $9.95

Save!
398 calories and $7.36!

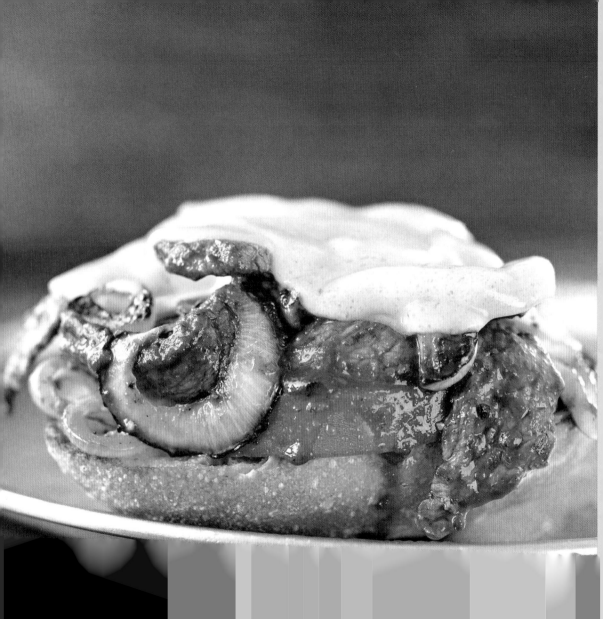

Caprese Sandwich

The pairing of creamy fresh mozzarella, juicy ripe tomatoes, and fat leaves of sweet basil is so good that you'd be crazy not to exploit it as often as possible to make yourself look like a culinary genius. This recipe requires absolutely no effort, save for about 2 minutes of slicing and 2 minutes of toasting. Plus, it morphs easily into other dishes. Not in the mood for a sandwich? Ditch the bread and eat this as a salad for dinner. Need a quick appetizer for a crowd? Slice the baguette into rounds; toast; and layer slices of tomato and mozz and a basil leaf on top of each. This is versatility at its most delicious.

You'll Need:

- 1 baguette, sliced in half lengthwise
- 1 clove garlic, peeled and cut in half
- 2 large heirloom tomatoes, sliced
- 4 oz fresh mozzarella, sliced
- 15–20 fresh basil leaves
- Salt and black pepper to taste
- 1 Tbsp olive oil
- 1 Tbsp balsamic vinegar

How to Make It:

- Preheat the broiler. Broil the baguette, cut sides up, 6" from heat, for about 2 minutes, until the inside is lightly toasted. Rub each half with a half clove of garlic; the crusty bread will release the garlic's essential oils, giving you instant garlic bread.
- Layer the bottom half of the baguette, alternating with slices of tomato, mozzarella, and basil leaves. Season evenly with salt and lots of fresh black pepper. Finish with a drizzle of olive oil and vinegar, then top with the other baguette half. Cut the whole package into four pieces.

Makes 4 sandwiches / Cost per serving: $2.96

This sandwich is best made in the summer months, when tomatoes are at their peak. If you can't find heirlooms, very ripe beefsteak tomatoes are your next best bet.

300 calories
17 g fat
(4.5 g saturated)
410 mg sodium

770 calories
29 g fat
(10 g saturated)
1,290 mg sodium

Not That!
Panera Tomato Mozzarella Hot Panini
Price: $6.89

Save!
470 calories
and $3.93!

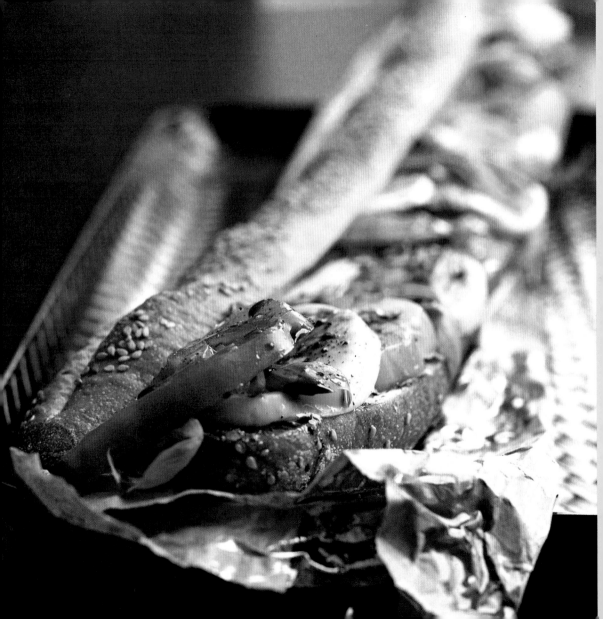

Grilled Chicken
Sandwich with Chimichurri

No chain menu in America is without a chicken sandwich or two. Eighty percent of the time, it is breaded and fried, and when it isn't (as in the case with Panera's Chipotle Chicken), it's so overloaded with condiments and bulky bread that you'll be lucky to escape consuming fewer than 1,000 calories. So much for being a healthy alternative to a hamburger. This sandwich delivers heroic flavor by employing chimichurri, an Argentine herb-based sauce that would make shoe leather taste like fine dining, along with a solid supporting cast of sweet peppers, sharp raw onions, and peppery greens. Good luck finding a side salad, let alone a real sandwich, at a restaurant for 310 calories.

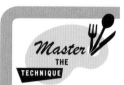

Master THE TECHNIQUE

Roasting peppers

You can buy bottled roasted red peppers in any supermarket, but save a few bucks and roast them yourself instead. Cook the bell peppers (red and yellow are best) at 400°F until the skin blackens and the flesh softens, about 25 minutes (you can also do this on a grill or even over a low flame on a gas stovetop). Place the peppers in a bowl, cover with plastic wrap, and let them sit for 10 minutes. Remove the plastic wrap and peel off the dark skin (the steam created by covering the peppers makes this easy). Discard the stems and seeds and they're ready to eat.

You'll Need:

- 4 **boneless skinless chicken thighs (6 oz each)**
- **Salt and black pepper to taste**
- 2 cups **mixed baby greens**
- 4 **whole-wheat sesame buns, split and lightly toasted**
- ½ **red onion, thinly sliced**
- ½ cup **jarred roasted red peppers**
- ½ cup **Chimichurri (see page 266)**

How to Make It:

- Preheat a grill, grill pan, or cast-iron skillet. Season the chicken all over with salt and pepper and grill or sear for 3 to 4 minutes per side, until firm and cooked through.
- Divide the mixed greens among the bun bottoms. Top each bun with a chicken thigh, then pile on the onion and peppers. Spoon on the chimichurri, then top with the other bun halves.

Makes 4 sandwiches / Cost per serving: $1.81

Want to save yourself the trouble of cooking the chicken? Use the meat from a store-bought rotisserie bird instead.

310 calories
8 g fat
(3 g saturated)
475 mg sodium

990 calories
56 g fat
(15 g saturated,
1 g trans)
2,370 mg sodium

Not That!
Panera Bread Chipotle Chicken on Artisan French
Price: $7.09

Save!
680 calories
and $5.28!

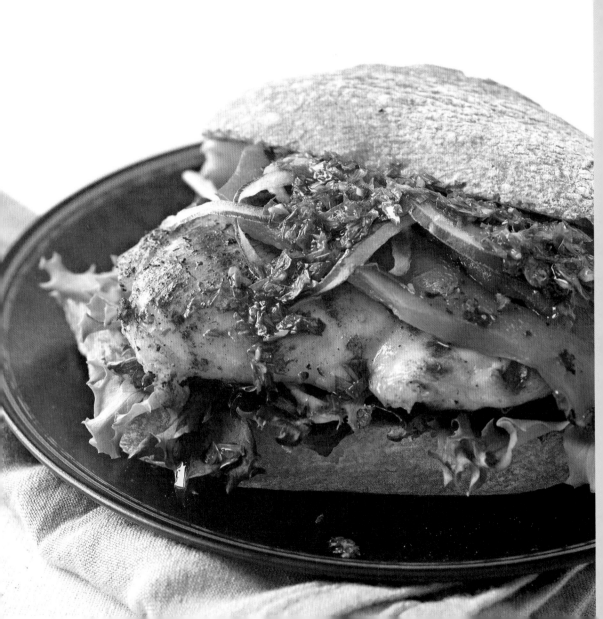

Portobello Cheesesteak

The mark of a great vegetarian dish is one that will be eagerly devoured by a diehard carnivore. This one fits the bill in spades: meaty slices of portobello sautéed with a thicket of peppers and onions, then tucked into a toasted roll and topped with a cap of melted provolone. But unlike so many vegetarian dishes out there masquerading as healthier than the meaty creations they replace (we're looking at you, 1,377-calorie portobello burger from The Cheesecake Factory), you could eat this cheesesteak 7 days a week and end up skinnier than when you started.

You'll Need:

- 1 Tbsp canola or olive oil
- 2 large portobello mushrooms, stems and gills removed, sliced
- 1 medium yellow onion, sliced
- 1 red bell pepper, sliced
- 1 Tbsp low-sodium soy sauce
- 1 Tbsp Worcestershire sauce
- Salt and black pepper to taste
- 4 slices provolone
- 4 soft whole-wheat hoagie rolls, split and toasted

How to Make It:

- Heat ½ tablespoon oil in a large sauté pan over medium-high heat. Add the portobello slices and cook, stirring occasionally, for about 5 minutes, until nicely caramelized. Transfer to a plate. Heat the remaining ½ tablespoon oil in the same pan. Add the onion and pepper and cook for about 5 minutes, until softened and beginning to brown.

- Return the mushrooms to the pan and stir in the soy sauce and Worcestershire. Cook for another 2 minutes, until the vegetables have absorbed most of the liquid. Remove from the heat and season with salt and pepper. Divide the vegetables into four piles in the pan and top each with a slice of cheese (the residual heat will help to melt it). Once the cheese has begun to melt, tuck the vegetable piles into the rolls.

Makes 4 sandwiches / Cost per serving: $2.33

The gills have little flavor and can give a dish a dark, muddy look. Remove them by taking a small spoon and scraping away the dark, thin flaps underneath the cap.

340 calories
14 g fat
(6 g saturated)
740 mg sodium

1,377 calories
22 g saturated fat
1362 mg sodium

Not That!

Cheesecake Factory Grilled Portobello on a Bun
Price: $10.95

Save!
1,037 calories and $8.62!

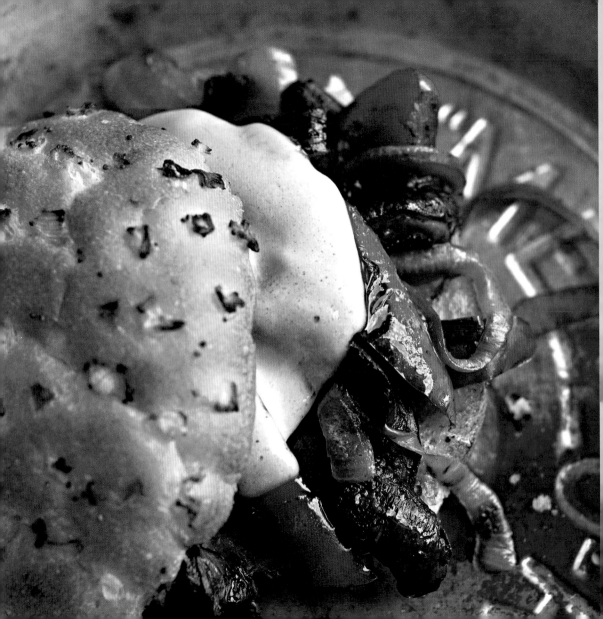

Cook This!
Italian Tuna Melt

Ahh, the tuna melt: Has any sandwich squandered more potential more consistently than this fishy fiasco? The recipe used by most establishments tells all: 2 parts mayo to 1 part tuna (which is why 59 percent of the calories in Quiznos' 1,000-calorie sandwich comes from fat). This recipe replaces the bulk of the mayo with a considerably healthier supporting cast: pesto, lemon juice, olives, and onions. That means you can taste something other than fat when you're eating it and feel something other than fat when you're through.

You'll Need:

- 2 cans (5 oz each) tuna, drained
- 1 small red onion, diced
- ¼ cup chopped green olives
- 2 Tbsp olive oil mayonnaise
- 2 Tbsp bottled pesto
- 1 Tbsp capers, rinsed and chopped
- Juice of 1 lemon
- 8 slices whole-wheat bread
- 2 oz fresh mozzarella, sliced (you can use low-fat shredded mozzarella, too)
- 1 large tomato, sliced
- About 1 tsp olive oil

How to Make It:

- In a mixing bowl, combine the tuna, onion, olives, mayo, pesto, capers, and lemon juice and stir to combine. Layer the bottom half of four slices of bread with mozzarella, then top with the tuna mixture, tomato slices, and remaining slices of bread.

- Preheat a cast-iron or nonstick pan over medium heat. Coat with a thin layer of olive oil and cook the sandwiches for 2 to 3 minutes per side, until the bread is toasted and the cheese is melted.

Makes 4 sandwiches /
Cost per serving: $2.38

When it comes to whole-wheat bread, nothing beats Martin's Whole Wheat Potato Bread.

$$(\Psi + \mathsf{I})^2$$

MEAL MULTIPLIER

"Tuna salad" is one of the biggest misnomers in the food world; both "tuna" and "salad" are healthy when on their own, but combined, they're nothing but trouble. Reinvent this troubled tandem with some more clever pairings from your pantry:

- Curry powder, shredded carrot, cashews, and golden raisins
- Salsa, sliced avocado, and Jack cheese
- Artichokes, sundried tomatoes, and provolone

340 calories
13 g fat
(2 g saturated)
980 mg sodium

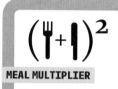

1,000 calories
66 g fat
(14 g saturated)
1,350 mg sodium

Not That!
Quiznos Regular Tuna Melt
Price: $4.49

Save!
*660 calories
and $2.11!*

140

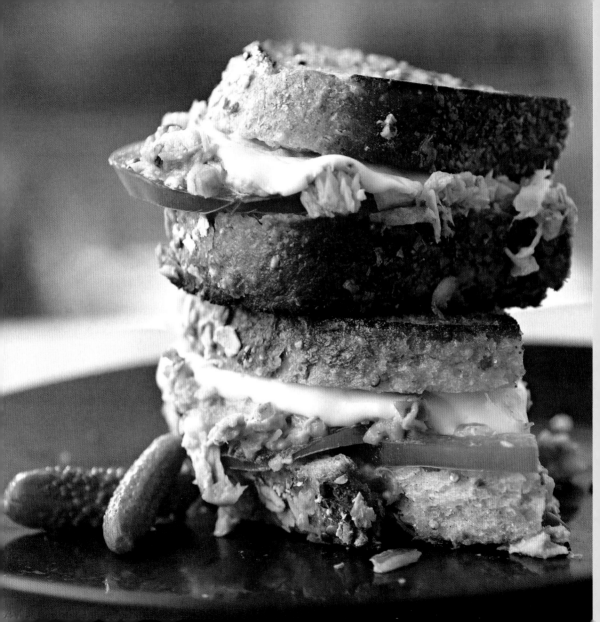

A.1. Swiss Burger

The United States is flush with quirky regional burgers, from the pastrami-topped burgers of Utah to the butter burgers of Wisconsin. Our favorite is the Midwestern smashed burger, which involves using a spatula to thwack a ball of ground beef into a thin patty while it cooks in a cast-iron skillet. Try it once and you may never go back to bulky grilled burgers again.

You'll Need:

- ½ Tbsp canola oil, plus more for the burgers
- 1 medium yellow onion, sliced
- 2 cups sliced white or cremini mushrooms
- Salt and black pepper to taste
- 1 lb ground sirloin
- 4 slices reduced-fat Swiss cheese
- 4 potato buns, split and lightly toasted
- 4 Tbsp A.1. Steak Sauce

How to Make It:

- Heat the oil in a large skillet or sauté pan over medium-low heat. Add the onion and cook for 3 to 4 minutes, until soft and translucent. Add the mushrooms and cook for 6 to 7 minutes, until the mushrooms and onions are browned and caramelized. Season with salt and pepper and remove from the heat.

- Heat a light film of oil in a large cast-iron skillet over medium-high heat. Form the sirloin into four loosely packed 1-inch balls, being careful not to overwork the meat. Season all over with salt and a bit of black pepper. Add to the pan and cook for a minute or two, then place a spatula on top of each patty and press down to flatten the meat into a burger about ⅓" thick. Cook for about 2 minutes, until a nice crust develops. Flip, using the spatula to scrape the burger free if necessary. Top with cheese and cook for 2 to 3 minutes more, until the meat is cooked through. Place the burgers on the toasted buns, then top with the mushrooms and onions. Finish by drizzling a tablespoon of A.1. on each.

Makes 4 burgers /
Cost per serving: $2.61

Save!
850 calories
and $7.38!

340 calories
15 g fat
(5 g saturated)
580 mg sodium

1,190 calories
82 g fat
(24 saturated,
2.5 trans)
2,070 mg sodium

Not That!
Applebee's Steakhouse Burger
with A.1. Steak Sauce
Price: $9.99

Smashed burger

This style of burger maximizes crust development and helps the beef retain a ton of juiciness. Heat a skillet, season the burger all over, and smash away.

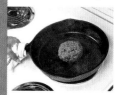

Step 1: *Place a 4-6 oz ball of beef in a hot skillet*

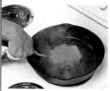

Step 2: *After a minute, smash the ball into a patty*

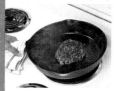

Step 3: *Cook for 2 minutes, flip, and continue cooking*

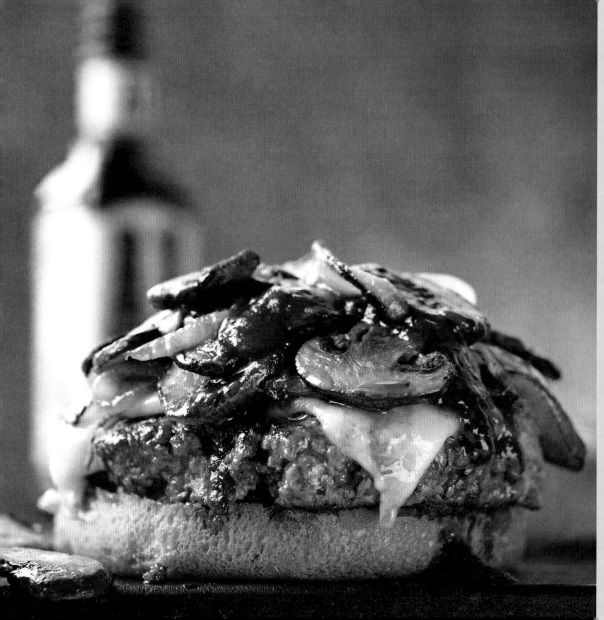

Off the Grill

Sizzling steaks, succulent fish, and everything in between

The Rules of the Grill

No matter who you are and how often you cook, these timeless adages of meat and fire will help you tame the flame once and for all.

1. Forget the fork.

Grill tool sets usually come with a spatula, a pair of tongs, and a scary, oversized fork for probing and pronging your food. First thing you should do is open the package and throw the fork out. The last tool you ever want to use is one that will break the surface of your food, creating an escape route for all the precious juices that are trapped inside. Spatula and tongs only.

2. Ditch the lighter fluid.

Have you ever smelled the stuff? If you have, you'd know that even the faintest residue of fluid on your food is bound to be a bad thing. Put down the squeeze bottle and pick up a charcoal chimney, a simple device that houses charcoal on top, newspaper on the bottom, and sets the whole pile ablaze with a simple flick from a lighter. Weber sells charcoal chimneys for about $15.

3. Know your zones.

A wildly hot grill can be a dangerous proposition, especially when you have larger cuts of meat that take time to grill. Put a chicken leg or a substantial steak directly over a raging flame and you'll char the outside before the center ever breaks room

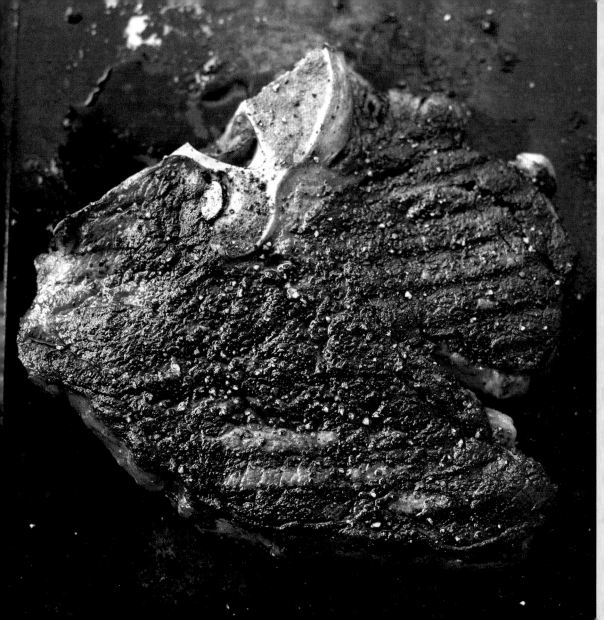

temperature. Always try to set up your grill with two temperature zones, one very hot area for searing and charring, and one cooler zone where you can cook thicker cuts slowly and thoroughly. If using a charcoal grill, gather the majority of the briquettes on one side of the grill (a technique called banking), leaving the other relatively free of direct heat. If gas is your go-to grill option, simply turn one burner on medium or high and keep another all the way down on low.

4. Rest your meat.

As tempting as it may be to take your grilled goodies from grate to plate, all meat needs time to rest before you go cutting into it. The heat of the grill has put all of the meat's internal juices in motion; slice it open prematurely and those juices will end up on your cutting board or your plate and not in your eagerly awaiting mouth.

By allowing poultry and red meat to cool, you give the juices a chance to stop swirling wildly about and eventually be reabsorbed back into the food. Big cuts of meat (thick steaks, roasts, whole chickens) need 10 minutes to rest; thinner cuts (chicken breasts, flank steak, pork tenderloin) will be ready to eat after 5.

5. Tame the temperature.

More than marinades, spice rubs, and fancy sauces, the most important skill a budding grill master needs to learn is how to cook meat and fish to its proper doneness. Cook enough and you'll learn to gauge a steak's internal temperature with a simple touch of the meat, as if your finger were some magical divining rod. But even the pros carry instant-read thermometers to ensure they've cooked their precious goods perfectly.

Harness the Heat

To get the most accurate read, insert the thermometer into the deepest part of the meat. Chicken should be cooked to an internal temperature of 160°F and pork to 140–145°F. For beef and lamb, the answers lie in the chart:

Doneness	Internal Temperature	What It Looks Like	What It Feels Like
Rare	120–125°F	Red from the center to the crust	Soft and squishy, like a sponge
Medium Rare	130–135°F	Red at the center, pink everywhere else	Slightly firm but yields to gentle pressure, like a Nerf football
Medium	140–145°F	Pink throughout	Barely yielding, like a racquetball
Medium Well	150–155°F	Slightly pink in the center, gray everywhere else	Firm and springy, like a tennis ball
Well	160°F and above	Gray throughout	Hard, like a basketball

CHAPTER 6

Master the Marinade

Marinades pack your food with flavor without the gut-busting calories of heavy sauces. They also break down tough muscle fibers and infuse your food with moisture, turning even pedestrian cuts of meat into the type of succulent fare you pay serious cash for in restaurants with linen and china. But, perhaps most importantly of all, marinades have an important health function: Research from the Food Science Institute of Kansas found that the polyphenols in marinade, drawn from a pool of herbs and spices, cut carcinogen deposits in grilled foods by up to 88 percent. That's all the motivation we need. Seal the deal with one of these five flavor-boosting, moisture-imparting, carcinogen-killing marinades.

THE SMOKY SOLUTION

Juice of 2 limes
- 1 cup orange juice
- 2 cloves garlic, minced
- 2 Tbsp pureed chipotle peppers
- ½ cup chopped cilantro

Best for:

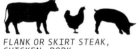

FLANK OR SKIRT STEAK, CHICKEN, PORK

THE EASTERN EXPRESS

- ½ cup rice wine vinegar
- 1 cup low-sodium soy sauce
- 2 Tbsp fresh grated ginger
- 2 Tbsp brown sugar

Best for:

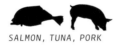

SALMON, TUNA, PORK

THE UTILITY PLAYER

- ½ cup balsamic vinegar
- 2 Tbsp Dijon mustard
- 2 cloves garlic, minced
- ¼ cup olive oil
- 2 Tbsp chopped fresh rosemary

Best for:

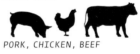

PORK, CHICKEN, BEEF

THE BOOZE HOUND

- 2 cups red wine
- 3 cloves garlic, minced
- 4 bay leaves
- 1 tsp black pepper

Best for:

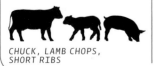

CHUCK, LAMB CHOPS, SHORT RIBS

THE CLUB MED

- 1 cup olive oil
Juice of 1 lemon
- 1 Tbsp fresh thyme
- 2 cloves garlic, minced
- ½ tsp red pepper flakes

Best for:

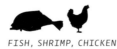

FISH, SHRIMP, CHICKEN

KEY

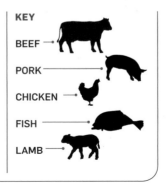

BEEF →

PORK →

CHICKEN →

FISH →

LAMB →

Chicken under a Brick

Drop the bottled barbecue sauce! The Italians figured out a magical way to grill chicken that involves no special sauces or condiments; in fact, all you really need is a brick or two and some aluminum foil. Whoever first placed brick to backbone was smart enough to recognize that the extra weight helped press the bird evenly—and forcefully—against the grill, which translates into a juicier bird with a crisper skin—a win-win in our book.

You'll Need:

- ¼ cup olive oil
- Grated zest and juice of 1 lemon
- 1 tsp red pepper flakes
- 1 tsp salt
- ½ tsp black pepper
- 1 whole chicken, back removed, split in half
- 2 lemons, halved
- 2 bricks, covered in aluminum foil

Ask the butcher at the meat counter to do this for you.

How to Make It:

- Combine the olive oil, lemon zest and juice, pepper flakes, salt, and pepper in a large bowl, baking dish, or sealable plastic bag. Add the chicken and turn to coat. Cover the bowl or seal the bag and marinate in the refrigerator for at least 30 minutes and up to 4 hours.

- Preheat a grill (you want a nice medium-low heat). Remove the chicken from the marinade and place on the grate, skin side up. Cover the grill and cook for 10 minutes, until the chicken is lightly charred. Flip the chicken over, then place a brick on top of each half so that it presses the chicken firmly and evenly against the grate. Cook for another 15 to 20 minutes, until the skin is thoroughly browned and crisp and the meat pulls away easily from the bone. (If the grill flares up, move the chicken to a cooler part of the grill.) While the chicken cooks, toss on the lemon halves, cut side down, and grill until charred and juicy.

- Separate each breast from the chicken leg by making a cut right at the thigh bone. Serve each of the four pieces of chicken with a grilled lemon half.

Makes 4 servings /
Cost per serving: $2.40

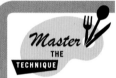

Master **THE** `TECHNIQUE`

Brick cooking

It may be the crudest, most rudimentary of tools, but a sturdy, foil-wrapped brick comes in handy in the kitchen. Try placing it on top of a pork chop or a flank steak in a cast-iron pan—the extra pressure will yield a beautifully caramelized crust. Better yet, it's perfect for making a panini: Simply place the sandwich in a hot cast-iron skillet, top with a brick, cook for 2 or 3 minutes, then flip and repeat.

280 calories
8 g fat
(2 g saturated)
780 mg sodium

1,100 calories
82 g fat
(16 g saturated)
1,960 mg sodium

Not That!
Uno Chicago Grill Lemon Herb Chicken (Grilled)
Price: $12.49

Save!
820 calories and $10.09!

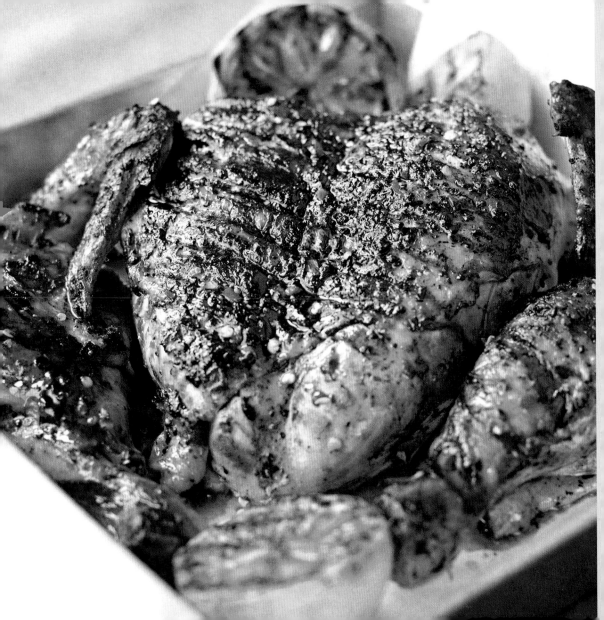

Bloody Mary Skirt Steak

As delicious as a Bloody Mary is as a drink, it makes an even better marinade. That's because the mix of sweet and salty from the tomato juice, the heat from the horseradish and Tabasco, and the acid from the lemon work together to both tenderize and energize an otherwise normal piece of beef. This marinade could do magic on chicken and pork as well, but the bold flavors of a Bloody seem to pair best with a hunk of grilled beef. Serve with grilled asparagus and roasted potatoes for a near-perfect meal.

You'll Need:

- **2 cups tomato juice (spicy V8 works best)**
- **2 Tbsp prepared horseradish**
- **4 cloves garlic, minced**

Juice of 1 lemon

- **½ Tbsp Worcestershire sauce**
- **10–15 shakes Tabasco sauce**

Black pepper to taste

- **1 lb skirt or flank steak**

How to Make It:

- Combine the tomato juice, horseradish, garlic, lemon juice, Worcestershire, Tabasco, and pepper in a baking dish and use a whisk to thoroughly mix. Add the steak and turn to coat. Cover with plastic wrap. Marinate in the refrigerator for at least 2 hours or up to 12.

- Preheat a grill. Pour off the marinade and discard. Use a paper towel to pat most of the marinade from the steak. When the grill is very hot, add the steak and cook for 3 to 4 minutes per side for medium rare. Let the meat rest for at least 5 minutes before cutting into thin slices against the grain of the meat.

Makes 4 servings / Cost per serving: $2.96

Both of these thin cuts of beef offer huge flavor and a pleasantly chewy texture at a relatively cheap price tag. Because they're thin, you'll want a very hot grill to ensure you develop a nice char before the interior is overcooked.

270 calories
11 g fat
(4.5 g saturated)
450 mg sodium

840 calories

Not That!

T.G.I. Friday's Flat Iron Steak
Price: $13.79

Save!

570 calories
and $10.83!

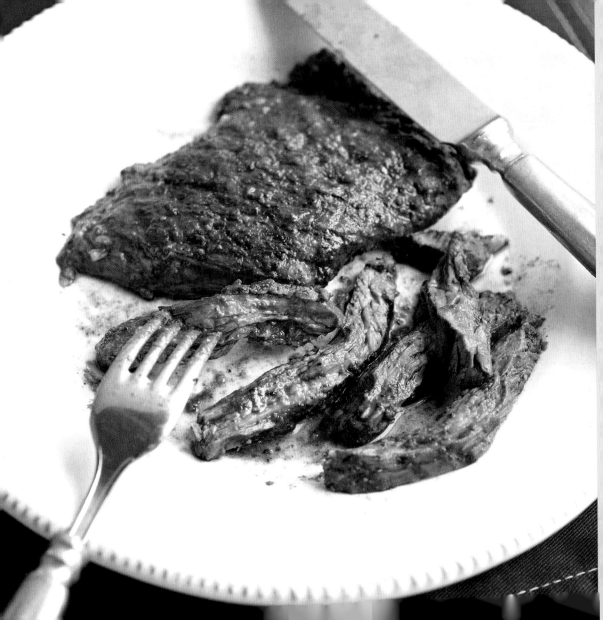

Pork Chop with Balsamic-Honey Glaze

When it comes to quality ingredients worth splurging on, heirloom pork is at the top of our list. Supermarket pork comes from a handful of mega-producers who have a near monopoly on the industry and who put out an inferior, tasteless product. (Hence the predictable complaints of pork being dry and boring.) Luckily, many small farmers are starting to raise heirloom varieties of pigs like Red Wattle, Berkshire, and Mangalitsa. If you can't find a local farmer selling pristine pig at the farmers' market, then try ordering a few chops from Niman Ranch (nimanranch.com) for a special occasion. One bite will banish any misconstrued belief that pork is "the other white meat."

You'll Need:

- ¼ cup balsamic vinegar
- 2 Tbsp butter
- 2 Tbsp honey
- 1 tsp chopped fresh rosemary
- ¼ tsp red pepper flakes
- 4 thick-cut pork chops
- Salt and black pepper to taste

How to Make It:

- Cook the balsamic vinegar, butter, honey, rosemary, and pepper flakes in a small saucepan over medium heat until the butter is melted and the mixture begins to bubble lightly. Remove from the heat.
- Preheat a grill or grill pan. Transfer about 2 tablespoons of the balsamic glaze to a small bowl and set aside. Season the pork chops all over with salt and pepper and brush with the remaining glaze. When the grill is medium-hot, add the pork and cook for 3 to 4 minutes each side, depending on thickness. (For perfect medium pork, a thermometer inserted into the thickest part of the chop will read 140°F.) Remove the chops and, with a clean brush, brush with the reserved glaze.

Makes 4 servings / Cost per serving: $2.06

Not all fresh herbs can be substituted with dried ones. A good rule of thumb is if the recipe involves cooking the herb (as is the case here), it's fine to use dried if no fresh is available (or if you'd rather not buy).

300 calories
19 g fat
(9 g saturated)
340 mg sodium

1,928 calories
57 g saturated fat
1,685 mg sodium

Not That!
Cheesecake Factory Grilled Pork Chops
Price: $18.95

Save!
1,628 calories
and $16.89!

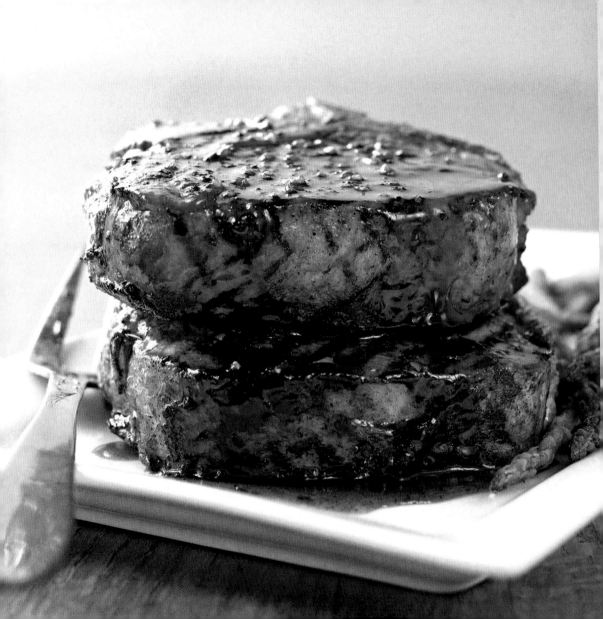

Cook This!
Grilled Calamari Salad

Squid is one of the most abundant forms of seafood in the global market, yet few Americans have ever enjoyed it in any other way than breaded and deep-fried, with a marinara chaser. With that type of treatment, it could be a Blooming Onion and you wouldn't know the difference. This salad has all the trappings of the much-adored appetizer—crunch from the peanuts, tomatoes, a bit of spice— but so much more. We don't want to promise that you'll never go back to the fried stuff after this, but it's a distinct possibility.

You'll Need:

- 1 lb squid, cleaned, tentacles reserved for another use
- ½ Tbsp peanut or canola oil
- Salt and black pepper to taste
- Juice of 1 lime
- 1 Tbsp fish sauce
- 1 Tbsp sugar
- ½ Tbsp chili garlic sauce (preferably sambal oleek)
- 4 cups watercress
- 1 small cucumber, peeled, seeded, and cut into matchsticks
- 1 medium tomato, chopped
- ½ red onion, very thinly sliced
- ¼ cup roasted peanuts

How to Make It:

- Preheat a grill. Toss the squid bodies with the oil and generously season with salt and lots of black pepper. When the grill is very hot, add the squid and grill for about 5 minutes, until lightly charred all over.
- Combine the lime juice, fish sauce, sugar, and chili sauce in a mixing bowl and whisk to blend. Slice the grilled squid into ½" rings. In a salad bowl, toss the squid, watercress, cucumber, tomato, onion, and peanuts with the dressing. Divide the salad among 4 plates.

Makes 4 servings / Cost per serving: $3.04

Watercress isn't always easy to find. Baby arugula, or even a few big handfuls of fresh basil leaves, can easily take its place here.

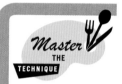

Master THE **TECHNIQUE**

Cooking calamari

Grilling squid ranks right up there next to tying your shoes and making your bed in the difficulty category, yet most people are terrified of the prospect. Purchase whole squid bodies (available fully cleaned, fresh or frozen, at any decent fish market or quality grocery store) and either grill them whole over high heat for no more than 5 minutes, or cut them into rings and sauté in olive oil for the same amount of time.

220 calories
8 g fat
(1.5 g saturated)
590 mg sodium

1,050 calories
93 g fat
(10.5 g saturated)
2,070 mg sodium

Not That!
Uno Chicago Grill Calamari Appetizer
Price: $10.79

Save!
830 calories and $7.75!

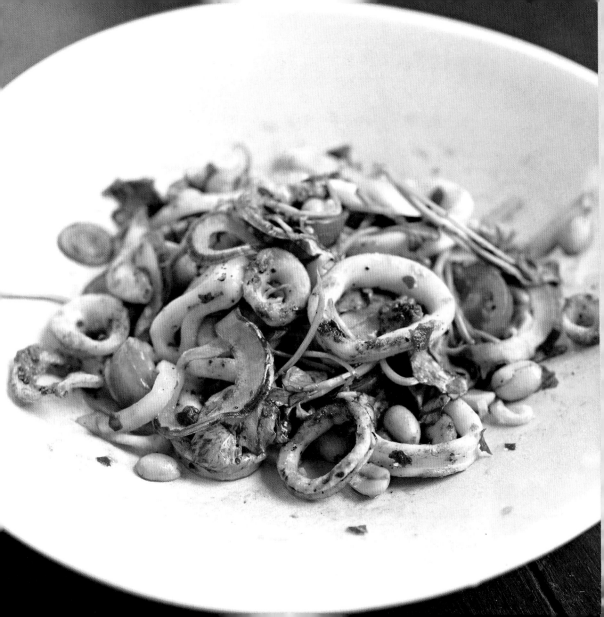

Grilled Chile Relleno

Traditionally, chiles rellenos require an amazing amount of work: roasting and peeling peppers, stuffing them, dipping them in egg wash, then deep-frying the pepper packages in a pot of oil. This recipe simplifies matters tremendously. Rather than go through all that labor, just cut off the tops, scoop in the stuffing, and pop them on the grill. You'll save about 90 minutes of prep work, 20 minutes of cleanup, and a few hundred calories per pepper.

You'll Need:

- 2 ears corn, shucked
- ½ Tbsp canola oil
- 8 oz cooked shrimp, chopped into ½" pieces
- ½ (14–16 oz) can black beans, drained
- 1 cup shredded Monterey Jack cheese
- Juice of 1 lime
- ½ cup chopped cilantro
- ½ tsp cumin
- Salt and black pepper to taste
- 8 poblano peppers
- Salsa (optional)

How to Make It:

- Stand each ear of corn up vertically on a cutting board and run your knife along the ear to remove the kernels. Heat the oil in a large nonstick pan over medium heat. Add the corn and cook for about 5 minutes, until lightly toasted. Remove from the heat, then combine with the shrimp, beans, cheese, lime juice, cilantro, and cumin, plus salt and pepper.
- Preheat a grill or grill pan. Remove the tops of the peppers and scoop out the seeds. Use a spoon to stuff the shrimp mixture into each pepper cavity, being careful not to overfill.
- Place the peppers directly on the grill and cook for about 10 minutes, until the skins have lightly blistered and the flesh has softened. Serve with a bit of salsa, if you like.

Makes 4 servings /
Cost per serving: $2.43

SECRET WEAPON

Poblano peppers

These slender, knobby peppers are the reliable Goldilocks of the capsicum world, spicier than a green bell pepper, but sweeter and more subtle than a jalapeño. The balanced heat level makes them perfect for dozens of dishes: omelets, fajitas, stir-fries. Poblanos are available at most major supermarkets these days, but if you can't find them or just don't trust them, any bell pepper will do for this recipe.

Save!

1,000 calories and $4.57!

360 calories
16 g fat
(6 g saturated)
400 mg sodium

1,360 calories
114 g fat
(10 g saturated)
2,380 mg sodium

Not That!

On the Border Cheese-Stuffed Chile Relleno (2) with Ranchero Sauce
Price: $7

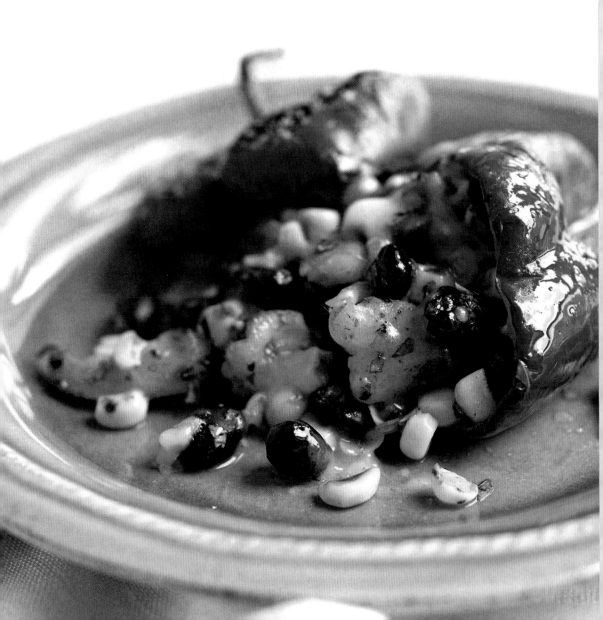

Cook This!
Red Curry Pork Kebab

One of the biggest trends to hit chain restaurants in the past year is the sudden proliferation of skewers and kebabs at places like Macaroni Grill, Olive Garden, and Red Lobster. It's a move we fully applaud, since it means that the heavy carbs and fatty sauces that end up on most restaurant plates are being replaced with lean protein and vegetables. These kebabs have plenty of both, all punched up with an addictive Thai curry sauce that you'll find yourself dipping everything in. Pineapple chunks would be a welcome addition here.

You'll Need:

- ½ cup light coconut milk
- 2 Tbsp Thai red curry paste
- 1 Tbsp peanut butter
- 1 lb pork loin, cut into ¾" pieces
- 1 red or yellow bell pepper, chopped into large pieces
- 1 large red onion, chopped into large pieces
- 8 wooden skewers, soaked in water for 20 minutes

Soaking the skewers will keep them from catching fire on the hot grill.

How to Make It:

- Preheat a grill. Combine the coconut milk, curry paste, and peanut butter in a mixing bowl and stir to thoroughly blend. Transfer half to a separate bowl and reserve.
- Thread the pork, bell pepper, and onion onto the skewers, alternating between the meat and vegetables. Use a brush to paint the skewers with some of the remaining curry sauce. When the grill is hot, add the skewers and cook for 3 to 4 minutes per side, basting with a bit more of the sauce as you go. The skewers are done when the meat and vegetables are lightly charred and the pork is firm but still slightly yielding to the touch.
- Brush the kebabs with the reserved sauce before serving.

Makes 8 skewers / Cost per serving: $1.43

240 calories
8 g fat
(3.5 g saturated)
380 mg sodium

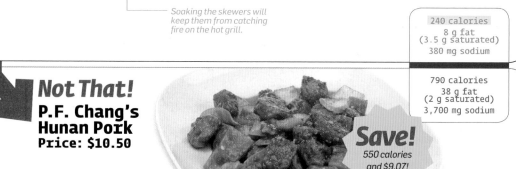

Not That!
P.F. Chang's Hunan Pork
Price: $10.50

790 calories
38 g fat
(2 g saturated)
3,700 mg sodium

Save!
550 calories
and $9.07!

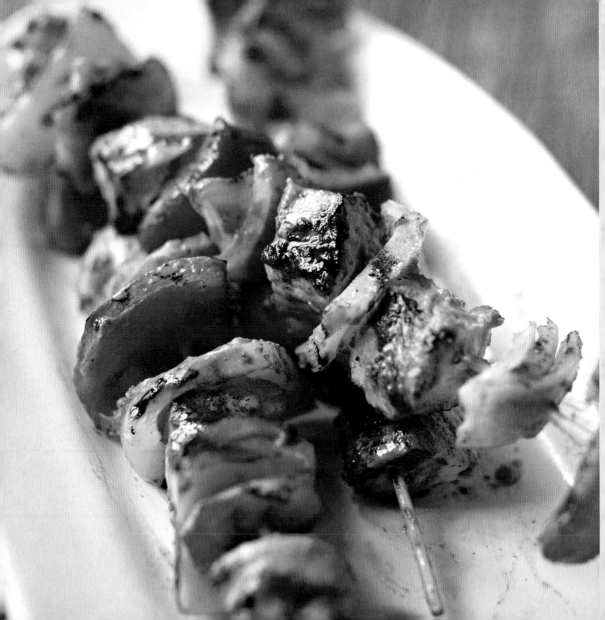

Cook This!
Grilled Mahi Mahi with Salsa Verde

Confusingly enough, both Mexicans and Italians have their own salsa verde, and both are ridiculously good condiments that can be used in a staggering number of dishes. This, the Italian version, is based on parsley, anchovies, capers, and lemon juice, a bright herbal punch that pairs especially well with the smoke and char of a grill. Like Mexico's version, this is equally good on meat as it is on fish. It's no slouch on vegetables either. So make a big batch and keep it in the fridge for instant flavor upgrades.

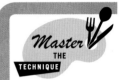

Master THE TECHNIQUE

Crispy fish skin
Too often we peel off the skin from fish fillets and toss it, discarding one of the healthiest and tastiest parts of the fish. When properly cooked, skin provides a crisp textural counterpoint to the fish's soft flesh. Whether cooking skin-on fillets on a grill or in a hot pan, start skin side down and cook for nearly 75 percent of time on that side, then flip and finish on the flesh side. Not all fish have skin made to be crisped. While the skin of salmon, sea bass, and mahi are great eats, halibut, tilapia, and swordfish skin should be discarded (either before or after cooking).

You'll Need:

¾ cup chopped fresh parsley

¼ cup chopped fresh mint (optional)

Juice of 1 lemon

¼ cup olive oil, plus more for grilling

2-3 anchovy fillets, minced

2 Tbsp capers, rinsed and chopped

2 cloves garlic, finely minced

Pinch of red pepper flakes

Salt and black pepper to taste

4 mahi mahi fillets, or other firm white fish like halibut, sea bass, or swordfish (about 6 oz each)

How to Make It:

● Preheat a grill. Make sure the grate is cleaned and oiled.

● Combine the parsley, mint if using, lemon juice, olive oil, anchovies, capers, garlic, and pepper flakes in a mixing bowl. Season with black pepper. Set the salsa verde aside.

● Rub the fish with a thin layer of oil, then season all over with salt and pepper. Place the fillets on the grill skin side down and grill for 5 minutes, until the skin is lightly charred and crisp and pulls away freely (if you mess with the fish before it's ready to flip, it's likely to stick). Flip and cook on the other side for 2 to 3 minutes longer, until the fish flakes with gentle pressure from your fingertip. Serve the fillets with the salsa verde spooned over the top.

Makes 4 servings /
Cost per serving: $4.08

280 calories
15 g fat
(2.5 g saturated)
390 mg sodium

1,194 calories
24 g saturated fat
1,967 mg sodium

Not That!
Cheesecake Factory Mahi Mahi Mediterranean
Price: $19.95

Save!
914 calories and $15.87!

162

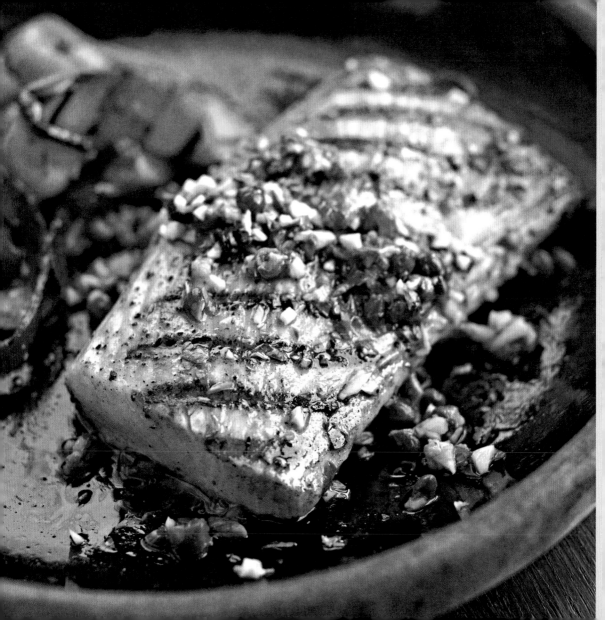

Grilled Steak Taco

Tacos should be a sure bet, regardless of the restaurant. Alas, not even this humble handheld street food is safe when caught in the clutches of the corporate chef. Excessive cheese and superfluous sauces ruin both the simple beauty of a taco and the nutritional integrity of a meal that should never top 500 calories. Our tacos get you back to the basics, with little more than a fiery marinade, toasted tortillas, and a scoop of salsa.

You'll Need:

- 2 chipotle peppers in adobo
- 1 cup orange juice
- 1 tsp ground cumin
- 2 cloves garlic
- 2 cups chopped fresh cilantro, plus more for garnish
- 1 lb flank steak
- ½ tsp salt
- ½ tsp pepper
- 8 corn tortillas
- ¼ cup guacamole

Salsa

- 1 red onion, minced
- 2 limes, quartered

How to Make It:

- Combine the chipotle, orange juice, cumin, garlic, and cilantro in a blender and puree. Place the steak and marinade in a resealable plastic bag and refrigerate for 30 minutes or up to 8 hours.
- Remove the steak from the marinade. Season with salt and pepper. Heat a grill, stovetop grill pan, or cast-iron skillet until hot. Cook the steak for 3 to 4 minutes per side (for medium rare).
- Heat the tortillas until warm and pliable. It's best to do this on a hot grill or cast-iron skillet, but in a pinch, wrap the tortillas in a damp paper towel and microwave for 45 seconds.
- Slice the steak across the grain into thin pieces and divide among the tortillas. Top with guacamole, salsa, onion, extra cilantro, and a squirt of lime juice.

Makes 4 servings / Cost per serving: $3.69

Cumin has been shown to help decrease the risk of colon, stomach, and liver cancers.

250 calories
7 g fat
(1.5 g saturated)
310 mg sodium

1,110 calories
44 g fat
(13 g saturated)
2,490 mg sodium

Not That!
Chevys Grilled Steak Tacos
Price: $10.99

Save!
860 calories
and $7.30!

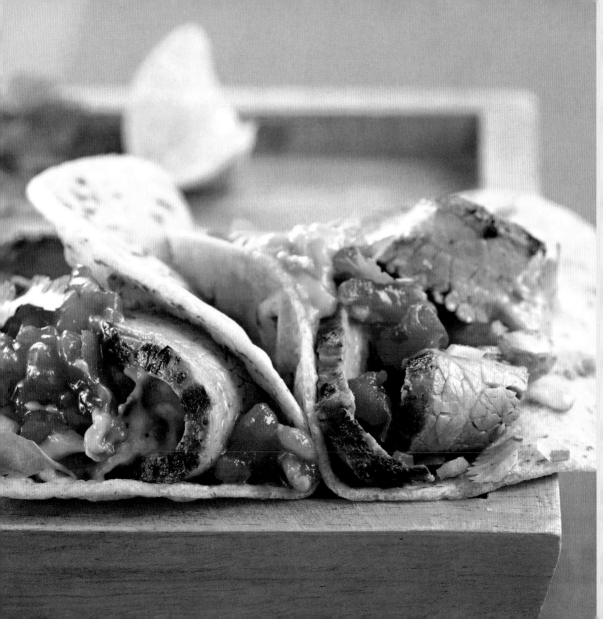

Pork Tenderloin Grilled with Pineapple Salsa

Chicken breast may still be king of the American meat market, but pork tenderloin is no less worthy of the crown. Besides being nearly as lean as white meat chicken (a 3-ounce portion of cooked pork tenderloin has only 3 grams of fat), pork also boasts an impressive array of nutrients, including more than a third of a day's dose of selenium, a trace mineral shown to be effective in cancer prevention. Another reason to love pork is its ability to stand up to big, gutsy flavors. Here, a heady rub of mustard and chili powder and a powerful salsa of pineapple and jalapeño help skyrocket the flavor quotient while adding only about 25 calories—plus a tide of first-rate nutrients—to the bottom line.

You'll Need:

- 1 Tbsp Dijon or grainy mustard
- ½ Tbsp honey
- ½ Tbsp chili powder
- Salt and black pepper to taste
- 1 lb pork tenderloin
- 4 (½"-thick) slices pineapple, core removed
- 1 red onion, minced
- 1 jalapeño pepper, minced
- ½ cup chopped fresh cilantro
- Juice of 1 lime

How to Make It:

- Preheat the grill. Combine the mustard, honey, chili powder, and a good sprinkle of salt and pepper and rub all over the pork. Place the pork and pineapple slices on the grill. Grill the pineapple for 2 to 3 minutes per side, until lightly charred and softened. Grill the tenderloin, turning once or twice, for about 10 minutes, until lightly charred and firm (but yielding) to the touch (an internal thermometer should read no more than 160°F). Let the pork rest for at least 5 minutes.

- While the pork rests, chop the pineapple into bite-size pieces. Combine with the onion, jalapeño, cilantro, and lime juice. Season with a bit of salt and pepper. Slice the pork and serve with the salsa.

Makes 4 servings /
Cost per serving: $2.28

210 calories
4 g fat
(1.5 g saturated)
390 mg sodium

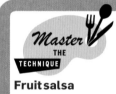

Master THE **TECHNIQUE**

Fruit salsa

Nothing impresses more and requires less than a fruit salsa. Start with the same base—1 minced onion, 1 minced jalapeño, ½ cup chopped cilantro, and the juice of a lime—and then add the fruit of your choice. Mango and papaya are obvious choices, but apples, melon, and even strawberries work beautifully as well.

Not That!
T.G.I. Friday's Pepper-Crusted Pork Chop
Price: $10.99

1,190 calories

Save!
980 calories and $8.71!

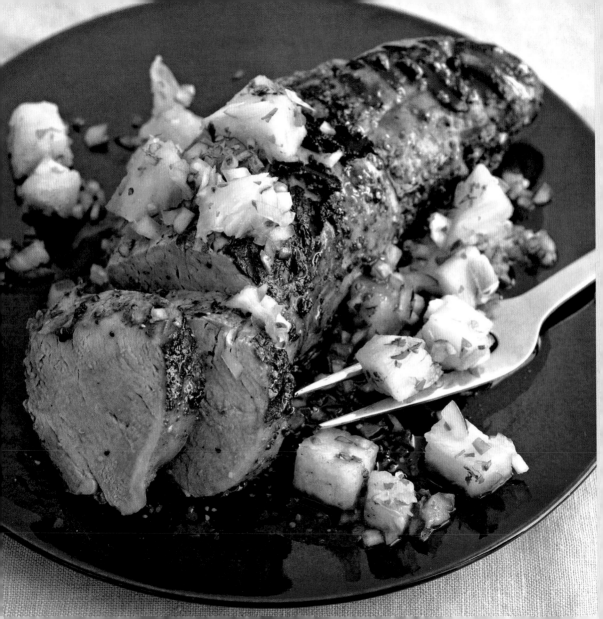

Cook This!
Lamb with Tzatziki

Lamb has long been a second-class citizen in American households, a meat you turn to maybe once a year when you've grown tired of chicken and beef. Too bad, since lamb is not only jam-packed with flavor and easy to cook, but surprisingly lean when you work with the right cuts. (The notion that lamb is "gamey" doesn't hold true anymore, partially because most lamb is so lean.) Though tzatziki, a Greek-style yogurt sauce, matches perfectly with a charred lamb chop, it also can—and should—be applied to grilled chicken, pork, and fish on a frequent basis.

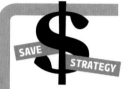

SAVE $ STRATEGY

You'll Need:

1 cucumber, peeled, halved, and seeded

1 cup Greek-style yogurt (we like Fage)

Juice of 1 lemon

2 Tbsp olive oil

2 cloves garlic, finely minced

2 tsp minced fresh dill

Salt and black pepper to taste

4 loin or shoulder lamb chops (about 4 oz each)

How to Make It:

- Preheat a grill. Grate the cucumber with a cheese grater, then use your (clean!) hands to wring out all the excess water. Combine the cucumber with the yogurt, lemon juice, half the olive oil, garlic, dill, and a good pinch of salt and pepper. Set the tzatziki aside.

- Rub the lamb with the remaining olive oil, then season all over with salt and pepper. Grill, turning once, until a meat thermometer inserted into the deepest part of a chop reads 135°F, 10 to 12 minutes, depending on the thickness of the cut. Serve with the tzatziki.

Makes 4 servings / Cost per serving: $3.75

Beautiful, perfectly trimmed loin lamb chops come with a steep price tag, often fetching up to $15 or more a pound. Many supermarkets sell individual shoulder chops, though, for about half the price, and they work every bit as well in this recipe. The same could be said about leg of lamb, which goes for about $6 a pound and proves to be an amazing cut for both roasting in the oven and tossing on the grill. Bottom line: Don't pass on lamb because you can't afford the priciest cut.

260 calories
15 g fat
(4 g saturated)
390 mg sodium

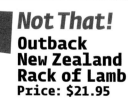

Not That!
Outback New Zealand Rack of Lamb
Price: $21.95

1,303 calories
112 g fat
(58 g saturated)
1,473 mg sodium

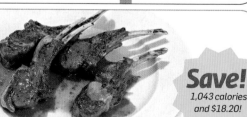

Save!
1,043 calories
and $18.20!

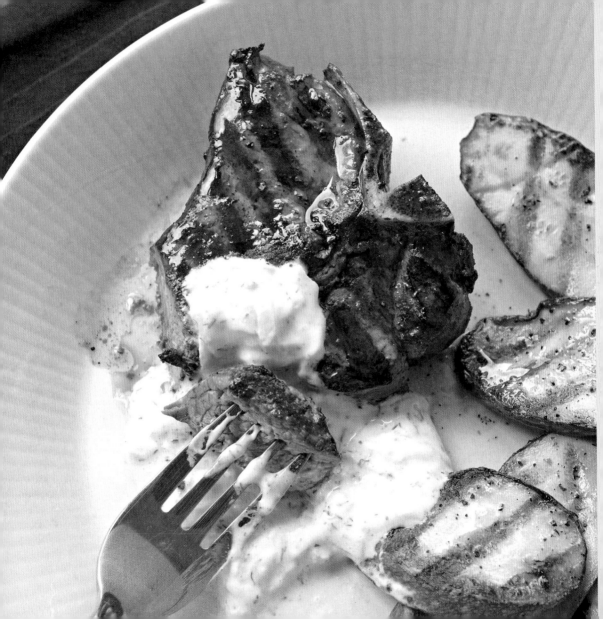

Pesto-Grilled Swordfish

No fridge should be without a bottle of premade pesto. It pairs perfectly with pasta, of course, but also works as an excellent sandwich spread, salad dressing enhancer, and instant marinade. This recipe takes the latter tack, slathering meaty swordfish steaks in pesto before grilling, then topping them with quick-sautéed tomatoes. The burst of sweetness from the tomatoes joins forces with the garlicky punch of the pesto, making for a dish that tastes every bit the creation of a restaurant chef.

You'll Need:

- 2 Tbsp bottled pesto
- 4 swordfish steaks (4–6 oz each)
- 1 Tbsp olive oil
- 2 cloves garlic, peeled and lightly crushed
- 2 cups cherry tomatoes
- Salt and black pepper to taste

How to Make It:

- Spread the pesto all over the swordfish steaks, cover, and marinate in the fridge for 30 minutes.

- While the fish marinates, heat the olive oil in a sauté pan over medium heat. Add the garlic and cook for a minute or two, until lightly browned. Add the tomatoes and sauté until the skins are lightly blistered and about to pop, about 5 minutes. Season with salt and pepper.

- Preheat a grill or grill pan. Season the fish all over with salt and pepper. When the grill is hot, cook the swordfish for 4 to 5 minutes per side, until the fish is cooked all the way through and the flesh flakes with gentle pressure. Reheat the tomatoes and top each steak with a scoop.

Makes 4 servings / Cost per serving: $5.05

Swordfish steaks are bulky, between 10 and 16 ounces, so plan on buying 2 smallish steaks and cutting them in half.

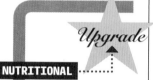

Upgrade

NUTRITIONAL

Greater grains

American eating traditions dictate that every homecooked meal come with a starch, which usually means potatoes or rice, neither of which add much to a meal other than empty carbs. But a new class of global grains has flooded the market that can boost nutrition and cut calories. Quinoa, from South America, is our favorite, but also try amaranth, couscous, and farro. All are excellent high-fiber rice and potato alternatives.

250 calories
13 g fat
(3 g saturated)
390 mg sodium

730 calories
29 g fat
(6 g saturated)
1,020 mg sodium

Not That!
Red Lobster Grilled Arctic Char
with Spicy Glaze
Price: $15.99

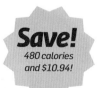

Save!
480 calories and $10.94!

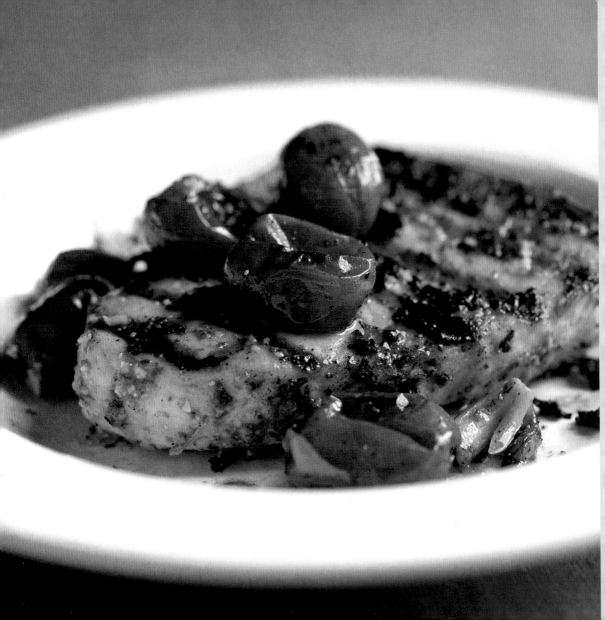

Cook This!
Hoisin Beef Kebab

In the Shinjuku district of Tokyo, behind the central train station (the busiest in the world), you'll find a long, narrow alleyway—appropriately dubbed Yakitori Alley—that is lined with dozens of tiny bars and stands billowing savory smoke into the air. Humble grill masters expertly char skewered food of all shapes and sizes: plump meatballs, tiny cherry tomatoes, even pure chicken skin that crisps up like potato chips. Though we never had this exact kebab there, the flavors are true to the spirit of Yakitori Alley; we hope the grill masters would approve.

You'll Need:

- 2 Tbsp hoisin sauce
- 1 Tbsp low-sodium soy sauce
- 2 tsp dark or toasted sesame oil
- 1 tsp chili sauce or paste, such as sriracha
- 1 lb sirloin, cut into ¾" pieces
- 8 scallion whites, chopped into ½" chunks
- 20 small mushroom caps
- 20 cherry tomatoes
- 8 wooden skewers, soaked in water for 20 minutes

How to Make It:

- Preheat a grill. Combine the hoisin, soy sauce, sesame oil, and chili sauce in a bowl and mix thoroughly. Transfer half to a separate bowl and reserve.
- Thread the beef, scallion whites, mushrooms, and cherry tomatoes onto the skewers, alternating between the meat and vegetables. Use a brush to paint the skewers with some of the remaining hoisin glaze. When the grill is hot, add the skewers and cook for 3 to 4 minutes per side, basting with a bit more of the sauce as you go. The skewers are done when the meat and vegetables are lightly charred and the beef is firm but still yielding to the touch.
- Brush the kebabs with the reserved glaze before serving.

Makes 8 skewers /
Cost per serving: $1.61

290 calories
10 g fat
(3 g saturated)
870 mg sodium

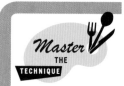

Master THE TECHNIQUE

Improvising sauces

Making a killer sauce for the grill on the fly is easier than most think. Start with a base with a well-rounded flavor: Ketchup, Dijon, hoisin all work. Then mix in other liquids or condiments that add strong single flavor notes: honey for sweetness, vinegar for acid, soy sauce for salt, sriracha for heat. Finally, turn to the spice cabinet to bring it all together. Chili powder, garlic and onion salt, cumin, brown sugar, mustard powder, and cayenne are all common elements of barbecue sauces and all could be the finishing touch for your next masterpiece.

Not That!
Uno Chicago Grill Sirloin Steak Tips
Price: $14.99

580 calories
28 g fat
(8 g saturated)
2,060 mg sodium

Save!
290 calories and $13.38!

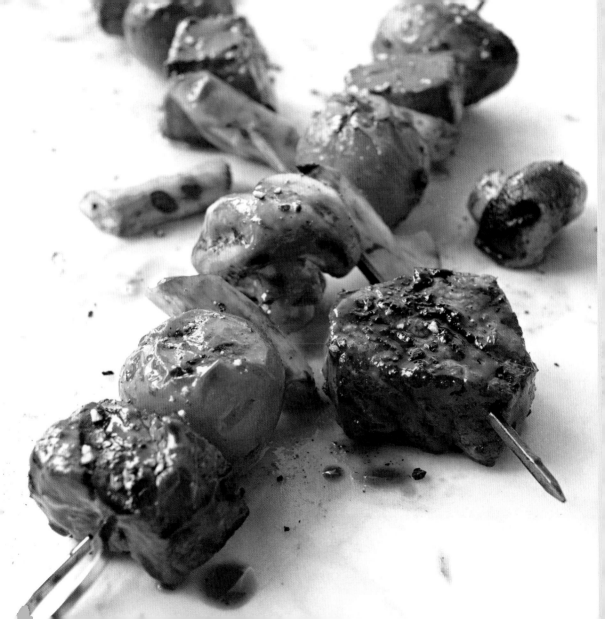

Cook This!
Jerk Pork

The supermarket is flooded with mediocre jerk marinades that lack the punch—the gutsiness—of real jerk cooking as done by the pit masters that pepper the Jamaican coastal communities. To get it right, one needs a small stash of fiery habanero or Scotch bonnet peppers, which, although they have become common-place in supermarkets, still need to be treated with caution when prepping and eating. To give you an idea of their power, a jala-peño is rated at 5,000 Scoville units (the accepted measurement for spiciness); a habanero rates at 350,000. Proceed with caution.

You'll Need:

- 2 **habanero or Scotch bonnet peppers, stemmed and roughly chopped**
- 8 **scallions, roughly chopped**
- Juice of 2 limes
- 2 **Tbsp canola oil**
- 3 **cloves garlic, chopped**
- 1 **tsp allspice**
- ¼ **tsp nutmeg**
- Salt and black pepper to taste
- 1 **lb pork loin**

How to Make It:

- Place the habaneros, scallions, lime juice, oil, garlic, all-spice, nutmeg, and a good pinch of salt and pepper in a food processor. Pulse until the mixture forms a paste with the consistency of pesto, adding a bit of water if it's too dry.
- Place the pork (chicken drumsticks work great, too) in a sealable plastic bag and pour the jerk marinade over it. Squeeze out the air, seal the bag, and rub the pork around to make sure it's evenly coated. Marinate in the refrigerator for at least 1 hour, but preferably overnight.
- Preheat a grill. Remove the pork from the marinade and season with a bit more salt and pepper. Grill, cooking on all sides, for about 10 minutes, until lightly charred and cooked through. (An internal thermometer inserted into the center of the pork will read 140°F.)

Makes 4 servings /
Cost per serving: $2.23

Either use gloves or limit exposure to skin by using tongs to help you handle the peppers.

LEFTOVER LOVE

This is the type of recipe you want to make a lot of, not just because its fiery bite is addictive right off the grill, but also because leftovers straight from the fridge make incredible dishes the next day. Toss hunks of cold pork with romaine, mango, shred-ded carrot, peanuts, and a simple vinaigrette. Or make a sandwich filling for the ages: Slice the pork thinly, then top with slowly cara-melized onions, roasted peppers, and melted Swiss cheese.

240 calories
11 g fat
(2 g saturated)
510 mg sodium

670 calories
24 g fat
(6 g saturated)
1,820 mg sodium

Not That!
Macaroni Grill Prime Pork Loin
Price: $14.99

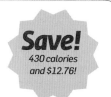

Save!
430 calories and $12.76!

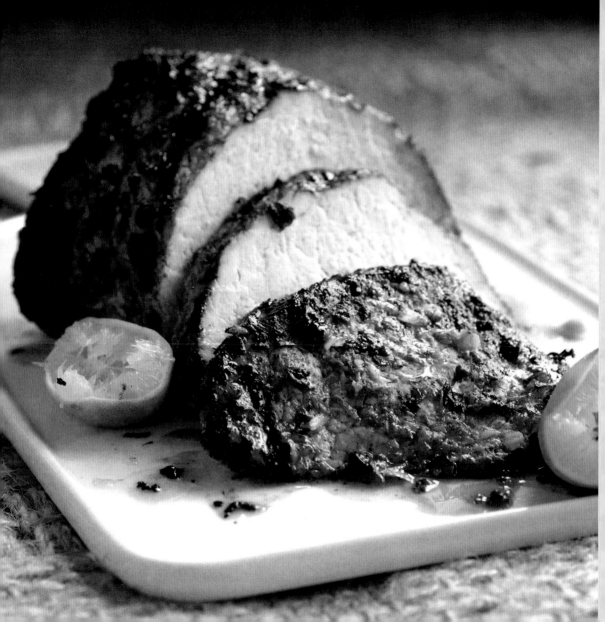

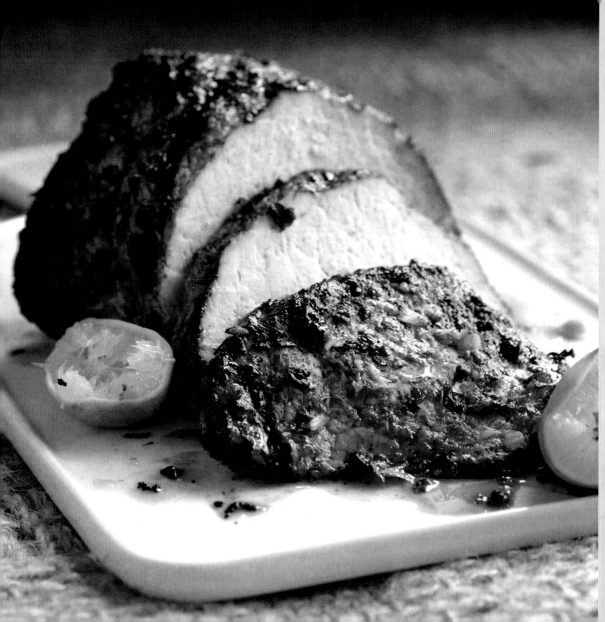

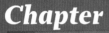
Chapter

7

Pizza & Pasta
Hearty Italian classics made
healthy at home

Cook This!
The Pizza Matrix

As crazy as Americans are for pizza, few ever dare to make it at home. That's truly a shame, because the pizza we turn to is overpriced, awash in empty calories, and ultimately not all that delicious. Anyone can do better in their home by combining a handful of fresh ingredients and following a few simple steps. And believe it or not, pizza made the right way can make for a truly well-balanced meal. Preheat the oven and follow along.

Four Near-Perfect Pizzas

We love pizza of all shapes, sizes, sauces, and toppings. These four wildly different pies show you just how versatile pizza can be.

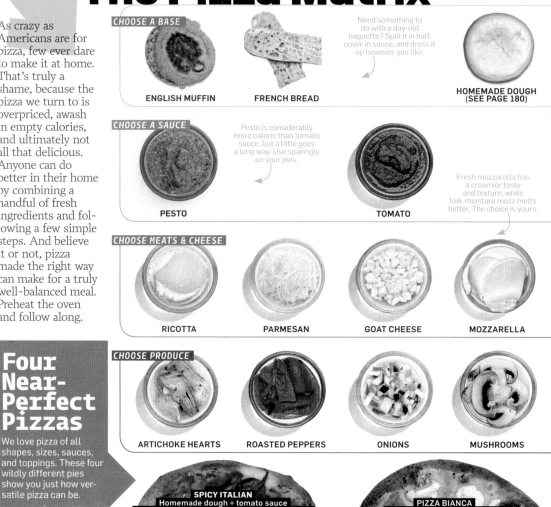

CHOOSE A BASE

ENGLISH MUFFIN

FRENCH BREAD

Need something to do with a day-old baguette? Split it in half, cover in sauce, and dress it up however you like.

HOMEMADE DOUGH (SEE PAGE 180)

CHOOSE A SAUCE

Pesto is considerably more caloric than tomato sauce, but a little goes a long way. Use sparingly on your pies.

PESTO

TOMATO

Fresh mozzarella has a creamier taste and texture, while low-moisture mozz melts better. The choice is yours.

CHOOSE MEATS & CHEESE

RICOTTA

PARMESAN

GOAT CHEESE

MOZZARELLA

CHOOSE PRODUCE

ARTICHOKE HEARTS

ROASTED PEPPERS

ONIONS

MUSHROOMS

SPICY ITALIAN
Homemade dough + tomato sauce + mozzarella + sopressata or turkey pepperoni + sliced onion + peppers

PIZZA BIANCA
Homemade dough + garlic and olive oil + ricotta + fresh rosemary

CHAPTER 7

Rules of the Pizza

Rule 1

The higher the heat, the better. True Italian pizzas are cooked in about 2 minutes in 1,000°F ovens. Preheat your oven for 30 minutes at 500°F (the max temp for most home ovens) for a light, crispy crust.

Rule 2

Nothing better approximates the smoky char of an wood-burning oven than a grill. Have your ingredients ready, slide the raw dough directly onto the hot grates, and grill until lightly charred, about 4 minutes. Flip and immediately add sauce and cheese, then cover the grill and wait for the cheese to melt.

Rule 3

Pizza isn't about how much cheese you can cram onto a slice; it's about the subtle interplay of bread, sauce, cheese and toppings. Don't use more than 2 ounces of cheese and a few pieces of meat or vegetable per slice.

Rule 4

Break out of the box. Nontraditional ingredients—barbecue sauce, chorizo, pistachios—can elevate a humble pie to new heights.

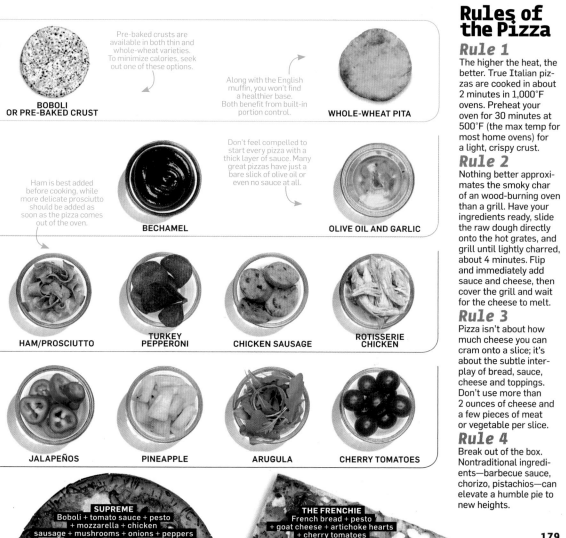

Pre-baked crusts are available in both thin and whole-wheat varieties. To minimize calories, seek out one of these options.

BOBOLI OR PRE-BAKED CRUST

Along with the English muffin, you won't find a healthier base. Both benefit from built-in portion control.

WHOLE-WHEAT PITA

Don't feel compelled to start every pizza with a thick layer of sauce. Many great pizzas have just a bare slick of olive oil or even no sauce at all.

BECHAMEL

OLIVE OIL AND GARLIC

Ham is best added before cooking, while more delicate prosciutto should be added as soon as the pizza comes out of the oven.

HAM/PROSCIUTTO

TURKEY PEPPERONI

CHICKEN SAUSAGE

ROTISSERIE CHICKEN

JALAPEÑOS

PINEAPPLE

ARUGULA

CHERRY TOMATOES

SUPREME
Boboli + tomato sauce + pesto + mozzarella + chicken sausage + mushrooms + onions + peppers

THE FRENCHIE
French bread + pesto + goat cheese + artichoke hearts + cherry tomatoes

179

Barbecue Chicken Pizza

California Pizza Kitchen made its bones slinging unconventional pizzas topped with ingredients like pear and gorgonzola, Jamaican jerk chicken, and even a full-blown salad. But none is more famous, or strangely satisfying, than the Original BBQ Chicken Pizza, which launched CPK into the national conscience in the '80s. As good as theirs is, we're confident ours is better. Plus, it's 10 bucks cheaper and has just a third of the calories.

Pizza Dough

You'll Need:

1 package instant yeast

1 cup hot water

½ tsp salt

1 Tbsp sugar or honey

½ Tbsp olive oil

2½ cups flour, plus more for kneading and rolling

How to Make It:

Combine yeast with the water, salt, and sugar or honey. Allow to sit for 10 minutes while the hot water activates the yeast. Stir in the olive oil and flour, using a wooden spoon to incorporate. When the dough is no longer sticky, place on a cutting board, cover with more flour, and knead for 5 minutes. Return to the bowl, cover with plastic wrap, and let the dough rise at room temperature for at least 90 minutes. Keeps covered in the refrigerator for up to 2 days.

You'll Need:

Pizza Dough (see left), 12 oz store-bought pizza dough, or 2 thin-crust prebaked pizza crusts (like Boboli)

¾ cup barbecue sauce

1½ cups shredded smoked gouda

½ red onion, thinly sliced

½ jalapeño pepper, thinly sliced

1 cup cooked chicken

Fresh cilantro leaves

How to Make It:

- Preheat the oven to 500°F. Place a pizza stone in the oven, if you have one.

- Using your hands, a rolling pin, and enough flour to keep it from sticking, stretch the dough into two thin circles, 10" to 12" in diameter. Spread each with a thin layer of barbecue sauce, then divide the gouda, onion, jalapeño, and chicken between the two.

- If using a pizza stone, bake one pie at a time by carefully sliding the pizza (preferably with a pizza peel) onto the pizza stone; if you don't have a stone, cook the pizzas on a baking sheet. The pizza is done when the crust is golden and the cheese is fully melted. Top with fresh cilantro, and cut into six or eight slices.

Makes 4 servings /
Cost per serving: $2.82

380 calories
14 g fat
(6 g saturated)
850 mg sodium

1,136 calories
19 g saturated fat
2,568 mg sodium

Not That!

California Pizza Kitchen The Original BBQ Chicken Pizza
Price: $12.99

Save!
756 calories
and $10.17!

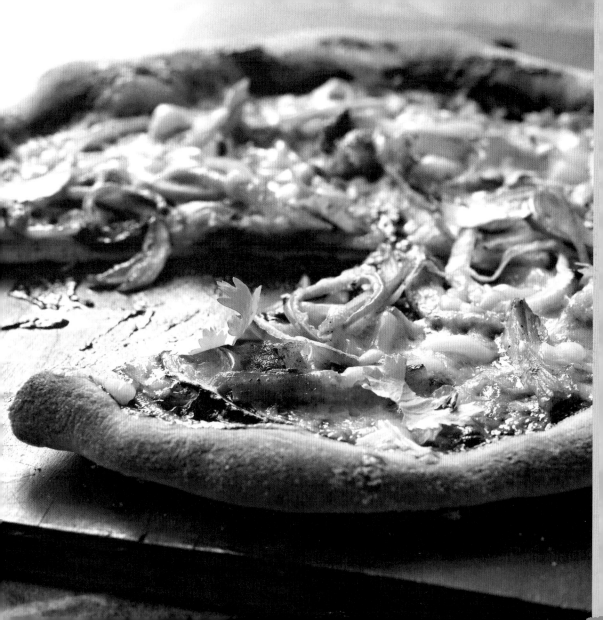

Pizza with Arugula, Cherry Tomatoes, and Prosciutto

This pie is based on a pizza once eaten at a trattoria high above the ocean in the impossibly scenic village of Positano, which clings to the cliffs above Italy's Amalfi Coast. Though you'll have a tough time re-creating the setting, this combination of ingredients flirts with those magical flavors. The cherry tomatoes roast down into sweet little orbs of sauce, the prosciutto adds a salty punch, and the arugula, which wilts gently from the residual heat of the pizza, brings a fresh, peppery note to the pie. *Bellissima!*

You'll Need:

Pizza Dough (see page 180), 12 oz store-bought pizza dough, or 1 large pre-baked crust, such as Boboli

1 **cup Pizza Sauce (see page 184)**

1 ½ **cups shredded part-skim mozzarella**

2 **cups cherry tomatoes**

2 **cups arugula**

6 **slices prosciutto, cut or torn into thin strips**

Shaved Parmesan

How to Make It:

- Preheat the oven to 500°F. If you have a pizza stone, place on the bottom rack of the oven.

- Divide the dough into 2 equal pieces (unless you're using a pre-baked crust). On a well-floured surface, use a rolling pin to work the dough into two thin circles, about 12" in diameter.

- If you have a pizza stone, place one circle of dough on a pizza peel, cover with a light layer of pizza sauce, then top with half the mozzarella and cherry tomatoes. Slide directly onto the pizza stone and bake for about 8 minutes, until the edge of the dough is lightly browned. If you don't have a pizza stone, cook the pizzas on a baking sheet instead.

- Remove the pizza to a cutting board and immediately top with half the arugula (which will wilt lightly from the heat), half the prosciutto, and a good measure of shaved or grated Parmesan. (If you have a large block of Parmesan, simply use a vegetable peeler to shave thin slices of cheese over the top.) Cut the pizza into six or eight slices.

- Repeat with the other circle of dough and the remaining ingredients.

Makes two 12" pizzas, or 4 servings / Cost per serving: $2.96

$$(\Psi+I)^2$$

MEAL MULTIPLIER

The beauty of pizza is its boundlessness; if you can imagine it, you can make it. Here are three out-of-the-ordinary ideas worth trying:

- Pesto base topped with grilled chicken, roasted peppers, and goat cheese
- Roasted asparagus spears, smoked mozzarella, and a fried egg
- Mascarpone or ricotta as the base, topped with grilled peaches and balsamic. Dessert!

400 calories
12 g fat
(5 g saturated)
980 mg sodium

900 calories
34 g fat
(15 g saturated)
2,290 mg sodium

Not That!

Romano's Macaroni Grill Prosciutto e Arugula Pizza
Price: $10.99

Save!
500 calories and $8.03!

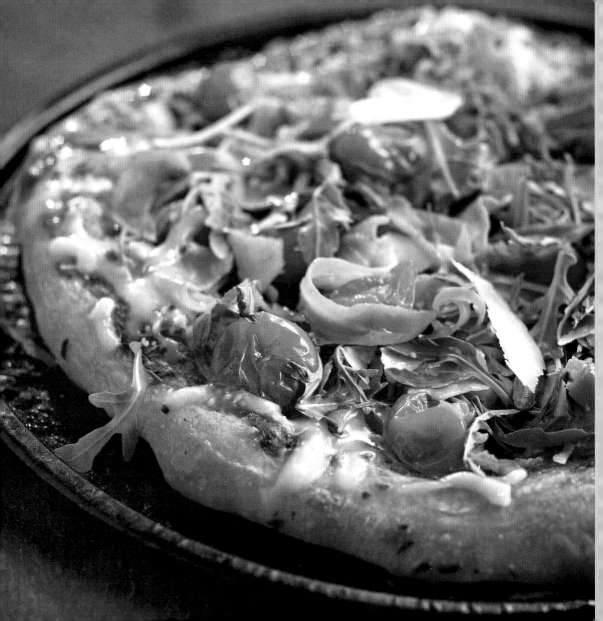

Bacon Pizza with Caramelized Onions and Goat Cheese

True artisanal pizza eschews floppy, sloppy slices in favor of a thin, delicate crust and a careful balance of sauce and toppings. The result is a pizza with a fraction of the calories and a surplus of flavor, which is exactly what this recipe re-creates.

Pizza Sauce

You'll Need:

- 1 can (28 oz) whole peeled tomatoes, drained
- ½ tsp salt
- 1 Tbsp olive oil
- 1 clove garlic, finely minced

How to Make It:

Place the ingredients in a blender and puree for a few seconds, until the tomatoes have broken down but still retain some chunky texture. Makes about 3 cups of sauce.

Pizza

You'll Need:

Pizza Dough (see page 180), 12 oz store-bought pizza dough, or 1 pre-baked pizza crust, such as Boboli
- 1 cup Pizza Sauce (see left)
- 1 cup fresh goat cheese
- 1 cup Caramelized Onions (see page 305)
- 4 strips bacon, cooked and crumbled
- ½ tsp chopped fresh rosemary (optional)

Red pepper flakes

How to Make It:

- Preheat the oven to 500°F. If you have a pizza stone, place on the bottom rack.
- Divide the dough into two equal pieces (unless you're using a pre-baked crust). On a well-floured surface, use a rolling pin to work the dough into two thin circles, about 12" in diameter. If you have a pizza stone, place one circle of dough on a pizza peel, cover with a light layer of sauce, then top with half the goat cheese, onions, bacon, and rosemary (if using), plus pepper flakes. Slide directly onto the stone and bake for about 8 minutes, until the edges are lightly browned. (If you don't have a stone, cook on a baking sheet placed directly on the oven floor, instead.)
- Cut the pizza into six or eight slices.

Makes two 12" pizzas, or 4 servings / Cost per serving: $2.76

370 calories
13 g fat
(6 g saturated)
880 mg sodium

1,380 calories
54 g fat
(24 g saturated)
3,030 mg sodium

Not That!

Domino's Small Hand-Tossed Pizza

with Onions and Bacon
Price: $7.99

Save!
1,010 calories and $5.23!

STEP-BY-STEP

Perfecting Pizza

The key to working dough is to keep everything well-floured: your hands, the rolling pin, the counter. Roll the dough as thin as you can without tearing it.

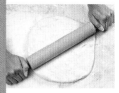

Step 1: *Apply weight to the pin to stretch the dough*

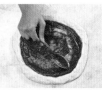

Step 2: *Lightly sauce, leaving a ¾-inch border*

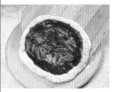

Step 3: *Slide off a floured peel onto a pizza stone*

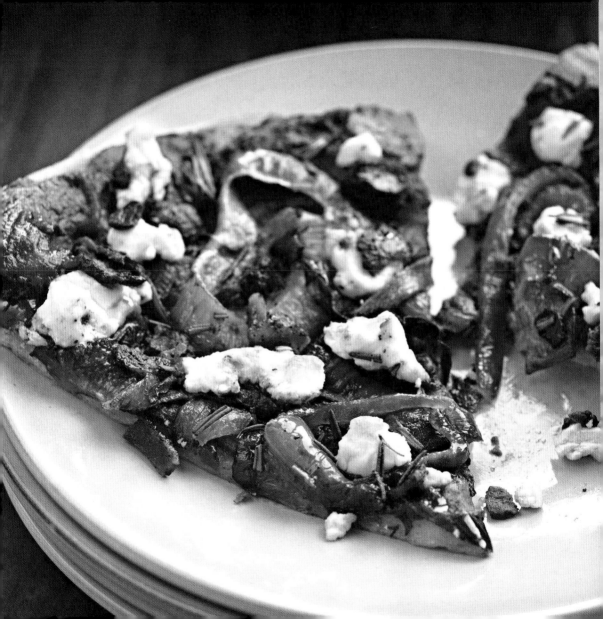

Spaghetti with Spicy Tomato Sauce

Bucatini alla Amatriciana is a staple in and around Rome and the type of dish Italian college kids cook when they miss Mama's cooking. The beauty of the dish is that just a few strips of bacon infuse an entire pot of pasta with a rich, meaty flavor, cut perfectly by the sweet of the tomatoes and the heat of the pepper flakes. No fatty sausage links, greasy ground beef, or fist-size meatballs necessary.

You'll Need:

- 4 strips bacon
- 1 small yellow onion, diced
- 4 cloves garlic, thinly sliced
- 1 tsp red pepper flakes (or more depending upon your heat preference)
- 1 can (28 oz) crushed tomatoes
- Salt and black pepper to taste
- 10 oz bucatini or spaghetti
- ½ cup chopped fresh parsley
- Pecorino Romano or Parmesan

How to Make It:

- Bring a large pot of salted water to a boil.

- Cook the bacon in a large skillet over medium heat until the fat is mostly rendered, about 5 minutes. Discard all but 1 tablespoon of the fat. Add the onion, garlic, and pepper flakes to the pan. Sauté for about 5 minutes, until the onion has begun to lightly brown. Add the tomatoes and season with salt and lots of black pepper. Bring to a simmer.

- Meanwhile, cook the pasta in the boiling water until al dente (usually about 30 seconds to a minute less than the package instructions recommend).

- Drain the pasta and add directly to the simmering tomato sauce. Stir together so that the sauce and noodles are evenly incorporated. Stir in the parsley. Divide among four warm pasta bowls and top with freshly grated cheese.

Makes 4 servings /
Cost per serving: $2.01

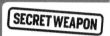

SECRET WEAPON

Pasta water

One of the most magical ingredients in the kitchen is also one of the most overlooked: the murky water you discard when draining pasta. The cloudiness is the result of starches released from the surface of the noodles, and even a few tablespoons can help you create a silky sauce that better sticks to pasta. Before draining the noodles, dip a coffee mug into the water and fish out a few ounces of liquid. Toss the pasta directly in the pan with the sauce and if the noodles look dry add the reserved water, a tablespoon at a time, until the sauce loosens and clings lightly to the pasta.

370 calories
5 g fat
(1.5 g saturated)
560 mg sodium

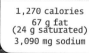

1,270 calories
67 g fat
(24 g saturated)
3,090 mg sodium

Not That!
Olive Garden Spaghetti & Italian Sausage
Price: $14.75

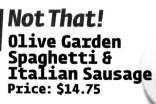

Save!
900 calories and $12.74!

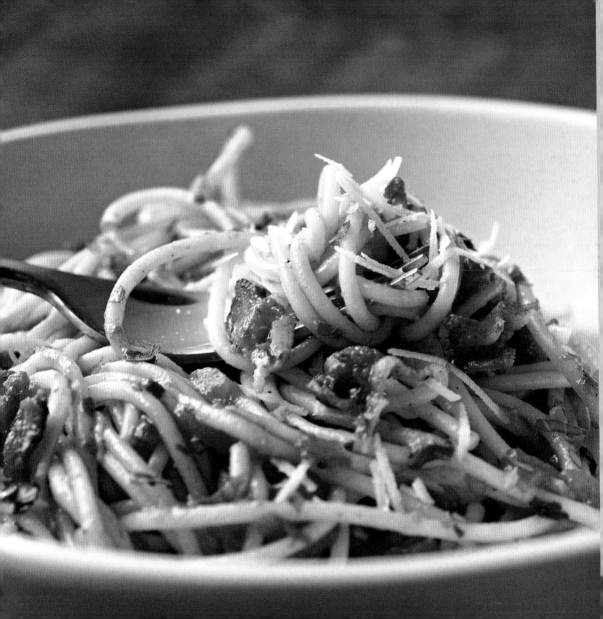

Cook This!
Orecchiette with Broccoli Rabe and Turkey Sausage

American chain restaurants are two-trick ponies when it comes to pasta. The first pasta they love involves noodles covered in a red sauce spiked with ground meat, meatballs, or Italian sausage. The second, more dangerous, go-to is pasta studded with chicken and shrimp, maybe a few vegetables, then drowned in butter and cream. The former is better than the latter, but both ignore the amazing diversity—and fundamental healthfulness—of regional Italian pasta cookery. This classic combines slightly bitter, peppery broccoli rabe (or, if you can't find rabe, regular broccoli) and lean crumbled sausage with orecchiette, little ear-shape pasta shells that cup the sauce beautifully.

You'll Need:

- 1 bunch broccoli rabe, bottom 1" removed
- 10 oz orecchiette pasta
- ½ Tbsp olive oil
- 2 links uncooked turkey or chicken sausage, casings removed
- 4 cloves garlic, minced
- ¼ tsp red pepper flakes
- ¾ cup low-sodium chicken stock
- Salt and black pepper to taste
- Pecorino Romano or Parmesan

How to Make It:

- Bring a large pot of salted water to a boil. Drop in the broccoli rabe and cook for 3 minutes. Use tongs to remove the greens and the chop into ½" pieces. Return the water to a boil. Cook the pasta until al dente.

- While the pasta cooks, heat the olive oil in a large skillet over medium heat. Add the sausage and cook for about 5 minutes, until lightly browned, then add the garlic and pepper flakes and sauté for another 3 minutes. Stir in the chopped broccoli rabe and chicken stock and lower the heat to a simmer. Season with salt and pepper.

- Drain the pasta and toss immediately into the pan with the sausage and greens. Toss the pasta (if the mix looks dry, use a bit of the pasta cooking water to loosen it up). Serve immediately with freshly grated cheese.

Makes 4 servings /
Cost per serving: $2.31

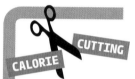

CALORIE CUTTING

A serving size of pasta in Italy is about 6 ounces; here, many restaurant noodle bowls top 2 pounds. We've used more modest serving sizes for the noodles in the book's pasta recipes, but kept the sauce portions more substantial. That means the pasta-to-sauce ratio will skew toward the latter, which makes for a more satisfying meal for fewer calories.

345 calories
8 g fat
(1.5 g saturated)
410 mg sodium

1,513 calories
95 g fat
3,177 mg sodium

Not That!
Ruby Tuesday Chicken & Broccoli Pasta
Price: $11.99

Save!
1,168 calories
and $9.68!

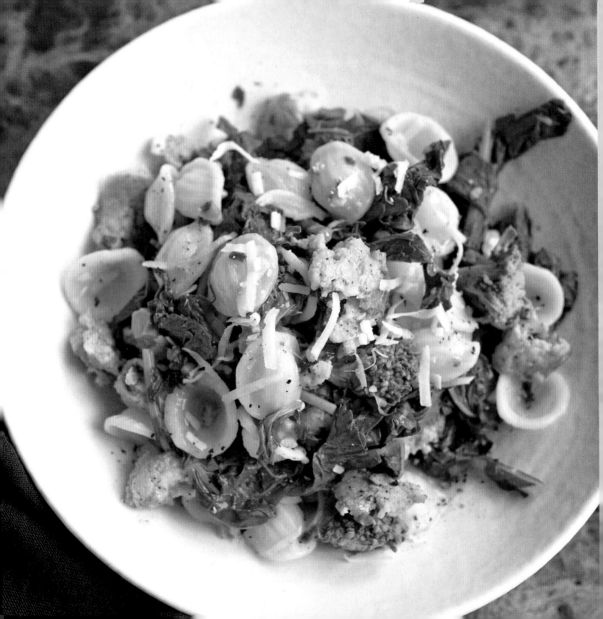

Baked Ziti

Long a staple of red-sauce loving Italian-American housewives, baked ziti is only a rung below mac and cheese on the comfort-food ladder. It's a simple formula—noodles covered in red sauce, speckled with cheese, maybe a bit of meat—but places like Olive Garden get it so wrong: No bowl of pasta should provide the saturated fat equivalent of 26 strips of bacon. And nobody in their right mind should pay to eat it. Save your cash, and your ticker, and eat this version instead.

You'll Need:

- 10 oz ziti, preferably whole-wheat if you can find it
- 1 Tbsp olive oil
- 2 links precooked chicken or turkey sausage, diced
- 1 medium yellow onion, diced
- 2 cloves garlic, minced
- 1 tsp red pepper flakes
- 1 can (28 oz) tomato puree
- Salt and black pepper to taste
- 1 cup fresh basil leaves, plus more for garnish
- ¾ cup cubed mozzarella (preferably fresh)
- Parmesan for grating

How to Make It:

- Preheat the oven to 400°F. Bring a pot of salted water to a boil. Cook the pasta until a minute shy of being done (it'll finish cooking in the oven).

- Meanwhile, heat the oil in a large skillet or sauté pan over medium heat. Add the sausage and cook for about 2 minutes, until lightly browned. Add the onion, garlic, and pepper flakes and cook until the onion is soft and translucent. Stir in the tomato puree, plus a good pinch of salt and black pepper. Reduce the heat and simmer for at least 10 minutes.

- Drain the pasta. Add to the skillet and toss with the sauce. Remove from the heat and stir in the basil and mozzarella. Dump the pasta into a 12" x 9" baking dish, sprinkle the top with a bit of Parmesan, and cover with foil. Bake for 15 minutes, then remove the foil and bake for another 10 minutes, until the top is crusty and browned. Garnish with basil leaves and serve.

Makes 4 servings /
Cost per serving: $3.01

410 calories
12 g fat
(5 g saturated)
600 mg sodium

Upgrade

NUTRITIONAL

Pad Your Pasta

The reason most pasta dishes fail is that the bulk of their volume comes from noodles, which means high calories, empty carbs, and little nutrition. To improve matters, cut the noodles down to 8 ounces and fill out the dish by adding any of the following to the pasta before baking: 2 cups cooked broccoli; 1 box thawed frozen spinach; 8 ounces sautéed mushrooms.

1,050 calories
48 g fat
(26 g saturated)
2,370 mg sodium

Not That!

Olive Garden Five Cheese Ziti al Forno
Price: $13.50

Save!
640 calories
and $10.49!

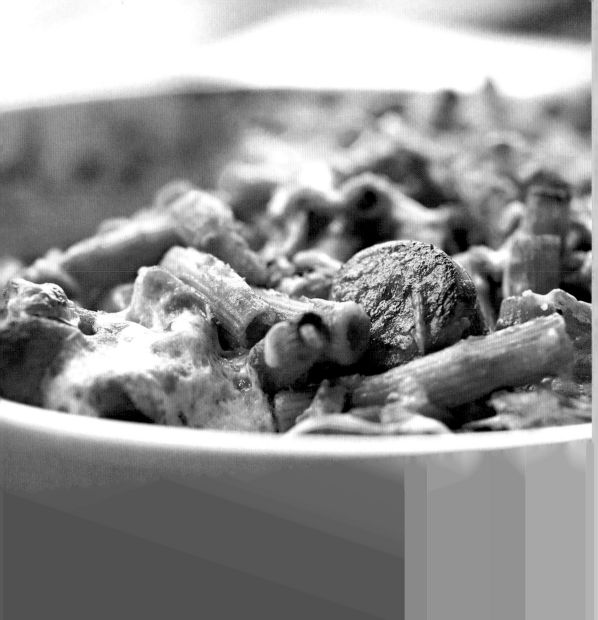

Cook This!
Zucchini Carbonara

Spaghetti carbonara is the Italians' take on bacon and eggs. It's comfort food at its finest: simple, unpretentious, soul-nourishing. Only problem is that a pile of bacon-strewn pasta won't win any nutrition awards. Add to that the fact that most American restaurants add heavy cream to carbonara—a huge no-no in Italy—and things get even worse. To lighten the dish, we've added a good amount of zucchini, which is cut in long, thin ribbons to mimic the shape of the pasta and help you cut back on the overall quantity of noodles. Beyond cutting calories, though, it adds a nutty sweetness to this classic that just makes a lot of sense. (Just don't tell the Italians, okay?)

You'll Need:

- 10 oz spaghetti
- 6 strips bacon, cut into ½" pieces
- 1 medium yellow onion, diced
- 1 large zucchini, sliced into thin ribbons
- 2 cloves garlic, sliced
- Salt and black pepper to taste
- 2 eggs
- Pecorino or Parmesan for grating
- 1 handful chopped fresh parsley

How to Make It:

- Bring a large pot of salted water to a boil. Add the pasta and cook until al dente (usually about 30 seconds to a minute less than the package instructions recommend).
- While the pasta cooks, heat a large sauté pan over medium heat. Add the bacon and cook until crispy, about 5 minutes. Transfer the bacon to a plate lined with paper towels. Discard all but a thin film of the fat from the pan. Add the onion, zucchini, and garlic and cook for 5 to 7 minutes, until soft and lightly browned. Stir back in the bacon and season with a bit of salt and plenty of coarse black pepper.
- Drain the pasta, using a coffee cup to save a few ounces of the cooking water. Add the pasta directly to the sauté pan and toss to coat. Stir in enough of the pasta water so that a thin layer of moisture clings to the noodles. Remove from the heat and crack the two eggs directly into the pasta, using tongs or two forks to toss for even distribution. Divide the pasta among four warm bowls or plates and top with grated cheese and parsley.

Makes 4 servings / Cost per serving: $1.72

370 calories
8 g fat
(3 g saturated)
960 mg sodium

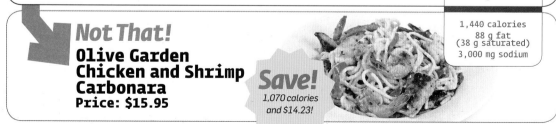

Not That!
Olive Garden Chicken and Shrimp Carbonara
Price: $15.95

Save!
1,070 calories and $14.23!

1,440 calories
88 g fat
(38 g saturated)
3,000 mg sodium

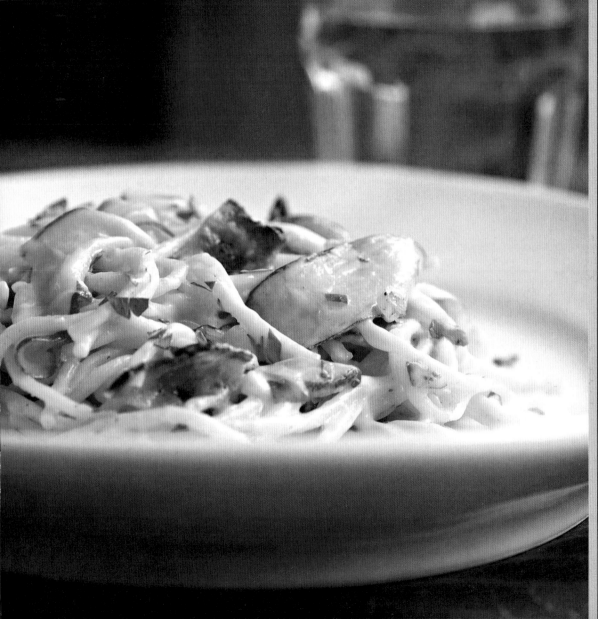

Cook This!

Gnocchi with Peas and Prosciutto

Packaged gnocchi—Italian dumplings made with potato and flour—makes for a solid base for a quick weeknight meal. Boil until they float to the surface, then fish them out and add directly to a pan of sautéed vegetables and maybe a bit of broth—or even toss with pesto or your favorite bottled marinara. Here, we take the classic Italian pasta pairing of peas and prosciutto, replace the noodles with dumplings, and throw in plenty of asparagus to round out the creation. You can make it richer with a drizzle of cream or half and half or a bit of butter, but this one is great as is.

You'll Need:

- 2 Tbsp butter
- ½ bunch (about 10 spears) asparagus, woody ends removed, chopped into 1" pieces
- 1 cup frozen peas
- 3 oz prosciutto or other high-quality ham, sliced into thin strips
- 1 cup low-sodium chicken or vegetable stock
- Salt and black pepper to taste
- 12 oz packaged gnocchi
- Parmesan for grating

How to Make It:

- Heat half the butter in a large skillet over medium heat. Add the asparagus and sauté for 2 to 3 minutes, then stir in the peas, prosciutto, and stock. Cook for 3 to 4 minutes, until the asparagus is tender and the peas are soft. Season with salt and black pepper; keep warm.
- Cook the gnocchi in a large pot of boiling water until they float to the top, no more than 5 minutes. Drain and add to the skillet with the vegetables, along with the other tablespoon of butter. Cook together for 1 minute, so that the sauce and gnocchi have time to mingle. Serve with freshly grated Parmesan.

Makes 4 servings / Cost per serving: $2.40

Most supermarket deli counters sell prosciutto of some sort these days. Prosciutto di Parma or San Danielle is the best, but for recipes that involve cooking the cured ham, a less expensive version will do.

275 calories
15 g fat
(6 g saturated)
770 mg sodium

1,220 calories
33 g saturated fat
3,740 mg sodium

Not That!

Maggiano's Little Italy Gnocchi
with Tomato Vodka Sauce
Price: $12.95

Save!
945 calories and $10.55!

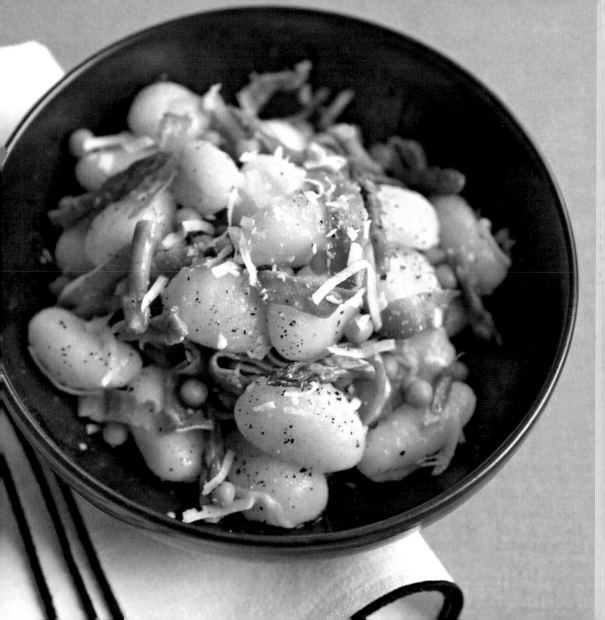

Lasagna Rolls

The idea of building a multi-tiered, multi-component lasagna can be dizzying for most cooks. For them, we offer this simplified form, the lasagna roll: a tight pasta bundle containing all the same flavors as the traditional baked pasta, but without the daunting architecture. It's basic shape helps you avoid creating one of those cheesy, soupy catastrophes so common in Italian-American restaurants, the ones where it's impossible to discern where the pasta stops and the sauce begins. The structure is sound, the flavors are clear and pronounced, and the calories are greatly reduced. What more could you want?

You'll Need:

- 10–12 long, thin lasagna noodles (about 6 oz)
- 6 oz Italian-style chicken or turkey sausage, casings removed
- 1 bag frozen spinach, thawed
- ¼ tsp red pepper flakes

Pinch of nutmeg

Salt and black pepper to taste

- 1 cup low-fat ricotta cheese
- 2 cups bottled marinara
- ¾ cup shredded low-fat mozzarella

How to Make It:

- Bring a large pot of salted water to a boil. Add the lasagna noodles and cook until al dente (usually about 30 seconds to a minute less than the package instructions recommend). Drain and toss with just enough oil to coat (to keep them from sticking).

- While the pasta cooks, brown the sausage in a large sauté pan over medium heat until cooked through. Add the spinach, pepper flakes, and nutmeg and cook until the spinach is warmed through. Season with salt and pepper. Remove from heat and let cool slightly. Combine with the ricotta in a large mixing bowl.

- Preheat the oven to 400°F. Spread a thin layer of the marinara on the bottom of a 13" x 9" baking dish. Lay out the noodles on a cutting board and cut each in half crosswise. Working one strip at a time, place a large spoonful of the spinach-ricotta mixture at the end of the noodle, then roll into a tight package (but not too tight or the filling will squeeze out). Continue until you've run out of the ricotta-spinach mixture, about 20 lasagna rolls. Place the rolls in the pan as you complete each one.

- Top the lasagna rolls with the remaining marinara, then with the mozzarella. Cover with foil and bake for 15 minutes. Remove the foil and bake for another 10 minutes, until the cheese and sauce are bubbling.

Makes 6 servings /
Cost per serving: $2.31

Save!
790 calories and $9.94!

380 calories
11 g fat
(3.5 g saturated)
950 mg sodium

1,170 calories
68 g fat
(39 g saturated)
2,510 mg sodium

Not That!
Olive Garden Lasagna Rollata al Forno
Price: $12.25

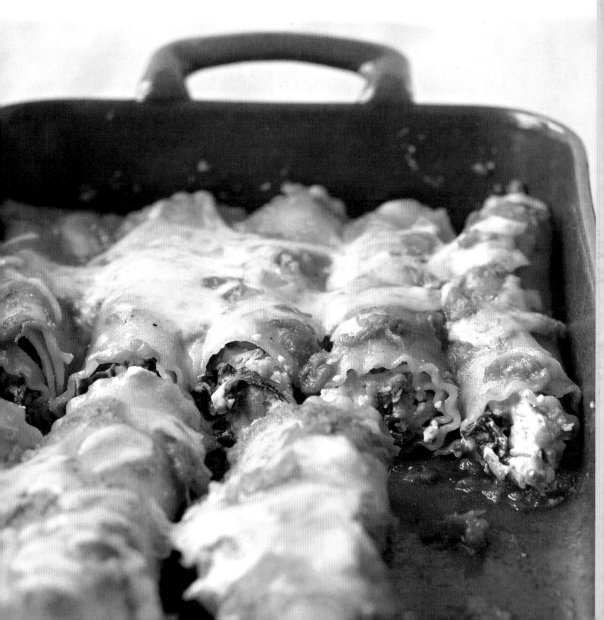

Cook This!
Red Pepper Alfredo

Fettuccine Alfredo, in its purest form, is nothing more than pasta, butter, and Parmesan cheese. It's far from a paradigm of sound nutrition, but considerably better than the pasta that appears on American menus the country over: a thick sludge of reduced heavy cream and a heap of noodles that, when combined, will chew up a full day of fat and the better part of your 24-hour caloric allowance. This version starts with a béchamel sauce, then blends that with roasted red peppers to make for a lighter, brighter, better Alfredo—for a quarter of the calories.

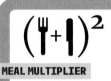

$$(\Psi + I)^2$$

MEAL MULTIPLIER

Consider this a base recipe, one that you can build on in dozens of different ways depending on your taste buds and mood. Any of these tweaks can be used to boost both flavor and nutrition:

- Stir 8 ounces of peeled raw shrimp into the sauce 2 minutes before adding the pasta, or 8 ounces of leftover chicken just as you add the pasta
- After tossing the pasta and sauce, stir in 4 cups baby spinach and cook just until it begins to wilt, about 1 minute
- Stir in 2 cups each sautéed mushrooms and roasted broccoli right before adding the pasta

You'll Need:

- 10 oz dried fettuccine
- 1½ Tbsp butter
- 1½ Tbsp flour
- 1 cup milk
- ½ cup half and half
- ¾ cup chopped bottled roasted red peppers
- 2 cloves garlic, halved
- ½ cup grated Parmesan
- Salt and black pepper to taste

How to Make It:

- Bring a large pot of salted water to a boil. Add the pasta and cook until al dente (usually about 30 seconds to a minute less than the package instructions recommend).
- Meanwhile, melt the butter in a medium saucepan over medium heat. Stir in the flour and cook for a minute, until the two are fully incorporated. Slowly add the milk and half and half, whisking to help prevent lumps from forming. Add the red pepper and garlic. Turn the heat to low and simmer for 10 minutes. Pour the mixture into a blender and puree until smooth and uniform in color. Return to the pan and stir in the Parmesan. Season with salt and pepper and simmer until the pasta is done cooking.
- Drain the pasta and add directly to the saucepan. Toss to coat evenly. Divide among 4 warm bowls or plates.

Makes 4 servings /
Cost per serving: $1.49

390 calories
12 g fat
(7 g saturated)
730 mg sodium

Not That!
Olive Garden Fettuccini Alfredo
Price: $11.50

1,220 calories
75 g fat
(47 g saturated)
1,350 mg sodium

Save!
830 calories
and $10.01!

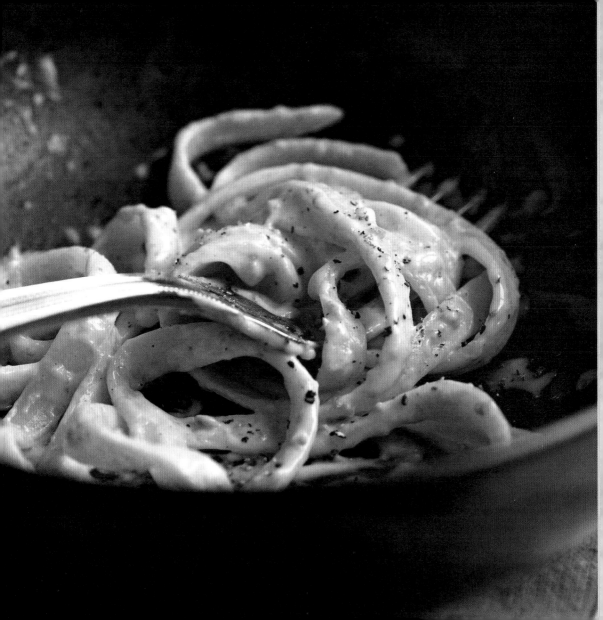

Cook This!
Meatballs with Polenta

Spaghetti and meatballs are inevitably a high-calorie affair. But the meatballs aren't the problem, it's the massive serving of pasta beneath them. At restaurants Romano's Macaroni Grill, Olive Garden, and Mom & Pop's Corner Italian Joint, more than half the calories are likely to come from the noodles alone. This recipe lightens up the meatball (using sirloin and turkey instead of veal and pork), but, more importantly, it ditches the spaghetti in favor of polenta, an Italian staple of stone-ground corn with a fraction of the calories.

You'll Need:

- 8 oz ground sirloin
- 8 oz ground turkey
- 1 egg
- ½ cup chopped fresh parsley, plus more for garnish
- ¼ cup grated Parmesan, plus more for garnish
- ½ tsp fennel seeds
- Salt and black pepper
- 1 slice white bread, torn into small pieces and briefly soaked in milk
- ½ Tbsp olive oil
- 1 small onion, minced
- 2 cloves garlic, minced
- Pinch of red pepper flakes
- 1 can (28 oz) crushed tomatoes
- 1 cup dried polenta, prepared according to package instructions

How to Make It:

- Preheat the oven to 450°F.
- Combine the sirloin, turkey, egg, parsley, Parmesan, fennel seeds, and ¾ teaspoon salt in a large mixing bowl. Squeeze the excess milk from the bread and add to the bowl. Use your (impeccably clean!) hands to gently mix the ingredients together. Form meatballs the size of golf balls, about 1" in diameter, being careful not to overwork the meat. Place the meatballs in a baking dish and bake for 25 minutes, until nicely browned all over.
- While the meatballs bake, heat the oil in a large sauté pan over medium heat. Add the onion, garlic, and pepper flakes and cook for about 3 minutes, until the onion is soft and translucent. Add the tomatoes, plus salt and pepper to taste, and simmer while the meatballs finish cooking.
- Transfer the meatballs straight from the oven to the sauce. Cook for at least 10 minutes (but preferably 20 to 30 minutes), turning the meatballs so that all parts have a chance to simmer in the sauce. Serve the meatballs and sauce over soft polenta, topped with a bit of chopped parsley and grated Parmesan.

Makes 4 servings /
Cost per serving: $2.99

380 calories
14 g fat
(4.5 g saturated)
1,010 mg sodium

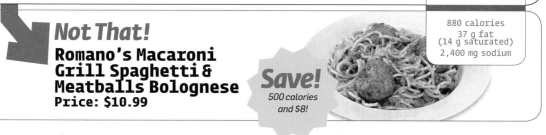

880 calories
37 g fat
(14 g saturated)
2,400 mg sodium

Not That!
Romano's Macaroni Grill Spaghetti & Meatballs Bolognese
Price: $10.99

Save!
500 calories
and $8!

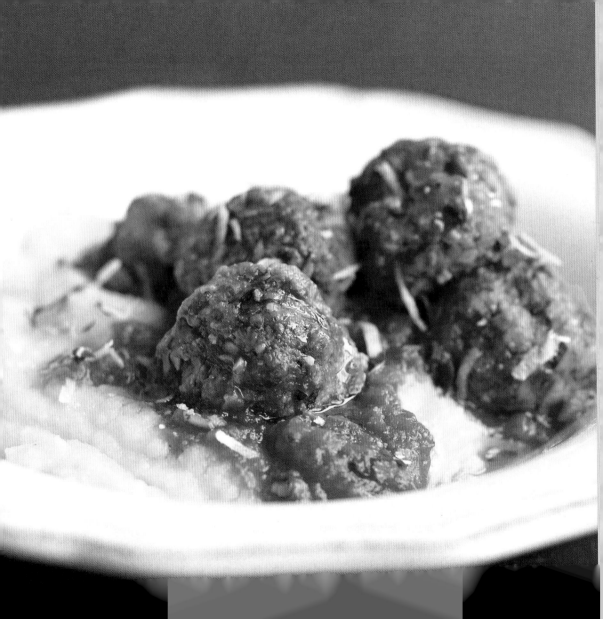

Loaded Calzone

Though it will never achieve the kind of superstar status enjoyed by its more celebrated cousin, a calzone is little more than a pizza folded over on itself and sealed. The potential for caloric overload is high, given the types (and quantities) of ingredients that typically find their way into the golden half moon: pepperoni, sausage, meatballs, 19 different types of cheese. But a calzone just as easily welcomes healthy vegetable fillings into its warm, doughy embrace. This version offers something for everyone: sautéed greens and roasted peppers for the produce proponents, and chunks of chicken sausage for the calorie-conscious carnivores.

You'll Need:

- ½ **bunch broccoli rabe or 1 bunch fresh spinach, trimmed**
- ½ **Tbsp olive oil**
- 1 **large link chicken sausage, casing removed**
- ½ **tsp red pepper flakes**
- ½ **cup bottled roasted red peppers**
- **Salt and black pepper to taste**
- **Pizza Dough (see page 180) or 12 oz store-bought pizza dough**
- 1 **cup ricotta cheese**
- 1 **cup Pizza Sauce (see page 184)**
- 1 **egg white, beaten**

How to Make It:

- Preheat the oven to 500°F.
- Bring a large pan of water to boil. Add the broccoli rabe and cook for 3 minutes. Drain. Return the pan to the stovetop and heat the oil over medium heat. Add the sausage meat and saute until cooked through. Stir in the broccoli rabe and pepper flakes and cook for another 3 to 4 minutes. Stir in the roasted peppers and season with salt and pepper.
- Divide the dough into two balls. On a clean, well-floured surface, roll each piece into a thin oval, about 14" long and 8" wide. Place the dough on two separate baking sheets. Spread half the ricotta across each, lengthwise, then top each with a ¼ cup of the pizza sauce and half of the broccoli rabe mixture. Fold the dough crosswise over the mixture, creating one large half moon, and pinch the dough to seal it completely. Brush the tops with the egg white.
- Bake the calzones for 12 to 15 minutes, until lightly browned and firm all over. Cut each calzone in half and serve with the remaining pizza sauce.

Makes 4 servings / Cost per serving: $2.53

395 calories
12 g fat
(3.5 g saturated)
750 mg sodium

1,420 calories
62 g fat
(28 g saturated, 2 g trans)
3,600 mg sodium

Not That!

Pizza Hut Meaty P'Zone Pizza
(full order)
Price: $6.99

Save!
1,025 calories and $4.46!

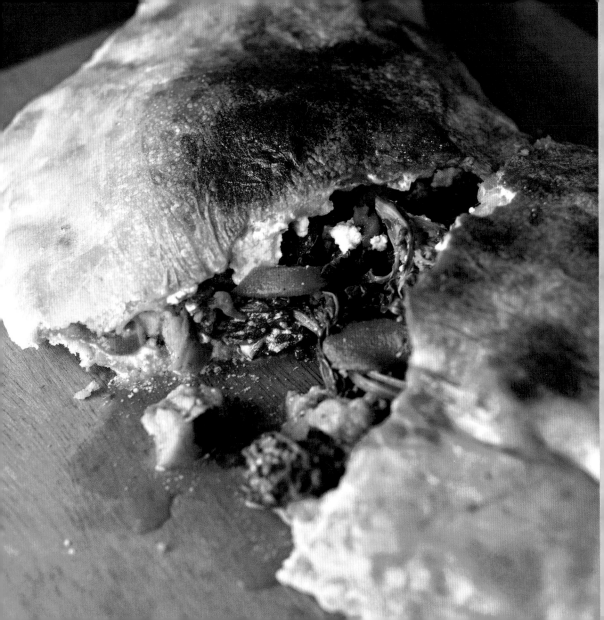

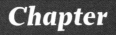

Chapter

American Classics

Eat all your favorite comfort foods
and watch the pounds melt away

205

11 Ways to Cook Chi

1

Grind almonds in a food processor until they're as fine as bread crumbs. Smear chicken cutlets all over with Dijon, then dip them into the almonds. Bake in a 425°F oven until crispy on the outside and cooked all the way through, about 12 minutes.

2

Use a paring knife to cut a pocket into the side of a chicken breast. Stuff with sundried tomatoes, toasted pine nuts, and feta. Roast in a 450°F oven for 10 to 12 minutes, until cooked through.

3

Pound a chicken breast until uniformly ¼" thick. Rub with salt, pepper, and olive oil and grill until lightly charred. Top with chopped figs, goat cheese, and arugula.

Combine 2 tablespoons red or green curry paste with a can of light coconut milk and 1 cup of chicken stock and simmer in a medium sauce pan. Stir in chunks of chicken breast, chopped bok choy, and sliced mushrooms and simmer for 10 minutes. Serve over brown rice with a wedge of lime.

4

Place a breast in the center of a large piece of aluminum foil. Top with artichoke hearts, sliced fennel, cherry tomatoes, pitted olives, and splash of olive oil and white wine. Fold up the foil to create a sealed packet and cook in a 400°F oven for 20 minutes.

5

cken Breast

6 *Combine 1 cup orange juice with ½ cup soy sauce and 1 tablespoon minced ginger. Boil until thick enough to coat the back of a spoon, about 10 minutes. Grill or broil chicken breasts until cooked through, and brush with sauce after.*

7
Combine 2 tablespoons Dijon with 1 tablespoon each of soy sauce, brown sugar, and melted butter. Brush it on the chicken before and during cooking.

8 Place bone-in, skin-on chicken breasts in a roasting pan with chunks of potato, onion, and carrot. Combine a ½ cup of olive oil with 3 cloves minced garlic and 1 tablespoon chopped rosemary. Pour this mixture over the chicken and vegetables, season with salt and pepper, and roast in a 400°F oven for 25 minutes.

9 *Bring 1 cup balsamic vinegar and 2 cups chicken broth to a simmer. Add chicken breasts and poach over very low heat until cooked through, about 10 minutes. Remove breasts, crank the heat, and boil until the liquid reduces in volume by half. Spoon over the chicken.*

11 Cook bone-in, skin-on chicken breasts in a skillet until crispy and cooked all the way through. Remove. Add minced shallots and mushrooms and cook until browned. Stir in 2 parts white wine and 1 part cream and cook until slightly thickened. Pour over chicken.

10 Soak breasts or thighs in lime juice, cumin, garlic, and some canned chipotle pepper for an hour. Grill until nicely charred and serve with guacamole, salsa, and hot corn tortillas.

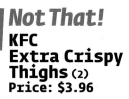

Cook This!
Oven-Fried Chicken

Southerners may grunt and grumble about the travesty of "fried" chicken not being cooked in big skillets of melted lard, but we'd bring this crispy, succulent bird to a church potluck in Savannah without batting an eye. A long soak in buttermilk spiked liberally with hot sauce both tenderizes and flavors the meat, while the spiced panko provides a layer of captivating crunch. We won't go as far as to say you won't taste the difference (properly fried chicken has a depth of flavor that stretches straight to your soul), but we can say with confidence that this chicken hits the spot.

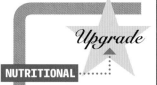

Upgrade

NUTRITIONAL

Better Bread Crumbs

No matter how little oil they absorb, bread crumbs are always empty calories, but breading on meat and fish doesn't need to be a total nutritional zero. Nuts make a perfect crunchy breading for chicken and fish fillets, coating them in a crunchy sheath rich in fiber and healthy fat. Almonds, pecans, and pine nuts make for the best coasting. Simply drop them in a food processor and blend until finely chopped.

You'll Need:

- 2 cups buttermilk
- ¼ cup Frank's Red Hot pepper sauce
- 1 lb chicken drumsticks and thighs
- 2 cups panko bread crumbs
- ½ tsp garlic salt
- ½ tsp smoked paprika
- ½ tsp salt
- ½ tsp black pepper
- ⅛ tsp cayenne

How to Make It:

- Combine the buttermilk and hot sauce in a large bowl or a sealable plastic bag. Add the chicken and turn to coat. Cover the bowl or seal the bag and marinate in the refrigerator for at least 1 hour and up to 12.

- Preheat the oven to 450°F. In a bowl, combine the bread crumbs with the spices. Working one piece at a time, remove the chicken from the buttermilk marinade and dip into the bread crumbs to thoroughly coat. (When breading food, it's best to use one hand for the dry element and one for the wet.)

- Place the breaded chicken on a nonstick baking sheet. Bake for about 20 minutes, until browned and crisp on the outside and cooked all the way through.

Makes 4 servings /
Cost per serving: $1.12

310 calories
7 g fat
(2.5 g saturated)
710 mg sodium

680 calories
48 g fat
(10 g saturated)
1,560 mg sodium

Not That!
KFC Extra Crispy Thighs (2)
Price: $3.96

Save!
370 calories and $2.84!

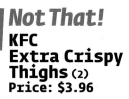

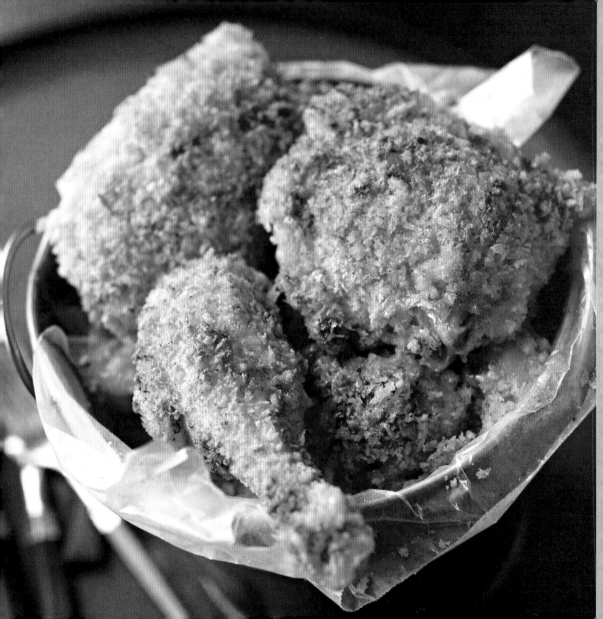

Serious Chili

Texans and New Mexicans—both of whom lay claim to the advent of chili—disagree on most matters when it comes to this divisive dish. Beans or no beans? Tomatoes? Chunks of chuck or ground? One truth all serious chili heads can agree on, though, is the fundamental importance of a good chili powder. That means skipping the bottled supermarket stuff and making your own secret spice powder. This is a beginner powder, requiring nothing more than toasting two different dried chiles, then pulverizing them in a coffee grinder. Use leftovers to rub on steaks, spike dips, and dust on slices of mango.

You'll Need:

- 3 ancho chiles
- 10 dried chiles de arbol
- 1 Tbsp oil or bacon grease
- 2 lb chuck roast, cut into ½" pieces
- Salt and black pepper to taste
- 2 medium onions, diced
- 2 poblano peppers, diced
- 2 cloves garlic, minced
- 1 tsp ground cumin
- 1 can (28 oz) tomato puree
- 2 cups low-sodium beef stock
- 1 can (14–16 oz) pinto beans, drained
- Diced onion, minced jalapeño, shredded cheese, chopped cilantro, and/or sour cream, for serving

How to Make It:

- Heat a cast-iron or stainless steel skillet over medium heat. Add the chiles and cook, turning occasionally, until lightly toasted and crispy. The chiles de arbol will take about 5 minutes; the anchos about 10. (Be careful not to inhale too deeply—chile smoke has been known to cause wild fits of coughing.) Discard the stems and seeds and place the chiles in a clean coffee grinder or food processor. Grind into a fine dust. That's your chili powder—the heart of this dish.

- Heat the oil in a large pot over medium-high heat. Season the beef with salt and pepper and add to the pan. Sear the meat until all sides are nicely browned, then add the onions, poblano peppers, garlic, cumin, and 2 tablespoons of the chili powder. Cook, stirring occasionally, for about 5 minutes, until the vegetables are softened. Stir in the tomatoes and stock. Lower the heat and simmer for at least 45 minutes (but preferably up to 90 minutes), until the beef is fork tender.

- Stir in the beans a few minutes before serving, and heat through. Serve with any of the garnishes.

Makes 8 servings /
Cost per serving: $1.89

380 calories
12 g fat
(4.5 mg saturated)
810 mg sodium

1,220 calories
54 g fat
(20 g saturated)
2,800 mg sodium

Not That!
Marie Callender's Bowl of Chili & Cornbread
Price: $7.99

Save!
840 calories
and $6.10!

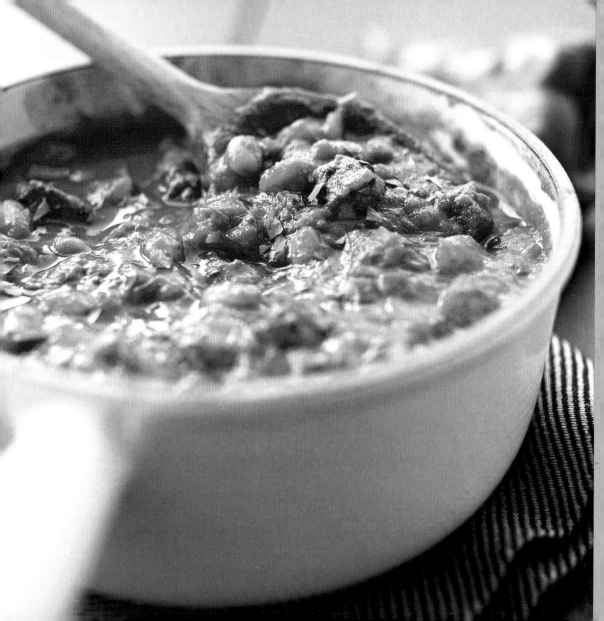

Cook This!

Teriyaki Pork Chop with Apple Chutney

This is a remake of the old Homer Simpson special: pork chops and applesauce. Only, this isn't some ordinary overcooked chop with a scoop of Mott's. The pork is soaked in a sweet, garlicky teriyaki marinade and the apples are sautéed with ginger and Chinese spices, making for a perfect yin-yang partnership (cue prolonged Homer drooling noise). It's easy enough to throw together on any given Tuesday night, but seemingly fancy enough to serve to dinner guests on a special Saturday.

You'll Need:

- 4 pork chops (about 6 oz each)
- 1 cup bottled teriyaki marinade (we like Soy Vay)
- ½ Tbsp peanut or canola oil
- ½ onion, diced
- 1 Tbsp grated fresh ginger
- 1 apple, peeled, cored, and diced
- ½ cup apple juice
- ¼ cup apple cider vinegar
- 1 tsp Chinese five-spice powder
- Salt and black pepper to taste

How to Make It:

- Combine the pork chops and teriyaki sauce in a shallow bowl or sealable plastic bag, turning the chops to coat. Cover the bowl or seal the bag and marinate in the refrigerator for at least 1 hour and up to 8.

- Preheat a grill, grill pan, or large cast-iron skillet. While the grill warms up, heat the oil in a medium saucepan over medium heat. Add the onion and ginger and cook for about 2 minutes, until the onion is translucent. Add the apple, apple juice, vinegar, and five-spice, and stir to combine. Lower the heat and simmer for about 10 minutes, until the fruit is softened (but not mushy) and the liquid has thickened enough to cling lightly to the apples.

- When the grill or pan is hot, remove the pork from the marinade, blotting off the excess with paper towels, and grill for 4 to 5 minutes per side, until lightly charred all over and firm but slightly yielding to the touch. (Be careful—if the grill is too hot, the sugars in the marinade will burn. Ultimately, you want a nice medium heat.) Serve each chop with a scoop of the apple chutney.

Makes 4 servings / Cost per serving: $2.44

315 calories
9 g fat
(3.5 g saturated)
890 mg sodium

1,928 calories
57 g saturated fat
1,685 mg sodium

Not That!
Cheesecake Factory Grilled Pork Chops
Price: $18.95

Save!
1,613 calories
and $16.51!

212

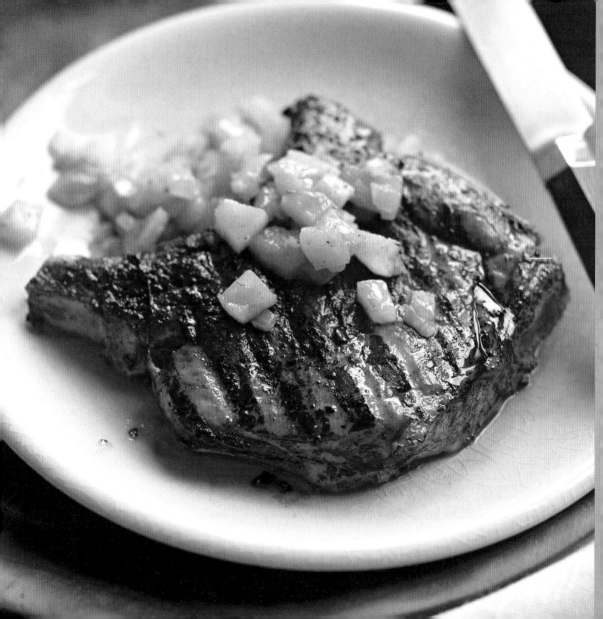

Cook This!
Chicken with Tomato, Olives, and Capers

Ever wonder why everything "tastes like chicken"? Because chicken doesn't taste like much in particular, making it a catch-all canvas for describing other things that don't taste like anything. The good news is this chicken does taste like something: Roasting it with tomatoes, capers, and olive oil bastes the chicken in a savory broth, keeping the meat moist and ultimately providing both a chunky, textured topping and an intensely satisfying sauce to dump over the top. You can pull this off in a single baking dish, but the foil is there to catch all the drippings—and spare you the post-dinner cleanup.

You'll Need:

4 boneless, skinless chicken breasts (4–6 oz each), pounded to uniform ¼" thickness

Salt and black pepper to taste

1 pint cherry tomatoes or 2 cups chopped tomatoes

½ red onion, diced

¼ cup green olives, pitted and chopped

¼ cup pine nuts

2 Tbsp capers

2 Tbsp olive oil

Thinly sliced fresh basil (optional)

How to Make It:

- Preheat the oven to 450°F. Season the chicken with salt and pepper. Take four large sheets of aluminum foil and fold each in half, then fold up about 1" of each side to create four trays, each large enough to comfortably hold a chicken breast. Place a breast on each piece of foil.
- Combine the tomatoes, onion, olives, pine nuts, capers, and olive oil with a few pinches of salt and pepper in a mixing bowl. Top the chicken breasts with the mixture.
- Place the chicken trays on a baking sheet and bake for about 15 minutes, until the chicken is cooked through. Serve with the tomato mixture and any accumulated juices from the foil drizzled on top. Garnish with basil if using.

Makes 4 servings / Cost per serving: $2.93

Many of the garnish ingredients in this book are optional because of cost, not taste. In a perfect world, you'd have them on hand, but if paying $3 for a few basil leaves feels unreasonable, the dish will survive well without it.

310 calories
18 g fat
(2.5 g saturated)
420 mg sodium

1,830 calories
52 g saturated fat
735 mg sodium

Not That!
Cheesecake Factory Chicken Piccata
Price: $15.95

Save!
1,520 calories and $13.02!

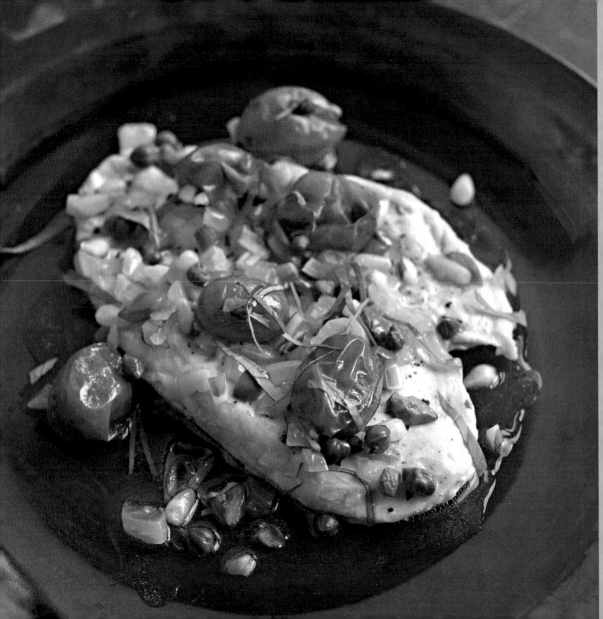

Cook This!

Beef Stroganoff

Beef stroganoff may be Russian in name and origin, but it's since become a global go-to, finding a home everywhere from Iran to Brazil to Australia. Only the best dishes inspire this type of universal love, and the ease and innate deliciousness of stroganoff is clearly why Americans have embraced it as their own. Though sour cream is normally stirred into the sauce at the last second, we tested this dish several different ways and found yogurt tasted every bit as good for fewer calories. Just make sure to remove the pan from the heat before adding, as high temperatures can cause the yogurt to break, jeopardizing the smooth, velvety sauce you really want.

You'll Need:

- ½ Tbsp canola oil, plus more if needed
- 12 oz white or cremini mushrooms, stems removed, halved
- 1 lb sirloin, cut into thin strips
- Salt and black pepper to taste
- 1 yellow onion, minced
- 2 cloves garlic, minced
- 1 Tbsp flour
- ¾ cup red wine
- ½ cup low-sodium beef stock
- 1 Tbsp tomato paste
- ¼ cup 2% plain Greek yogurt •
- Chopped fresh parsley

Don't try to substitute regular yogurt here. Greek yogurt has a distinct lactic tang that better approximates sour cream.

How to Make It:

- Heat the oil in large sauté pan over medium heat. Add the mushrooms and cook for about 5 minutes, until softened and caramelized. Remove and reserve.
- Season the beef with salt and pepper. In the same pan, adding more oil if necessary, cook the beef for about 5 minutes, until well-browned all over. Remove and reserve with the mushrooms. Add the onion and garlic to the pan and cook until the onion is translucent. Stir in the flour until it evenly coats the vegetables, then add the wine, stock, and tomato paste, scraping the pan to release any flavorful bits stuck to the bottom. Turn the heat down to low and simmer for about 12 minutes, until the liquid thickens and reduces by about half.
- Return the mushrooms and beef to the pan and heat through, then remove from the heat. After the liquid cools just slightly, stir in the yogurt. (If the heat is too high, the yogurt will separate.) Serve over buttered noodles or steamed rice and garnish with parsley.

Makes 4 servings / Cost per serving: $2.38

260 calories
7 g fat
(2 g saturated)
690 mg sodium

813 calories
43 g fat
(15 g saturated)
1,782 mg sodium

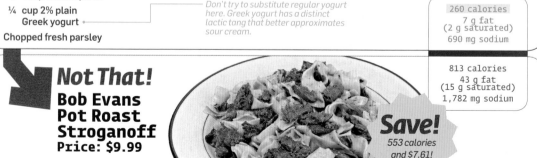

Not That!
Bob Evans Pot Roast Stroganoff
Price: $9.99

Save!
553 calories
and $7.61!

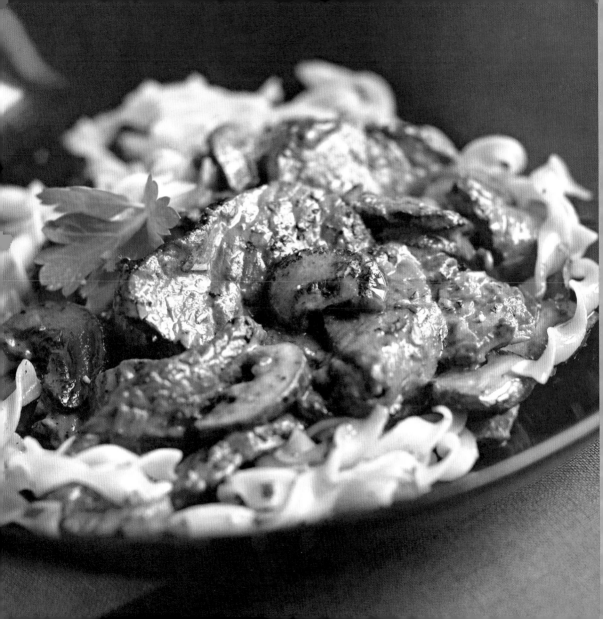

Seared Sirloin with Red Wine Mushrooms

Do you really want to go out and spend $20 or $30 on a steak dinner only to find out the beef was of dubious origin and the nutritionals look more like Dow Jones updates than calorie counts? That's what's in store for you when you seek out your beef fix at one of our country's largest national chains. We not only guarantee that this recipe will slash your bill by 75 percent, but that your taste buds will thank you many times over. Skip the grill and cook on cast iron instead—it not only gives your steak a marvelous crust in a matter of minutes, but it helps form the basis for this knockout mushroom sauce. Cook this when you need to impress someone—even if it's just yourself.

You'll Need:

- 1 Tbsp olive oil
- 4 sirloin steaks or petite filets (6 oz each)
- Salt and black pepper to taste
- 2 shallots, minced
- 2 cloves garlic, minced
- ½ lb white or cremini mushrooms, cleaned, stems removed, and sliced
- 1 cup red wine
- 1 cup low-sodium beef stock
- 2 tsp fresh rosemary, chopped

How to Make It:

- Preheat the oven to 400°F. Heat the oil in a large cast-iron or oven-safe skillet over high heat. Season the steaks with salt and plenty of black pepper and add to the hot pan. Sear the first side for 3 to 4 minutes, until a deep brown crust has developed, then flip. Place the pan in the oven to finish cooking (about 6 to 8 minutes for medium rare; an instant-read thermometer inserted into the thickest part will read 135°F). Remove from the oven and transfer the steaks to a cutting board to rest.

- Using a potholder, place the pan back on the stove over medium heat. Add the shallots, garlic, and mushrooms and cook for 3 to 4 minutes, until the mushrooms have begun to caramelize. Add the red wine and the stock, using a wooden spoon to scrape the bottom of the pan. Cook for another 2 to 3 minutes, until the alcohol has burned off and the liquid has reduced by about half. Stir in the rosemary.

- Divide the steaks among four plates, top with mushrooms, and spoon on the sauce.

*Makes 4 servings /
Cost per serving: $4.47*

405 calories
12 g fat
(5 g saturated)
677 mg sodium

Not That!

IHOP Sirloin Steak Tips Dinner
Price: $12.99

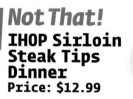

1,040 calories

Save!
635 calories
and $8.52!

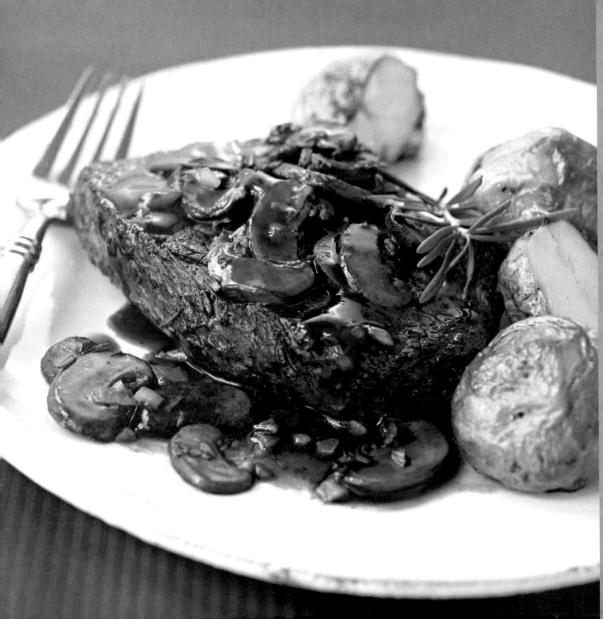

Cook This!

Turkey Sloppy Joes

It's amazing that multiple companies make a living selling packets, boxes, and cans of sloppy joe mix, many of them loaded with funky preservatives and fillers that even chemists would have a difficult time deciphering. All in the name of shaving 30 seconds from your total cooking time. The best part about sloppy joes is that everything you need is likely already in your pantry and spice cabinet, gathering dust, waiting for a chance to shine. Open a can, measure out a few spices (if you have children, employ them as your sous chefs), and you'll have a crowd-pleasing dinner on the table in about 15 minutes.

You'll Need:

- ½ Tbsp olive oil
- 1 large onion, diced
- 1 green bell pepper, diced
- 1 lb lean ground turkey
- 1½ cups tomato sauce
- 2 Tbsp tomato paste
- 2 Tbsp brown sugar
- 1 Tbsp red wine vinegar
- 1 Tbsp Worcestershire sauce
- ½ Tbsp chili powder
- 10–12 shakes Tabasco or other hot sauce
- Salt and black pepper to taste
- 4 whole-wheat or sesame rolls, split and toasted

How to Make It:

- Heat the oil in a large skillet or sauté pan over medium heat. Add the onion and bell pepper and cook for about 2 minutes, until softened. Add the turkey and cook, using a wooden spoon to break up the meat, until the turkey is lightly browned. Add the tomato sauce, tomato paste, sugar, vinegar, Worcestershire, chili powder, and hot sauce and season with salt and pepper.
- Turn the heat down to low. Simmer for 10 minutes, until the liquid has reduced and the sauce fully coats the meat. Divide the mixture among the rolls.

Makes 4 sandwiches / Cost per serving: $2.07

Lean ground sirloin or chicken works just as well here as turkey. As crazy as it sounds, so does a few fillets of finely chopped catfish—the perfect way to sneak fish into your family's diet.

340 calories
11 g fat
(2.5 g saturated)
820 mg sodium

580 calories
23 g fat
(9 g saturated)
1,530 mg sodium

Not That!

Subway
6-inch Meatball
Marinara Sandwich
Price: $3.45

Save!
240 calories and $1.38!

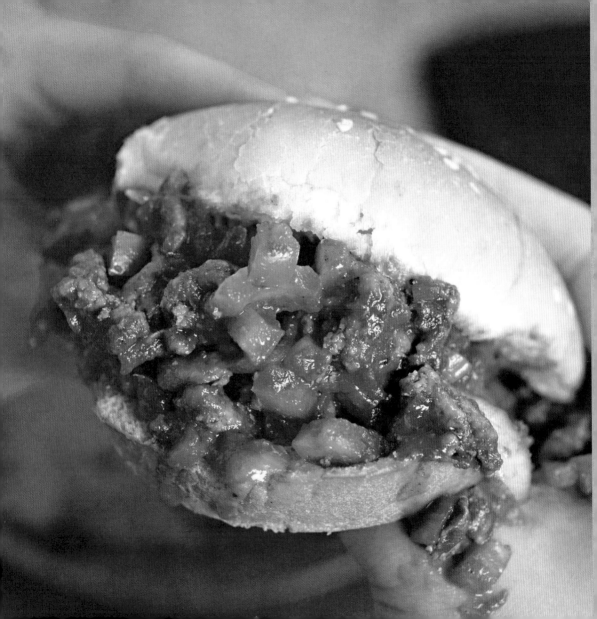

Chicken Pizzaioli

Chicken parmesan is not only one of the most popular dishes in America, but it may be the single dish that best encapsulates the Big Three behind our obesity epidemic: fried food, melted cheese, and massive portion sizes. Olive Garden's rendition represents the average plate of chicken parm—a scary proposition given the fact that it packs nearly an entire day's worth of saturated fat and enough salt to sustain a small colony for years. To lighten things up without losing flavor, we ditch the breading (which gets soggy underneath the sauce anyway) and sear the chicken rather than fry it. A ladle of red sauce and a thin layer of bubbling mozzarella rounds the dish out—without rounding you out.

You'll Need:

1 Tbsp olive oil

4 chicken breasts (6 oz each)

1 tsp dried thyme or rosemary

Salt and pepper to taste

1 medium yellow onion, sliced

½ cup chopped green olives

4 cloves garlic, minced

1 tsp red pepper flakes

1 can (28 oz) crushed tomatoes

1 cup grated mozzarella

How to Make It:

- Place the chicken breasts on a cutting board, cover with plastic wrap, and use a meat mallet or heavy-bottomed pan to pound the chicken into ½-inch thick cutlets. Season with thyme or rosemary and a healthy sprinkle of salt and pepper.

- Heat the oil in a large cast-iron skillet or oven-safe pan over medium high heat. When hot, add the chicken and cook for 3 to 4 minutes, until a nice crust has developed on the surface of the chicken, then flip and cook for another 3 to 4 minutes. Remove and reserve the chicken.

- Preheat the broiler. In the same pan, add the onions, olives, garlic, and red pepper flakes. Sauté until the onions have begun to lightly caramelize, about 5 minutes, then add the tomatoes. Cook for another 3 minutes, then slide the chicken back into the pan. Divide the mozzarella between the chicken breasts, then place the whole pan into the oven. Broil for 3 to 4 minutes, until the cheese is melted and bubbling. Serve the chicken with a generous scoop of the spicy red sauce.

Makes 4 servings /
Cost per serving: $3.56

360 calories
15 g fat
(3 g saturated)
812 mg sodium

Not That!
Olive Garden Chicken Parmigiana
Price: $13.50

1,090 calories
49 g fat
(18 g saturated)
3,380 mg sodium

Save!
730 calories
and $9.94!

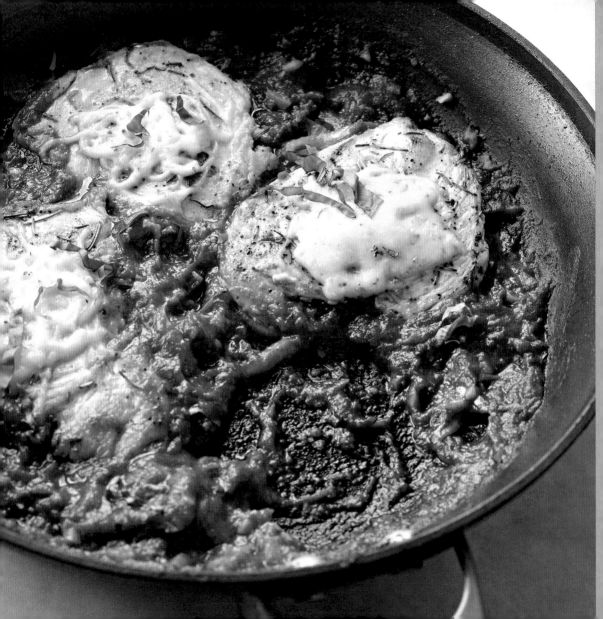

Cook This!
Chicken-White Bean Chili

We've never been shy in proclaiming our affection for chili. Fiber-rich beans, protein-packed meat, antioxidant-dense chiles and spices—it's an easy dish to love, especially when those three elements combine to make for an explosively flavorful bowl of goodness. Though not a classic bowl of red, this version deserves a place in your dinner roster.

You'll Need:

- 1 Tbsp olive oil
- 2 yellow onions, chopped
- 4 cloves garlic, minced
- 1 lb boneless, skinless chicken thighs, cut into small pieces
- 1 lb lean ground chicken
- 1 can (7 oz) roasted green chiles
- 1 tsp ground cumin
- 1 tsp dried oregano
- ¼ tsp cayenne pepper
- 4 cups low-sodium chicken stock
- 1 can (14–16 oz each) white kidney beans (also called cannellini and great northern beans), drained

Salt and black pepper to taste

Fresh cilantro, shredded cheese, diced onion, sour cream, and/or sliced jalapeños for serving

How to Make It:

- Heat the oil in a large pot over medium heat. Add the onion and garlic and cook for about 3 minutes, until the onion is translucent. Add the chicken thighs, ground chicken, chiles, cumin, oregano, and cayenne. Sauté until the chicken is mostly cooked through, about 8 minutes. Add the stock and beans. Turn the heat down to low.
- Simmer uncovered for at least 20 minutes, or longer if you have the patience. Taste the chili and adjust the seasoning with salt and pepper. Serve with any combination of the garnishes.

Makes 8 servings / Cost per serving: $1.84

The mix of ground and chopped chicken gives this chili a more interesting texture, but if you prefer one over the other, simply use 2 pounds of your chicken of choice.

380 calories
13 g fat
(3 g saturated)
860 mg sodium

847 calories
12 g saturated fat
1,843 mg sodium

Not That!
Cheesecake Factory White Chicken Chili
Price: $10.95

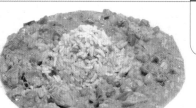

Save!
467 calories and $9.11!

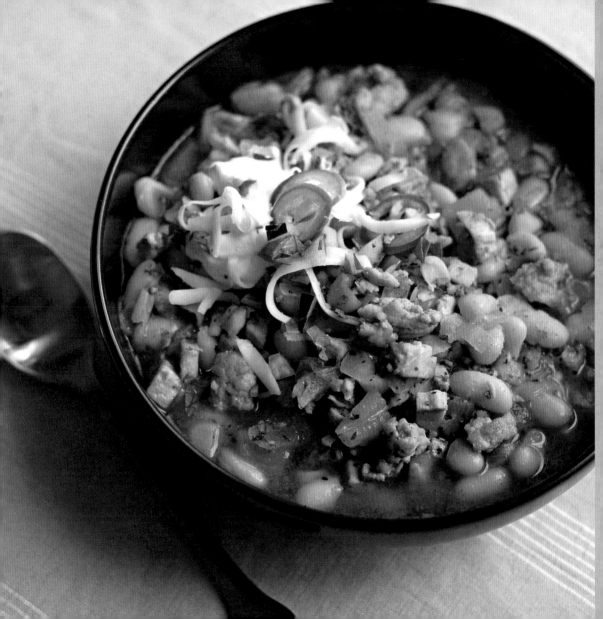

Cook This!
Fish with Herbed Bread Crumbs

Deep-frying is the ultimate equalizer: It takes any raw ingredient, regardless of how healthy it may be, and turns it into nutritional garbage. (Plus, have you ever noticed how fried food all tastes the same? Don't believe us? Order the 1,500-calorie Admiral's Feast at Red Lobster and see if you can tell the difference between one type of fried seafood and the next.) This butter-laced bread crumb topping gives you the satisfying crunch and richness of fried food without ruining the inherent flavor—or nutrition—of the fish itself.

You'll Need:

2 slices white bread or 1 English muffin, split

2 Tbsp chopped fresh parsley

1 tsp fresh thyme leaves

4 halibut fillets or other flaky white fish such as cod or swordfish (4–6 oz each)

Salt and black pepper to taste

2 Tbsp butter, softened

How to Make It:

- Preheat the oven to 450°F. Place the bread, parsley, and thyme in a food processor and pulse until you have small but not superfine bread crumbs. You want a bit of texture here.

- Lay the fish on a baking sheet and season all over with salt and pepper. Smear the tops with a thin layer of softened butter, then press the herbed bread crumbs into the butter so that they adhere to the fish. Bake for about 20 minutes, until the fish is cooked through and flakes with gentle pressure from your finger.

Makes 4 servings / Cost per serving: $4

Thinner fillets like catfish and tilapia are likely to overcook before the breadcrumbs are toasted, but any thick white fish fillet will be perfect.

320 calories
11 g fat
(4.5 g saturated)
390 mg sodium

990 calories
55 g fat
(18 g saturated)
1,290 mg sodium

Not That!
Romano's Macaroni Grill Crusted Sole
Price: $14.99

Save!
670 calories
and $10.99!

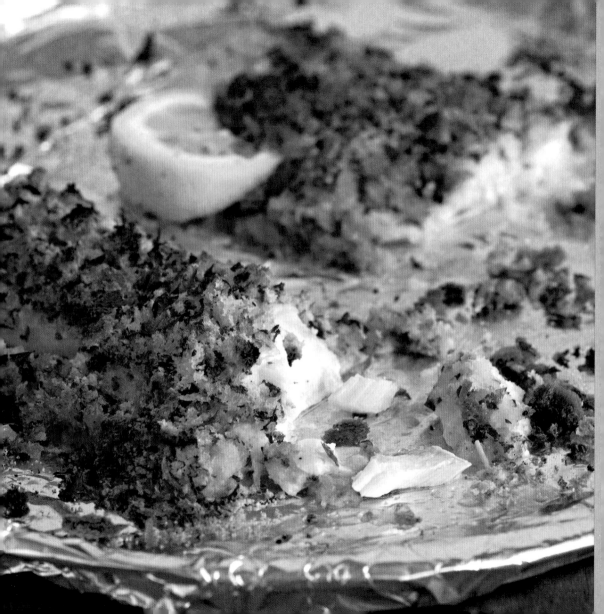

Cook This!
Turkey Breast Herb-Roasted

A recent study from the Harvard School of Public Health found that consuming processed meats—high in sodium and chemical preservatives—every day could boost your risk of heart disease by up to 42 percent. This turkey breast is not only low in sodium and nitrate-free, but it also makes the most delicious turkey sandwiches you've ever tasted.

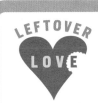

LEFTOVER LOVE

This dish was built for leftovers, so roast the turkey up on a lazy Sunday afternoon and use it all week as the foundation for some incredible meals:

- As a sandwich, stacked on sourdough with avocado, romaine, and whipped cream cheese cut with cranberry sauce
- As a salad, tossed with arugula or spinach and hard-boiled egg slices, olives, and cherry tomatoes
- As a taco, tossed with a few big spoonfuls of salsa verde, tucked into a warm tortilla, and topped with guacamole

You'll Need:

- 8 cups water
- ¾ cup salt
- 1 cup sugar
- 1 large boneless turkey breast (about 3 pounds)
- 2 cloves garlic, peeled
- Salt and black pepper to taste
- 1 Tbsp olive oil
- ½ Tbsp minced fresh rosemary

How to Make It:

- Combine the water, salt, and sugar in a pot large enough to hold the turkey and bring to a boil. Stir until the sugar and salt have fully dissolved. Remove from the heat and let cool to room temperature. Add the turkey breast, cover, and place in the fridge to brine for at least 4 hours, and up to overnight.

- Preheat the oven to 425°F. Remove the turkey from the brine, pat dry, and roll up into a tight log. Use butcher twine to tie three separate knots, about 2" apart, that will hold the turkey in this tight shape.

- Finely mince the garlic, using a pinch of salt and the back of your knife to mash it into a paste. Combine with the olive oil and rosemary, then rub all over the turkey, along with a good amount of black pepper. Place the turkey in a large roasting pan and roast until a thermometer inserted into the center of the meat reads 160°F, about 1 hour. Let the turkey rest before slicing.

- The turkey can be served as is with traditional sides, or will keep up to a week in the fridge for sandwiches.

Makes 12 servings / Cost per serving: $1.27

140 calories
2 g fat
(0 g saturated)
520 mg sodium

690 calories
30 g fat
(9 g saturated, 3 g trans)
3,093 mg sodium

Not That!
Bob Evans Turkey and Dressing
Price: $9.99

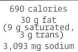

Save!
550 calories and $8.72!

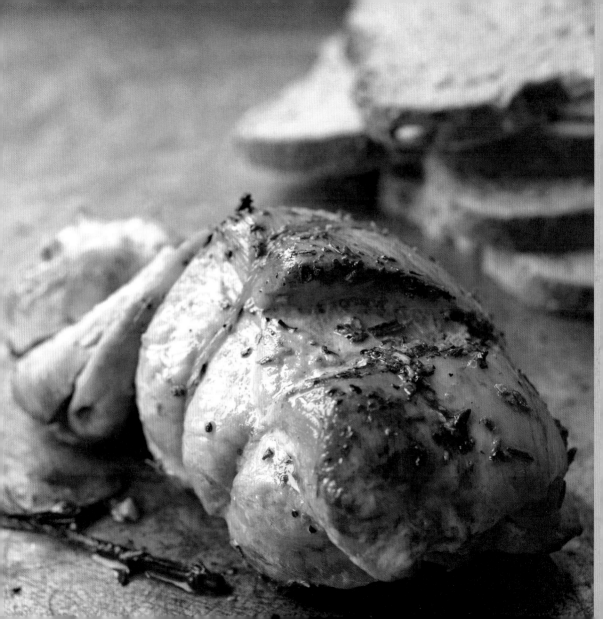

Cook This!
Crispy Duck Breast with Balsamic Cherries

Like lamb, buffalo, and rabbit, duck gets no love from the home cook. Problem is, duck is viewed as restaurant food, a fancy ingredient that requires a towering toque's deft touch to prepare. Not even close. All it takes is a hot pan and a bit of salt and pepper to cook up a moist, juicy duck breast that will rival any supermarket steak you might have instead. Seven ingredients and 15 minutes yield a dish chefs train 2 years to learn to prepare.

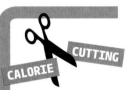

CALORIE CUTTING

You'll Need:

- **4 small duck breasts or 2 large breasts (about 1 pound total)**
- **Salt and black pepper to taste**
- **2 shallots, minced**
- **16 cherries, pitted and roughly chopped**
- **¼ cup low-sodium chicken stock**
- **¼ cup balsamic vinegar**

No duck in the supermarket? Try dartagnan.com.

How to Make It:

- Heat a large skillet over medium heat. Use a very sharp knife to score the skin on each duck breast, cutting ½" diamonds across the entire surface. Season all over with salt and black pepper. Add the duck breasts to the pan, skin side down, and cook for 5 to 6 minutes, until plenty of fat has rendered and the skin is a deep golden brown. Flip and cook for another 3 to 4 minutes, until the duck is firm but yielding, like a Nerf ball. Transfer to a cutting board and let rest for 5 minutes.

- While the duck rests, discard all but a thin film of the duck fat. (If you really want to indulge, roast your breakfast potatoes in some of the fat the next morning.) Add the shallots to the pan and cook for 1 minute before adding the cherries. Cook for 2 minutes, then pour in the stock and vinegar. Simmer for about 3 minutes, until the liquid has reduced by half. Season with black pepper.

- Thinly slice the duck and divide among four plates. Serve with the cherry-balsamic sauce spooned over the top.

Makes 4 servings /
Cost per serving: $3.75

Take comfort in the fact that most of the duck's fat is healthy fat. But healthy or not, every kind of fat, regardless of source, packs 9 calories per gram, more than twice what you'd take in from a gram of carbs or protein. If you're looking to take this dish as low as it goes, simply follow the recipe, but after the duck has rested on the cutting board, use a knife to cut away the top layer of crispy fat. Why not remove it before cooking? Because it will help insulate and baste the breast while it cooks, leaving you with juicier meat, even after the fat is gone.

270 calories
10 g fat
(3 g saturated)
290 mg sodium

1,300 calories
58 g fat
(16 g saturated)
3,760 mg sodium

Not That!
P.F. Chang's VIP Duck
Price: $18.50

Save!
1,030 calories and $14.75!

230

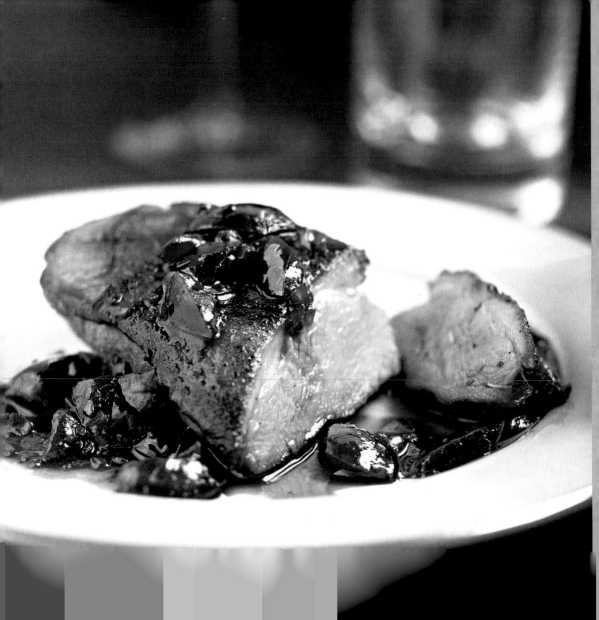

Cook This!
Chicken Cordon Bleu with Honey Mustard

It's French in name, but it feels American, right down to its molten cheese core. Normally, this chicken is stuffed, breaded, then deep-fried into submission. But our testing found that a high-heat oven provides all the crunch we want without all the calories we don't. If honey mustard feels a bit like gilding the lily, it is, but at 350 calories for the whole dish, why not?

You'll Need:

- 4 boneless, skinless chicken breasts (about 6 oz each), pounded to uniform ¼" thickness

Salt and black pepper to taste

- 8 thin slices deli ham
- 4 slices Swiss cheese
- 2 Tbsp flour
- 1 egg, beaten
- 1 cup panko bread crumbs

Juice of ½ lemon

- 2 Tbsp Dijon mustard
- 1 Tbsp honey
- ½ Tbsp olive oil mayonnaise

How to Make It:

- Preheat the oven to 450°F. Season the chicken all over with salt and pepper. Lay two slices of ham and one slice of cheese across each breast, then roll widthwise until you have a tight, jellyroll-like package.

- Place the flour, egg, and bread crumbs in separate shallow bowls. Working with one rolled-up breast at a time, dip first in the flour to lightly coat, then in the egg, then immediately in the bread crumbs. Use your fingers to make sure the chicken is evenly coated with crumbs.

- Arrange the chicken on a baking sheet and bake for 15 to 18 minutes, until the chicken is firm to the touch and cooked through and the bread crumbs are brown and crunchy.

- While the chicken bakes, stir together the lemon juice, mustard, honey, and mayo to make a smooth, uniform sauce. Serve the chicken with the honey mustard drizzled over the top.

*Makes 4 servings /
Cost per serving: $2.14*

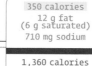

Save!
1,010 calories
and $12.12!

```
350 calories
12 g fat
(6 g saturated)
710 mg sodium
```

```
1,360 calories
81 g fat
(33 g saturated,
1 g trans)
3,007 mg sodium
```

Not That!
Mimi's Cafe Chicken Cordon Bleu
Price: $14.26

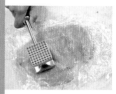
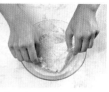
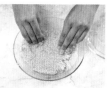

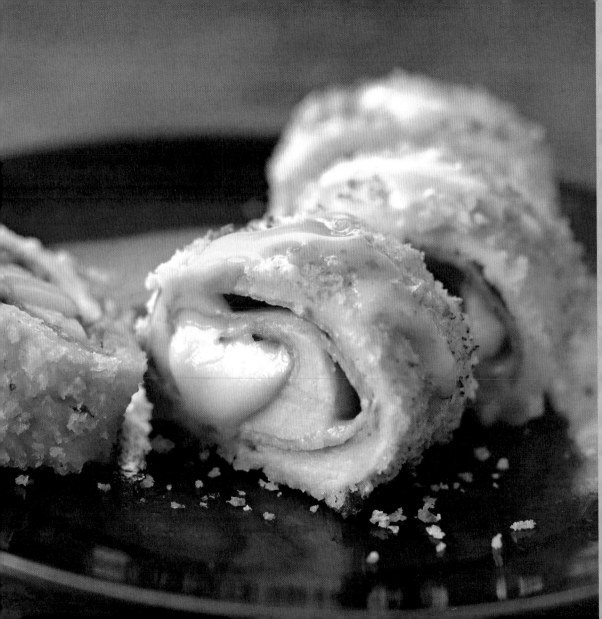

Jambalaya

No city or region in America lays claim to a richer, more influential lineup of culinary creations than New Orleans and the surrounding Creole country. Gumbo, étouffée, beignets, po' boys—all are part of Louisiana's incomparable culinary heritage. No dish, though, is more famous than jambalaya, the rice-based hodgepodge of meat, seafood, and vegetables, not unlike the Spanish paella. By decreasing the rice ratio and increasing the produce and protein, this recipe cuts the calories and carbs dramatically. But it still has enough soul to satisfy the most discerning Creole critics.

You'll Need:

- 1 tsp olive or canola oil
- 1 cup diced turkey kielbasa
- 1 medium onion, diced
- 1 medium green bell pepper, diced
- 2 cloves garlic, minced
- 8 oz boneless, skinless chicken breast, cut into ½" cubes
- 1 cup long-grain rice
- 2¼ cups low-sodium chicken stock
- 1 can (14 oz) diced tomatoes
- 1 Tbsp tomato paste
- ⅛ tsp cayenne pepper
- 2 bay leaves
- 8 oz medium shrimp, peeled and deveined
- Salt and black pepper to taste
- Frank's Red Hot, Tabasco, or other hot sauce
- Chopped scallions (optional)

How to Make It:

- Heat the oil in a large skillet or sauté pan over medium heat. Add the kielbasa and cook for about 3 minutes, until lightly browned. Add the onion, bell pepper, and garlic and cook, stirring occasionally, for 4 to 5 minutes, until the vegetables have softened.
- Push the vegetables and kielbasa to the perimeter, making a well in the center of the pan. Add the chicken and sauté until lightly browned but not cooked through, about 3 minutes. Stir in the rice, stock, tomatoes, tomato paste, cayenne, and bay leaves. Turn the heat to low, cover, and simmer for 17 minutes, until nearly all of the liquid has been absorbed by the rice. Uncover, add the shrimp, and cook for 2 to 3 minutes, until the rice is tender and the shrimp is cooked through. Discard the bay leaves. Season with salt, black pepper, and hot sauce and garnish with the scallions, if using.

Makes 4 servings / Cost per serving: $4.15

380 calories
15 g fat
(4.5 g saturated)
1,070 mg sodium

Save!
550 calories
and $8.84!

Not That!
Red Lobster Shrimp Jambalaya
Price: $12.99

930 calories
50 g fat
(19 g saturated)
3,000 mg sodium

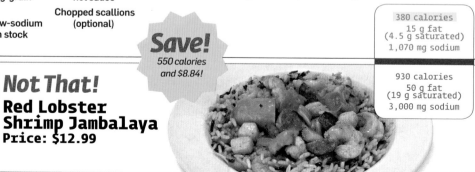

234

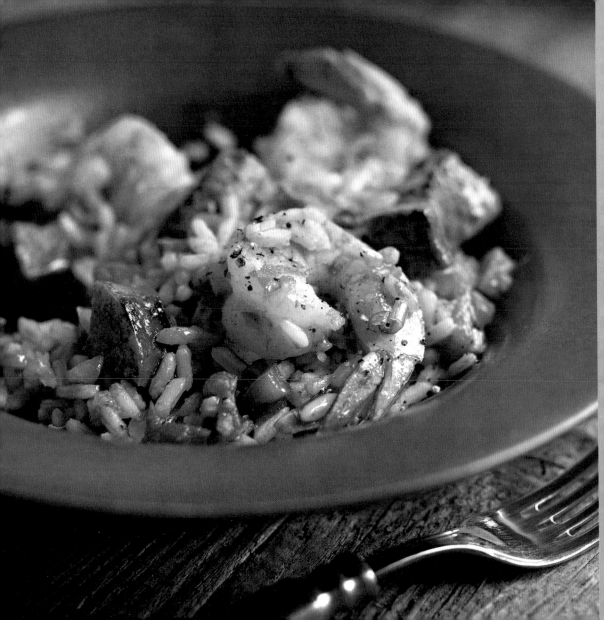

International Classics

The most delicious dishes from
around the world

The World's Best Cond

The global pantry is ripe for raiding. These 14 products will help you create high-flavor, low-calorie meals with a simple twist of the wrist.

Red Curry Paste

Curry can be interpreted in dozens of different ways, but classic red curry paste is the most versatile of them all. Made from a host of Southeast Asian staples—ginger, garlic, galangal, kaffir lime—red curry can be used in everything from slow-simmering sauces and stews to meat rubs and dips.

Cook This! Rub directly on chicken or pork before grilling or roasting; combine a few tablespoons with a can of light coconut milk and a cup of chicken stock, then simmer with fish or meat and plenty of vegetables; mix 2 tablespoons red curry and smooth peanut butter with a tablespoon of soy and the juice of a lime and use as a dipping sauce for pretty much anything.

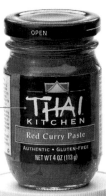

Kimchi

"Fermented cabbage" doesn't do much as a description to endear kimchi to first-time eaters, but this Korean staple, with its bold balance of chili spice and vinegar tang, has a profound ability to turn skeptics into lifelong devotees. While kimchi can be made from a variety of vegetables (radish and cucumber are particularly common), it's most often made by pickling Napa cabbage with red chiles, garlic, ginger, and a host of other rotating ingredients.

Cook This! Scatter kimchi on top of grilled hot dogs (instead of sauerkraut) or burgers; puree in a blender and serve alongside steak; stir-fry with strips of thinly sliced pork and onions.

Hoisin

To call hoisin the ketchup of Chinese cooking is a little reductive, but the similarities are tough to deny: ubiquity in their respective countries of origin, versatility to serve as part of a sauce or a standalone dip, and, most important, an uncanny ability to incorporate the full spectrum of flavors—sweet, spicy, sour, hot—into one little jar. Made from sweet potatoes, vinegar, garlic, red chiles, among other ingredients, use hoisin once and it's likely to get as much use in your kitchen as that bottle of Heinz.

Cook This! Brush on salmon or beef before grilling; combine with soy sauce and sriracha and use as a marinade for chicken drumsticks or wings; use as the major flavor component of a stir-fry.

iments→ASIA

Sriracha

Admittedly, we're addicted to this stuff, but so is anyone who's ever dabbed a bit on a hot dog, swirled it into a bowl of chili, or used a squirt to punch up a stir-fry. It's made primarily from pureed red chiles, but sriracha is more than just raw firepower: It adds a touch of sweetness, acidity, and a garlic bite to raw and cooked dishes alike.

Cook This! Mix with mayonnaise and spread onto grilled tuna or turkey burgers; squirt onto quesadillas or tacos; squeeze onto an egg sandwich.

Fish Sauce

Though its name might not evoke hunger pangs, fish sauce is nevertheless the backbone of a handful of the world's most delicious and healthy cuisines, including Thai and Vietnamese. Its strong smell may be off-putting at first, but its salty, savory punch is reminiscent of Worcestershire sauce, capable of amplifying flavor without ratcheting up the calories.

Cook This! Combine with lime juice, sugar, and a thinly sliced chili pepper to make a dipping sauce or dressing for grilled meats and vegetables; stir into a Bloody Mary instead of Worcestershire (a close relative of fish sauce); splash a tablespoon or two into a stir-fry instead of soy sauce.

Rice Wine Vinegar

Packing your pantry with a variety of vinegars is always a good idea. Too often what dishes lack is a high note, a tang that snaps your taste buds into focus and keeps you coming back for more. Rice wine makes a mellow, sweet vinegar that provides a nice contrast to dishes heavy on spice, fat, and/or salt.

Cook This! Float jalapeño, cucumber, or onion slices in rice wine vinegar for 30 minutes for quick pickles; add a tablespoon to stir-fries to sharpen their flavor; mix with soy, sesame oil, and sriracha for a dipping sauce for grilled meat, potstickers, and lettuce wraps.

Chili-Garlic Sauce

This coarse chili paste (often called *sambal oleek*) balances spice with a good dose of garlic funk. Whereas sriracha is most often used as a condiment put on food after it's been cooked, chili-garlic sauce forms the base of many stir-fries and cooked dishes.

Cook This! Add to any stir-fried green vegetable—spinach, broccoli, green beans, bok choy, asparagus; use as a dip for dumplings; combine with soy sauce and sesame oil and use as a stir-fry sauce for chicken or pork.

*If you can't find these products in your local grocery store or Asian market, all are available from *asianfoodgrocer.com*.

Salsa Verde

Though salsa is America's most used condiment (sorry, ketchup), this fiesty green rendition, made from a mix of tomatillos, jalapenos, cilantro, and lime juice, is still relatively unknown. It brings a bit of spice to your food, but more important, it brings acidity, a sharp and welcome contrast to grilled meat, melted cheese, and simmered beans.

Cook This! Dump onto nachos, tacos, and burritos; spoon a bit on top of fried eggs; use as a sandwich spread or salad dressing.

Herbes de Provence

Long before spice companies started overcharging for their mediocre spice blends, cooks in southern France were using this floral mix of fennel, thyme, lavender, tarragon, and bay to season everything from roasted meat to homemade tomato sauce. This will end up being one of the most useful members of your entire spice rack.

Cook This! Rub all over a whole chicken before roasting; toss with vegetables before grilling; stir into tomato sauce

Canned Chipotle

These powerful red chiles (pronounced chi-POHT-lay) are actually jalapeños that have been dried and smoked. You can get heat from a hundred different sources; what makes chipotle so special is the smokiness, coupled with the vinegar bite of the tomato adobo sauce these chiles are canned with. Blend a whole can until smooth, then keep covered in your fridge for up to a month.

Cook This! Mix with orange juice, olive oil, and garlic for an amazing meat marinade; stir a spoonful into sour cream to give the cool condiment some burn; blend a tablespoon with a 14-ounce can of tomatoes, cilantro, garlic, and chopped onion for instant salsa.

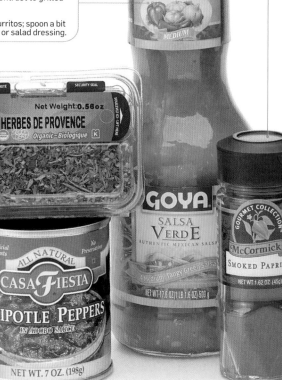

iments → The REST of the WORLD

Smoked Paprika

The Hungarians may be the world's largest paprika producers, but the Spaniards really got this red powder right. That's because they smoke their sweet red peppers over smoldering oak before grinding it, resulting in a spice with a rich, robust flavor to match its brilliant color.

Cook This! Mix with chili powder and rub onto steaks before grilling; add to simmering beans and pots of chili; dust onto scrambled and deviled eggs.

Tapenade

This heady paste, made from olives, garlic, capers, and anchovies, is used throughout southern France as a spread for crusty bread. But the gutsy flavor and abundance of healthy fats makes tapenade a condiment that can and should be used frequently in your kitchen.

Cook This! Mix with canned tuna and chopped hard-boiled egg for an amazing sandwich filling; spread on a baguette, top with goat cheese, and bake until the bread is crisp; dab directly on meat and fish after cooking.

Harissa

The hot sauce of choice in Northern African is a fiery red paste made from piri piri chiles, garlic, and, depending on who's making it, a variety of spices like cumin and coriander. As addictive as the burn may be, it's also good for you: Research has shown that capsaicin—the chemical in chiles that gives them fire—actually increases metabolism.

Cook This! Mix with yogurt and use as a dip, a sandwich spread, or a meat marinade; stir into curries or stir-fries.

Pesto

Pesto has become a catchall phrase used to describe any puree of nuts and herbs, but we're talking about pesto *Genovese*, that forest green concoction of fresh basil leaves, garlic, pine nuts, Parmesan, and olive oil. It can be made at home in minutes or bought by the bottle and kept in the fridge, but either way, have it on hand. Its payload of antioxidants and healthy fat is only bested by its formidable flavor.

Cook This! Rub pesto on meat or fish before grilling; mix with equal part mayonnaise and spread on sandwiches; toss with boiled green beans, chunks of red potatoes, and cherry tomatoes for a world-class salad.

*If you can't find these products at your local grocery store, all are available from *igourmet.com*.

241

Asian Chicken Meatballs

Meatballs are hardly the sole provenance of Italian grandmothers and their oversize vats of tomato "gravy." Most of the world has its own spin on the combination of ground meat and seasonings, and you'd be wise to embrace a few in your kitchen. These meatballs are inspired by street-corner grills in Vietnam and Thailand, where ginger, garlic, and chiles reign supreme. With those bold flavors, plus the char of a hot charcoal grill, you won't need a fat-heavy mix of meat, or a pile of spaghetti, to make an outstanding dinner. Serve them with steamed rice, cucumbers, maybe a bit of sauce, and big lettuce leaves for wrapping and let everyone make their own Asian-style burrito.

You'll Need:

- 1 lb ground chicken or pork
- 1 small red onion, minced
- 2 cloves garlic, minced
- 1 Tbsp minced fresh ginger
- 1 Tbsp minced lemongrass (optional)
- 1 jalapeño pepper, minced
- 2 tsp sugar
- 1 tsp salt
- 4–8 wooden skewers, soaked in water for 20 minutes

Boston lettuce, steamed rice, Pickled Cucumber Salad (see page 301), Ginger Scallion Sauce (see page 268), and/or sriracha for serving

How to Make It:

- Preheat a clean, lightly oiled grill or grill pan. In a large mixing bowl, combine the ground meat with the onion, garlic, ginger, lemongrass if desired, jalapeño, sugar, and salt, stirring gently to evenly distribute all the ingredients. Roll the mixture into golf ball–size orbs, then carefully thread 3 or 4 onto each skewer.

- When your grill is hot, add the meatball skewers and grill for 4 to 5 minutes per side, until a light char has developed on the outside and the meatballs are cooked through. When done, they should feel firm, but springy to the touch.

- Use the lettuce and rice to make little Asian-style wraps with the meatballs, topping with cucumbers and your choice of sauces.

Makes 4 servings /
Cost per serving: $2.11

230 calories
12 g fat
(3.5 g saturated)
670 mg sodium

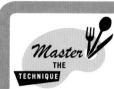

Master THE TECHNIQUE

Asian Wraps

Korean love to use large lettuce leaves to house grilled meats, rice, kimchi, and sauces. In fact, it could be anything: grilled steak, pork loin, chicken chunks, even grilled vegetables. It's like eating a delicious burrito for a quarter of the calories. Invent at will; just don't forget the sriracha.

Not That!

P.F. Chang's Mu Shu Pork
with Pancakes and Hoisin
Price: $12.50

1,210 calories
58 g fat
(14 g saturated)
5,820 mg sodium

Save!
980 calories and $10.39!

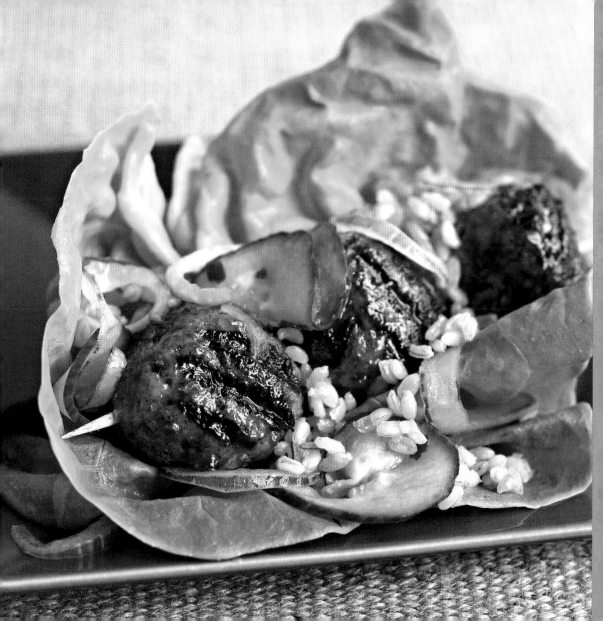

Cook This!
Sea Bass Packet

Why more people don't cook food in packets is one of the culinary world's great mysteries. Not only is it one of the healthiest, easiest ways to cook fish, chicken, and vegetables, but the abundance of flavorful steam trapped inside the packet means your food will still be delicious, even if you overcook it. Plus, there are no pots or pans to clean—just toss the foil in the trash and move on. Sure beats driving to a restaurant, waiting for a table, shelling out $22 for a 600-calorie piece of fish with more than a day's worth of sodium, and then driving home disappointed.

You'll Need:

4 sea bass, halibut, or other white fish fillets (6 oz each)

8 spears asparagus, ends removed, chopped

4 oz shitake mushrooms, stems removed

1 Tbsp grated fresh ginger

2 Tbsp low-sodium soy sauce

2 Tbsp mirin (sweetened sake), sake, or sweet white wine

Salt and black pepper to taste

How to Make It:

● Preheat the oven to 400°F.

● Lay 4 large (18" x 12") pieces of aluminum foil on the kitchen counter and fold each into thirds. Place a fish fillet in the center third of each piece, then scatter the asparagus, mushrooms, and ginger over each. Drizzle with the soy sauce and mirin and season with a small pinch of salt (remember, soy sauce already packs plenty of sodium) and black pepper. Fold the outer two sections of the foil over the fish, then roll up the ends toward the center to create fully sealed packets.

● Arrange the packets on a large baking sheet and bake for 15 for 20 minutes, depending on the thickness of the fish fillet. (If the fillets are ½ inch thick or less, it will take closer to 15 minutes; if they are almost a full inch, it will need 20 minutes.) Place each packet directly on a plate and serve.

Makes 4 servings / Cost per serving: $5.85

This is the most expensive recipe in the book because sea bass and halibut are pricey fish. To cut cost, use any affordable white fish, as long as it's super fresh. Even tilapia or catfish will work great here.

250 calories
4.5 g fat
(1 g saturated)
540 mg sodium

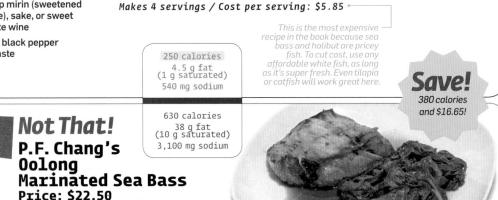

Save!
380 calories
and $16.65!

630 calories
38 g fat
(10 g saturated)
3,100 mg sodium

Not That!
P.F. Chang's Oolong Marinated Sea Bass
Price: $22.50

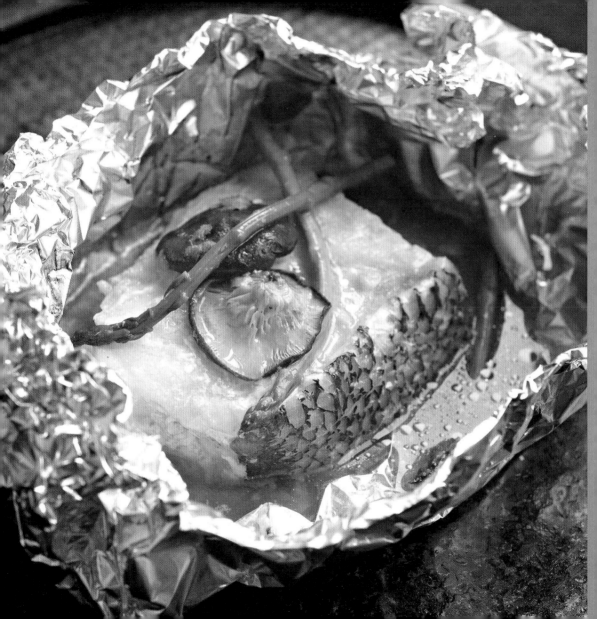

Chili-Mango Chicken

The combination of heat and sweet is a rollercoaster for our taste buds and a partnership that lurks behind—knowingly or not—our affection for so many Asian dishes: General Tso's, orange chicken, and mu shu pork, among others. Here, that combination upgrades a basic chicken stir-fry to something special with just two ingredients: The heat comes from a lashing of chili sauce (look for the bottle with the Red Rooster and a green screw-on cap) and the sweet from a thin coating of quick-cooked mango chunks.

You'll Need:

- 1 pound boneless, skinless chicken thighs, chopped into ½" pieces
- 1 Tbsp cornstarch
- 1 Tbsp low-sodium soy sauce
- ½ Tbsp sesame oil
- ½ Tbsp peanut or canola oil
- 1 red onion, chopped
- 1 Tbsp grated or minced fresh ginger
- 2 cups sugar snap peas
- 1 mango, peeled, pitted, and chopped
- 1 Tbsp chili garlic sauce (preferably sambal oleek)

Black pepper to taste

How to Make It:

- Combine the chicken, cornstarch, soy sauce, and sesame oil in a mixing bowl and let sit for 10 minutes.
- Heat the peanut oil in a wok or large skillet over high heat. Add the onion and ginger and cook for 1 to 2 minutes, until the onion is translucent. Add the sugar snaps and stir-fry for 1 minute, using a metal spatula to keep the vegetables in near-constant motion. Add the chicken, along with its marinade, and stir-fry for about 2 minutes, until the meat begins to brown on the outside. Add the mango, chili sauce, and black pepper and stir-fry for 1 minute longer, until the chicken is cooked through and the mango has softened into a near sauce-like consistency. Serve over brown rice.

Makes 4 servings / Cost per serving: $2.06

Sugar snaps can be expensive and difficult to find outside peak season (late spring to early summer). Snow peas, green beans, and even broccoli all make solid substitutes.

240 calories
8 g fat
(1 g saturated)
410 mg sodium

2,030 calories
80 g fat
(15 g saturated,
1 g trans)
4,480 mg sodium

Not That!

Applebee's Crispy Orange Chicken Bowl
Price: $12.99

Save!
1,790 calories
and $10.93!

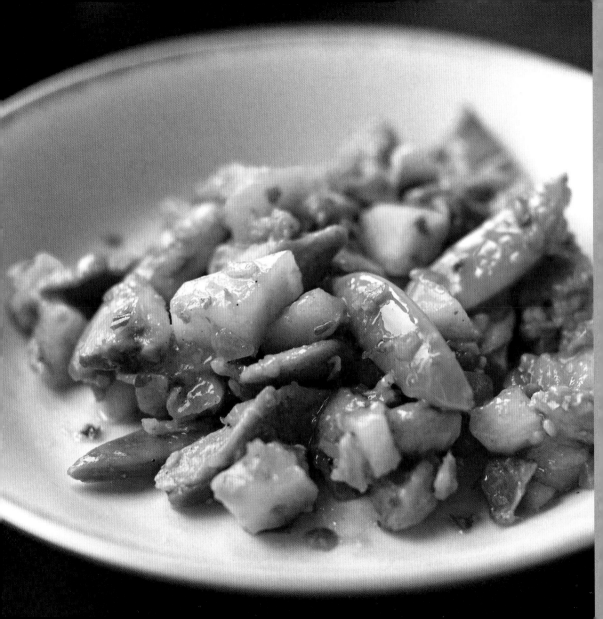

Beef & Beer

Not only do the Belgians drink the best beer in the world, they also cook with it. This recipe is inspired by a Belgian dish called carbonnade, a hearty stew of beef and onions braised in beer. It's the type of dish you want to come home to on a blustery winter night. Take 10 minutes to prep in the morning, then set a slow cooker on low and go about your day. By the time you come home, this bone-sticking beef stew will be ready.

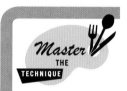

Master THE **TECHNIQUE**

You'll Need:

- 1 Tbsp canola or olive oil
- 3 lb chuck roast

Salt and black pepper to taste

- 2 Tbsp red wine vinegar
- 5 yellow onions, sliced
- 1 can dark beer (we like Guinness, but the Belgians don't), plus more if needed
- 2 cups low-sodium beef stock
- 1 Tbsp Worcestershire sauce
- 4 bay leaves
- 8 ounces button mushrooms, each cut in half (optional)

How to Make It:

- Heat the oil in a large skillet over high heat. Season the chuck all over with salt and pepper. Add the beef to the pan and sear until all sides are nicely browned, about 10 minutes. Remove the beef, then add the vinegar, onions, and beer to the pan, scraping up any bits that may cling to the bottom.

- Place the beef in the base of a slow cooker and pour the onions and beer over. Add the stock, Worcestershire, and bay leaves; if the liquid doesn't cover all or most of the beef, add a bit more beer. Cook on low for 6 hours (or on high for 4). (See "Stovetop Slow Cooking" on page 270, for tips on making this on the stovetop.) If using the mushrooms, add them in the last hour of cooking. Discard the bay leaves. Serve the beef with the vegetables and a good ladle of the braising juices, or a sauce made from the liquid (at right).

Makes 8 servings /
Cost per serving: $3.08

345 calories
13 g fat
(3.5 g saturated)
437 mg sodium

Restaurant-quality sauces

Fancy restaurants can charge $25 an entrée because they use a few simple strategies to concentrate flavor. Regardless of what you've braised—pot roast, osso buco, lamb shanks—the cooking liquid is pure gold that should never be wasted. Transfer a few ladles' worth to a small saucepan set over high heat. Boil vigorously until the liquid has reduced to a syrup-like consistency. Finish with a pat of cold butter swirled into the sauce, then pour it over the meat after you've plated it.

Not That!

IHOP
French Onion
Pot Roast
Price: $10.99

940 calories

Save!

595 calories
and $7.91!

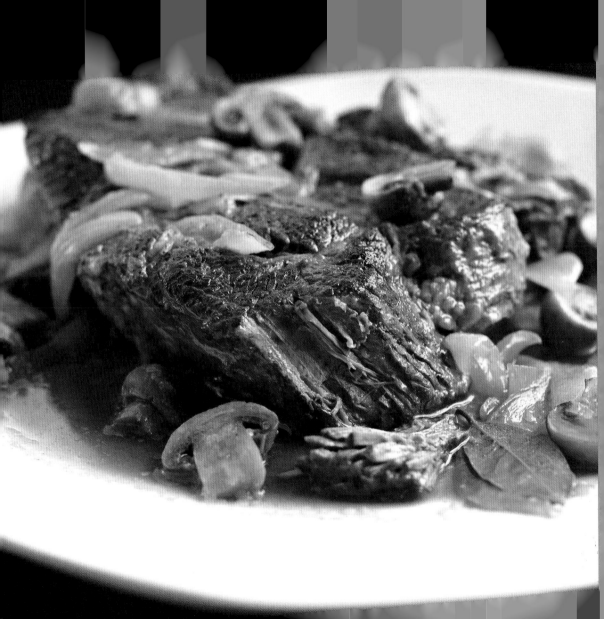

Cook This!

Curry with Cauliflower & Butternut Squash

Such is the food world we live in that even a simple vegetable stir-fry at a restaurant packs nearly 1,000 calories and a day's worth of sodium. It's a simple, unsuspecting dish that underscores just how vulnerable we are every time we decide to eat out. This Indian-style curry takes no more than 25 minutes to prepare, yet it will taste like it's been simmering away all day. The balance of the creamy coconut milk, the sweet cubes of squash, and the subtle heat of the curry powder could make the most dedicated meat eater forget he was eating only vegetables.

You'll Need:

- ½ Tbsp canola oil
- 1 medium onion, diced
- ½ Tbsp minced fresh ginger
- 2 cups cubed butternut squash
- 1 head cauliflower, cut into florets
- 1 can (14–16 oz) garbanzo beans (aka chickpeas), drained
- 1 jalapeño pepper, minced
- 1 Tbsp yellow curry powder
- 1 can (14 oz) diced tomatoes
- 1 can (14 oz) light coconut milk
- Juice of 1 lime
- Salt and black pepper to taste
- Chopped cilantro

How to Make It:

- Heat the oil in a large sauté pan or pot over medium heat. Add the onion and ginger and cook for about 2 minutes, until the onion is soft and translucent. Add the squash, cauliflower, garbanzos, jalapeño, and curry powder. Cook for 2 minutes, until the curry powder is fragrant and coats the vegetables evenly. Stir in the tomatoes and coconut milk and turn the heat down to low. Simmer for 15 to 20 minutes, until the vegetables are tender. Add the lime juice and season with salt and black pepper. Serve garnished with the chopped cilantro.

Makes 4 servings /
Cost per serving: $2.47

Carrots or potatoes would both be perfect substitutes for the squash, just in case butternut is not in season.

260 calories
8 g fat
(4.5 g saturated)
510 mg sodium

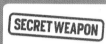

SECRET WEAPON

Curcumin

At the heart of Indian curry powder is one of the world's most potent elixirs: curcumin, an antioxidant known to fight cancer, inflammation, bacteria, cholesterol, and a list of other maladies—large and small—too long to publish here. Curcumin resides in turmeric, the bright yellow spice that gives curries their characteristic hue. Don't limit the healing powers to recipes like this, though. Stir curry powder into yogurt for a vegetable dip, slip it into mayonnaise for a powerful sandwich spread, or rub directly onto chicken or white fish before grilling.

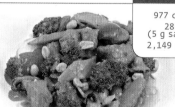

Not That!
Houlihan's Vegetable Stir Fry
Price: $10.99

977 calories
28 g fat
(5 g saturated)
2,149 mg sodium

Save!
717 calories and $8.52!

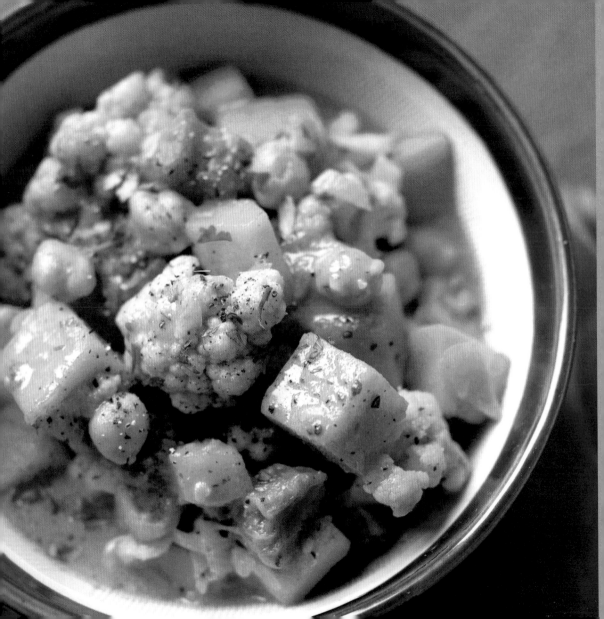

Chicken Adobo

This may be the easiest recipe in the entire book—only marginally more challenging than toasting bread or pouring yourself a bowl of cereal. Chicken adobo is a staple of the Philippines, a dish so delicious and simple that it's a wonder it's not a weekday standard in houses across America. The key is to reduce the sauce down to a syrup thick enough to cling to the chicken and infuse your meal with a huge jolt of savory garlic-soy flavor. If you prefer your chicken with a deep caramelized crust, try sliding it under the broiler for a few minutes just before serving. Crust or not, make sure to add a vegetable (roasted broccoli is great) and a scoop of brown rice before sitting down to chow.

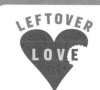

LEFTOVER LOVE

Chicken adobo is leftover gold, not just because it's pretty awesome cold straight from the refrigerator, but because it can be converted into an amazing array of dishes that will make you forget you're eating last night's dinner. Make an Asian-style wrap by stuffing tortillas or Bibb lettuce leaves with a few chunks of chicken adobo, along with steamed brown rice, chopped scallions, roasted vegetables, and a squirt of sriracha. Or scatter the chicken on a salad of greens, mandarin oranges, almonds, and red bell pepper strips dressed with soy sauce, peanut oil, and lime juice.

You'll Need:

- ½ cup rice wine vinegar
- ½ cup low-sodium soy sauce
- 4 cloves garlic, peeled and crushed
- 4 bay leaves
- 1 tsp coarsely ground black pepper
- 1 lb skinless chicken thighs
- 2 cups prepared brown rice

How to Make It:

- In a medium saucepan, combine all the ingredients. Bring to a bare simmer, cover, and cook for 20 to 25 minutes, until the chicken is very tender and cooked all the way through.
- Remove the chicken from the pot and bring the mixture to a vigorous boil. Continue to boil for about 10 minutes, until the cooking liquid reduces by half and is thick enough to cling easily to the back of a spoon.
- Return the chicken to the pot and heat through. Discard the bay leaves. Serve the chicken with the rice and the reduced sauce.

Makes 4 servings /
Cost per serving: $1.46

230 calories
2 g fat
(0.5 g saturated)
880 mg sodium

900 calories
48 g fat
(6 g saturated)
5,550 mg sodium

Not That!
P.F. Chang's Chicken with Black Bean Sauce
Price: $13.25

Save!
670 calories and $11.79!

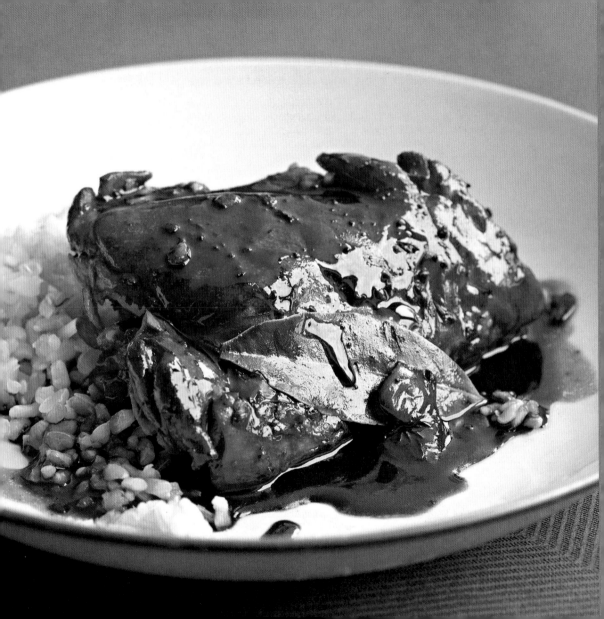

Miso-Marinated Scallops

Pureed fermented soybeans might not sound like good eats, but miso is one of the culinary world's greatest flavor enhancers. Credit goes to miso's huge dose of umami (see Secret Weapon below) that it contributes to soups, dressings, and marinades. You'll find a variety of miso pastes in the refrigerator section of upscale grocers such as Whole Foods. The more intense red miso can take a pedestrian steak to a new stratosphere, while the more mild white miso proves a perfect marinade for fish and seafood. If you can't find miso at a store near you, score some online at asianfoodgrocer.com.

You'll Need:

- ½ cup white miso paste
- ½ cup sake
- ¼ cup sugar
- ¼ cup canola oil
- 1 lb large scallops, tough membranes removed
- 2 cups sugar snap peas
- ½ Tbsp sesame oil
- Salt and black pepper to taste

How to Make It:

- Combine the miso, sake, sugar, and oil in a mixing bowl and whisk to thoroughly combine. Transfer one-fourth of the mixture to a small bowl, cover, and refrigerate. Add the scallops to the remaining miso, turn to coat, and marinate in the fridge for at least 2 hours and up to 12.

- Preheat the broiler. Place an oiled baking sheet or large cast-iron skillet 6" beneath the broiler. Remove the scallops from the marinade and pat dry. Toss the sugar snaps with the sesame oil and salt and pepper to taste. When the baking sheet is very hot, carefully remove and arrange the sugar snaps and scallops on the sheet. Return to the oven and broil for 5 to 6 minutes, until the scallops are thoroughly browned and firm and the sugar snaps are tender. Serve the scallops and snap peas with a drizzle of the reserved miso sauce.

Makes 4 servings / Cost per serving: $4.24

Make sure there is no milky liquid accumulated beneath the scallops in the fish case, a sign that the scallops have likely been dyed or pumped full of additives.

SECRET WEAPON

Umami

Salty, sour, sweet, bitter...umami? Considered the fifth main flavor group, umami can best be described as an intense savory flavor found in tomatoes, mushrooms, Parmesan, and more. The Japanese in particular prize umami, and many of their staples contain big doses of it, from soy sauce to dried seaweed to miso paste. A good rule of thumb: The more umami in your food, the better it will taste.

300 calories
15 g fat
(1.5 g saturated)
920 mg sodium

885 calories
45 g fat
(9 g saturated)
3,690 mg sodium

Not That!
P.F. Chang's Sichuan Scallops
Price: $15.50

Save!
585 calories
and $11.26!

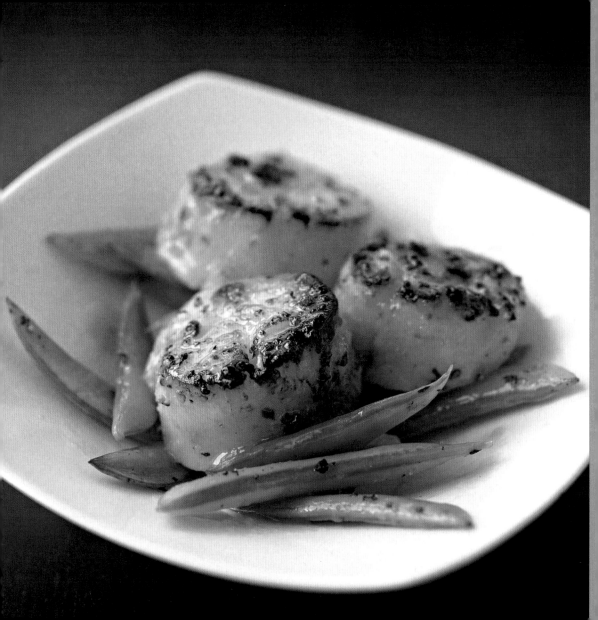

Chicken Scaloppine

Another Italian classic lost in translation. Too many cooks (including the toques at Macaroni Grill) interpret this dish—traditionally chicken or pork, lightly floured and cooked with sage and prosciutto—as a huge helping of meat, breaded and fried and covered in a murky, sodium-strewn gravy. Our lighter, more authentic version wraps chicken and sage in a layer of prosciutto, which then becomes a crispy skin that keeps the chicken moist while it sautés. A splash of wine and chicken stock directly into the cooking pan becomes your 2-minute sauce. Just the latest proof of why simpler is so often better.

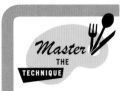

Master THE TECHNIQUE

Pounding Protein

A number of recipes throughout this book call on you to pound a chicken breast into a thinner cutlet. The reason being that meat—chicken, steak, pork—that has a uniform thickness cooks quicker and more evenly. The process is easy: Take out a large cutting board and lay the chicken on top. Cover with a few layers of plastic wrap and use a meat mallet (or a heavy-bottomed pan) to thwack the meat into submission. Of course, many supermarkets sell chicken and other meats in cutlet form, but, really, where's the fun in that?

You'll Need:

4 boneless, skinless chicken breasts or thighs (about 6 oz each), pounded to uniform ¼" thickness

Salt and black pepper to taste

8 fresh sage leaves

4 thin slices prosciutto

1 Tbsp olive oil

1 cup white wine

½ cup low-sodium chicken stock

1 Tbsp butter

Fresh parsley (optional)

How to Make It:

- Season the chicken with salt and pepper. Lay two sage leaves across each breast, then wrap each with a slice of prosciutto, using a toothpick or two to secure the wrap.
- Heat the oil in a large skillet over medium heat. When the oil shimmers, add the chicken and cook for 4 to 5 minutes per side, until the prosciutto is browned and crispy and the chicken is firm to the touch and cooked through. Transfer to 4 plates.
- Add the wine and stock to the pan and cook for about 2 minutes, until the liquid has reduced by half, scraping the bottom of the pan to loosen any cooked bits. Swirl in the butter and parsley (if using). Pour the sauce over the chicken and serve.

Makes 4 servings /
Cost per serving: $2.51

280 calories
11 g fat
(3.5 g saturated)
460 mg sodium

910 calories
59 g fat
(21 g saturated)
3,030 mg sodium

Not That!

Romano's Macaroni Grill Chicken Scaloppine
Price: $12.99

Save!
630 calories
and $10.48!

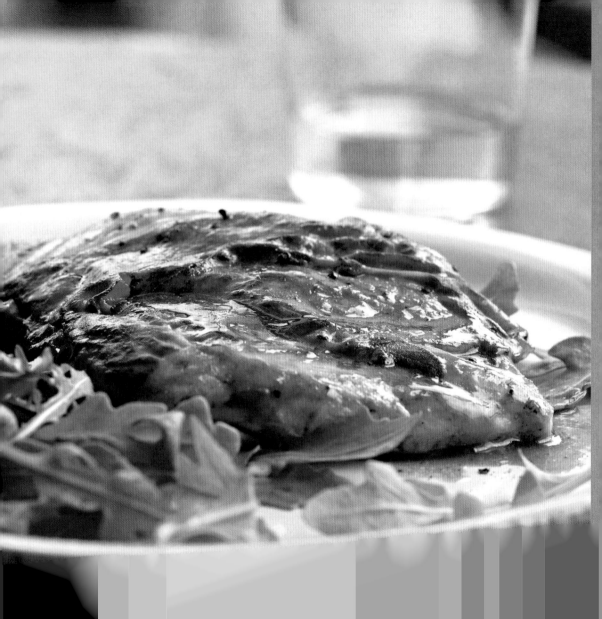

Cook This!
Hawaiian Crepe

Hawaiian pizza ranks as one of our favorite pies by the mere fact that no other combination packs as much flavor for so few calories. Same holds true with these crepes. The key to a good crepe is to let it properly brown and take on crispy patches; most cooks get anxious and remove them prematurely from the pan, yielding a pale, lifeless shell. Be patient.

You'll Need:

CREPE BATTER

- 1 cup flour
- 2 large eggs
- 2 Tbsp melted butter

Pinch of salt

- ¾ cup low-fat milk
- ½ cup water

CREPE FILLING

- ½ Tbsp butter, plus more for cooking the crepes
- 4 oz deli ham, cut into strips
- 2 cups diced pineapple
- 1 jalapeño pepper, minced
- 1 cup low-fat ricotta cheese

Salt and black pepper to taste

How to Make It:

- To make the batter: Combine the flour, eggs, melted butter, and salt in a large mixing bowl. Gradually add the milk, then the water, whisking to prevent any lumps.

- To make the filling: Heat the butter in a medium nonstick skillet over medium heat. Add the ham, pineapple, and jalapeño and cook for 4 to 5 minutes, until the ham is lightly browned on the edges and the pineapple is softened. Remove from the heat, stir in the ricotta, and season with salt and pepper.

- Heat a 12" nonstick skillet over medium heat. Add enough butter to coat, then pour in about 2 table-spoons of the crepe batter, swirling and tilting the pan so that the batter covers the entire surface with a thin film. Cook on the first side for 1 to 2 minutes, until the bottom takes on a deep brown color all over. Flip the crepe and spoon in some of the ricotta-ham mixture. Cook for 1 to 2 minutes, until brown and crisp on the bottom. Fold the crepe over the stuffing and slide onto a plate.

- Repeat to make three more crepes.

Makes 4 large crepes or 8 smaller crepes (made in an 8" pan) / Cost per serving: $1.66

370 calories
18 g fat
(8 g saturated)
390 mg sodium

880 calories

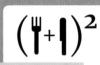

$(\Psi + \mathord{]})^2$

MEAL MULTIPLIER

Consider this recipe the base for all your crepe needs—sweet and savory. (If making the batter for dessert crepes, you can add 2 tablespoons of sugar to the batter to lightly sweeten it.) Here are a few approaches worth exploring:

- Sautéed mushrooms, onions, spinach, and crumbled feta cheese
- Smoked salmon, roasted asparagus, and ricotta or whipped cream cheese
- Sliced strawberries, mascarpone cheese, and honey

Not That!
IHOP Chicken Florentine Crepes
Price: $10.79

Save!
510 calories
and $9.13!

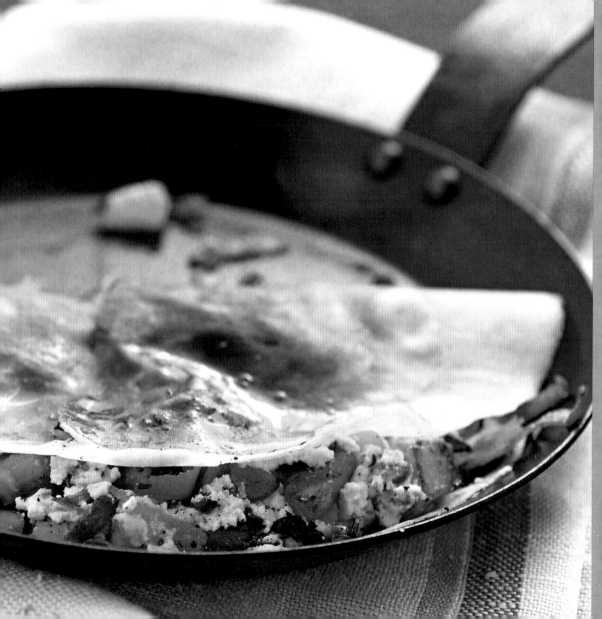

Margarita Chicken

Sizzling chicken and steak platters clutter the menus of nearly every major chain restaurant in this country, a testament to the enduring popularity of meat and melted cheese. We can't fault people for loving it—who wouldn't?—but we do take issue with the fact that these savory skillets rarely contain fewer than 1,000 calories, regardless of who's holding the spatula. That is, unless you are. Our version—a meal that you can have on the table in 20 minutes—contains all the same bells and whistles (Cheese! Salsa! Sizzle!) for a savings of $9 and nearly 900 calories *per portion*.

You'll Need:

½ can (14–16 oz) black beans, drained

¼ tsp cumin

Juice of 1 lime

Salt and black pepper to taste

½ Tbsp canola or olive oil

4 boneless, skinless chicken breasts (6 oz each)

1 cup prepared salsa, preferably salsa verde

1 cup shredded Pepper Jack cheese

Chopped fresh cilantro

How to Make It:

- Preheat the oven to 450°F. Combine the black beans and cumin in a saucepan and heat all the way through. Squeeze in the lime juice and adjust the seasoning with salt and pepper. Remove from heat, but warm before serving.

- Heat the oil in a large skillet over medium-high heat. Season the chicken all over with salt and pepper and sear in the hot pan for 3 to 4 minutes on the first side, until a nice crust develops, then flip. Cook for another 3 to 4 minutes, then spoon the salsa over the meat, top with the cheese, and place in the oven. Bake until the chicken is cooked through and the cheese is fully melted and bubbling, no more than 5 minutes. Divide the beans among 4 plates, top with the chicken, and garnish with cilantro.

Makes 4 servings / Cost per serving: $2.49

Made from tomatillos, onions, jalapeños, and lime, salsa verde strikes a perfect balance between acidity and spice, brightening and intensifying flavors in everything it touches.

330 calories
12 g fat
(4.5 g saturated)
480 mg sodium

1,200 calories

Not That!

T.G.I. Friday's Sizzling Chicken & Cheese
Price: $11.49

Save!
870 calories
and $9!

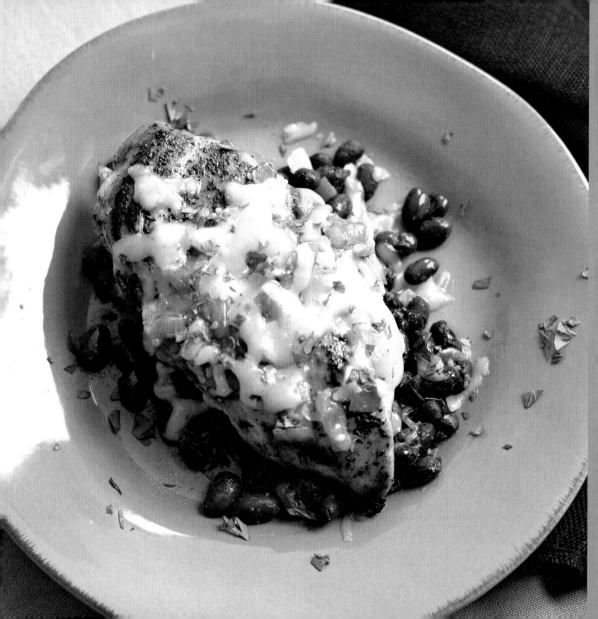

Moroccan Salmon with Quinoa Pilaf

The Moroccan pantry is one of the finest on the planet, overflowing with powerful spices, tantalizing condiments, and healthy whole grains. It's the perfect source for inspiration, yet so few restaurants—big or small—take cues from this North African culinary powerhouse. We won't make the same mistake. This sweet-savory combination of spices could be rubbed on chicken or pork, but it takes especially well to the (healthy) fattiness of the salmon.

You'll Need:

- 1 cup quinoa
- 1 ¼ cups chicken stock or more if needed
- ½ cup fresh parsley, chopped
- ¼ cup raisins (preferably golden), plumped in hot water for a few minutes
- 2 Tbsp pine nuts, toasted in a pan or the oven for a few minutes
- 1 tsp salt
- ½ tsp black pepper
- ¼ tsp cumin
- ⅛ tsp cinnamon
- ⅛ tsp cayenne
- 4 skinless salmon fillets (4–6 oz each)

How to Make It:

- Preheat the oven to 350°F. Prepare the quinoa according to package instructions, using chicken stock instead of water. Stir in the parsley, raisins, and pine nuts. Cover and keep warm.
- Combine the salt, black pepper, cumin, cinnamon, and cayenne and rub over the salmon fillets. Place on a baking sheet and bake until the fish flakes with gentle pressure from your finger, 10 to 12 minutes, depending on the thickness of the salmon. Serve each salmon fillet over a generous scoop of the quinoa pilaf.

Makes 4 servings /
Cost per serving: $4.82

310 calories
13 g fat
(2 g saturated)
780 mg sodium

Not That!

California Pizza Kitchen Ginger Salmon
Price: $17.49

980 calories
8 g saturated fat
2,299 mg sodium

Save!
670 calories
and $12.67!

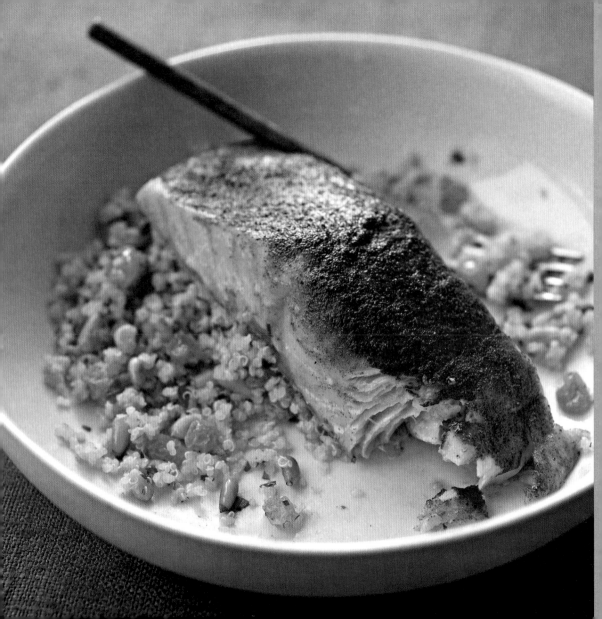

Sweet & Spicy Beef

Stir-fries, by their very nature—fresh vegetables, a bit of protein, a thin veneer of sauce—should be bona fide healthy eats. Unfortunately, America's adaptation of Chinese food involves less of the fresh vegetables, a fatty rather than lean protein, and an abundance of oily sauce that makes every dish taste just like the last. Hence the cavalry of 1,000-calorie meals swimming in sodium. This spicy-sweet beef treatment is exactly what a stir-fry should be: fast, flavorful, and incredibly good for you.

Master THE TECHNIQUE

Mise en place

"Mise en place" (pronounced meez a plas) is the fancy French phrase that basically means "have all your ingredients ready before you start cooking." For serious cooks, it's not just a suggestion, it's a religion. Nowhere is that dictum more essential than with stir-frying. Mince, dice, and chop your way through all the vegetables and proteins you'll need, then arrange on a plate or cutting board in the order you'll need them. Have sauces and condiments measured out. And, most importantly, always have salt and pepper at arm's length.

You'll Need:

- 2 Tbsp low-sodium soy sauce
- 2 tsp cornstarch
- 12 oz flank steak, thinly sliced against the grain
- ½ Tbsp peanut or vegetable oil
- 8 scallions, greens and whites separated, chopped
- 4 cloves garlic, thinly sliced
- 2 cups mushrooms, thinly sliced
- 4 cups green beans, ends removed, or sugar snap peas
- 2 Tbsp hoisin sauce
- 1 Tbsp chili garlic sauce

How to Make It:

- In a large shallow dish, stir together the soy sauce and cornstarch with a fork. Add the steak, toss to coat, and let sit for 10 minutes.
- Heat the oil in a wok or large sauté pan over high heat. When the wok is screaming hot, add the scallion whites and the garlic and cook for 30 seconds, until fragrant but not browned. Add the mushrooms and green beans and stir-fry for 3 to 4 minutes, using a metal spatula to keep the vegetables in near-constant motion.
- Add the beef, along with the soy sauce, and continue to stir-fry for 3 minutes, until the beef is fully browned on the outside. Stir in the hoisin and chili sauce and cook until the sauce lightly clings to the surface of the meat and vegetables. Garnish with the scallion greens.

Makes 4 servings /
Cost per serving: $2.64

300 calories
13 g fat
(5 g saturated)
570 mg sodium

1,011 calories
45 g fat
(12 g saturated)
4,020 mg sodium

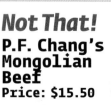

Not That!
P.F. Chang's Mongolian Beef
Price: $15.50

Save!
711 calories
and $12.86

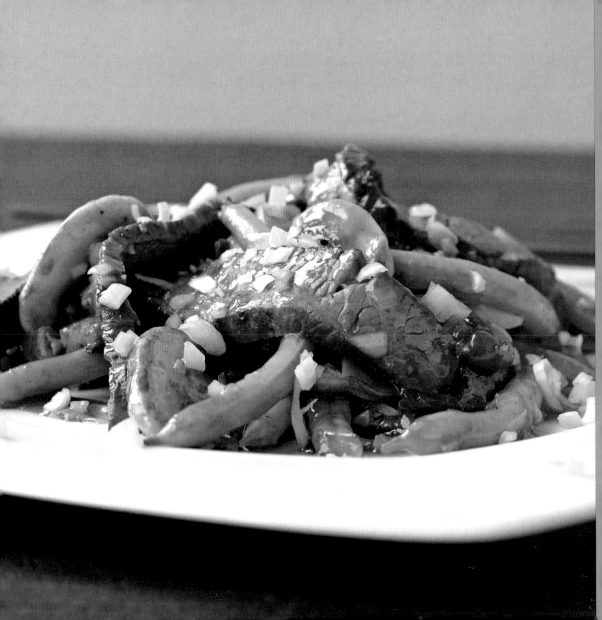

Cook This!
Scallops with Chimichurri

Chimichurri is an herb-based sauce from Argentina used to adorn and enhance a variety of different dishes, grilled meats and fish above all. After some careful reflection, we've decided that chimi is pretty much the world's greatest condiment, turning bad food good and making good food great. Once you make it, you'll have a hard time not painting it on everything you come across: sandwiches, grilled vegetables, eggs. So it's probably worthwhile to double the recipe and have a bit stashed in the fridge for when cravings strike, which will be often after you make this dish.

You'll Need:

½ cup water

Salt

2 Tbsp red wine vinegar

1 cup fresh parsley, chopped

2 cloves garlic, minced

Pinch red pepper flakes

3 Tbsp olive oil

1 lb large sea scallops

Black pepper to taste

How to Make It:

● Combine the water and ½ teaspoon salt in a bowl and microwave for 30 seconds. Stir so the salt thoroughly dissolves, then mix in the vinegar, parsley, garlic, and pepper flakes. Slowly drizzle in 2 tablespoons of the olive oil, whisking to incorporate. You can use the chimichurri now, but it's best to let the flavors marry for 20 minutes or more; it will keep covered in the fridge for 3 days.

● Heat the remaining 1 tablespoon oil in a large skillet over medium-high heat. Thoroughly dry the scallops with paper towels, then season on both sides with salt and pepper. When the oil is hot, add the scallops and cook for 2 to 3 minutes on the first side, without disturbing them, until a deep brown crust has developed. Flip and cook for 1 to 2 minutes longer, until firm but yielding to the touch. Serve drizzled with the chimichurri.

Makes 4 servings / Cost per serving: $3.98

Scallops are the most underrated of all seafood. They're incredibly lean, but with a sweet, meaty taste that makes them feel indulgent, Plus, they cook effortlessly in about 5 minutes.

200 calories
11 g fat
(1.5 g saturated)
480 mg sodium

550 calories

Not That!
Bonefish Grill
Grilled Jumbo Sea Scallops
with Chimichurri Sauce
Price: $16.20

Save!
350 calories
and $12.22!

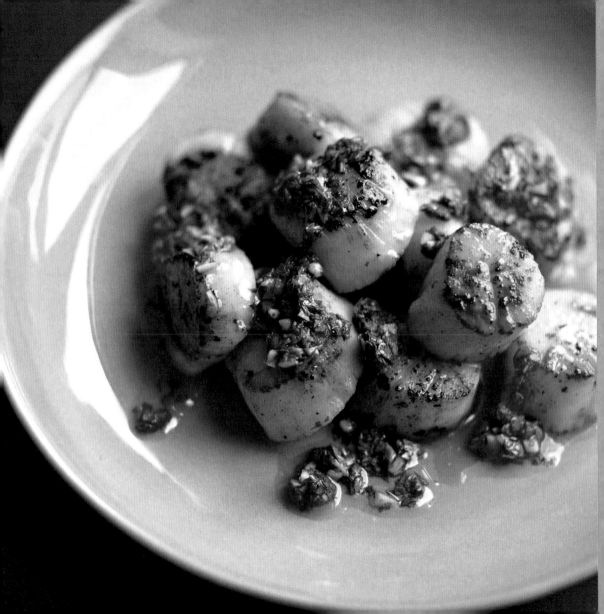

Cook This!
Seared Ahi with Ginger-Scallion Sauce

As much as we love ahi tuna for its profusion of lean protein and heart-strengthening, brain-boosting omega-3 fatty acids, what we love most about the fish is the fact that even a kitchen neophyte can cook it perfectly in less than 5 minutes. All it takes is a pan set over high heat, a touch of oil, and a sprinkle of salt and pepper. We add bok choy to make this a more nutritious, substantial dish, but any green vegetable (spinach, broccoli, asparagus) will do. Just don't skip the ginger-scallion sauce, a ubiquitous Chinatown condiment good enough to make a pair of old socks into a memorable meal.

You'll Need:

- 1 bunch scallions, bottoms removed, finely chopped
- 2 Tbsp fresh ginger, peeled and grated
- 1 Tbsp low-sodium soy sauce
- 3 Tbsp peanut oil
- 1 Tbsp rice wine vinegar
- 16 oz ahi or other high-quality tuna steaks

Salt and pepper to taste

- ½ lb shitake mushrooms, stems removed, sliced
- 1 lb baby bok choy, stems removed

How to Make It:

- Combine the scallions, ginger, soy sauce, 2 tablespoons of the oil, and vinegar in a mixing bowl and stir thoroughly to combine. Set aside. (Making this ahead and storing in the refrigerator is not only possible but advisable, as even 30 minutes of sitting allows the flavors to marry nicely.)
- Heat the remaining oil in a large cast-iron skillet or sauté pan. Season the tuna liberally with salt and lots of black pepper. When the oil is lightly smoking, add the tuna to the pan and sear for 2 minutes per side, until deeply browned. Remove.
- While the tuna rests, add the shitake mushrooms to the same hot pan (use another drizzle of oil if the pan is dry). Cook for 2 to 3 minutes, until lightly browned, then add the bok choy. Cook for another 2 to 3 minutes, until the bok choy is lightly wilted. Season to taste with salt and pepper.
- Slice the tuna into thick strips. Divide the bok choy and mushrooms among four warm plates. Top with slices of tuna, then drizzle with the ginger-scallion sauce.

Makes 4 servings /
Cost per serving: $5.38

301 calories
12 g fat
(2 g saturated)
271 mg sodium

1,610 calories
49 g saturated fat
1,075 mg sodium

Not That!
Cheesecake Factory Wasabi Crusted Ahi Tuna
Price: $11.95

Save!
1,309 calories and $6.57!

268

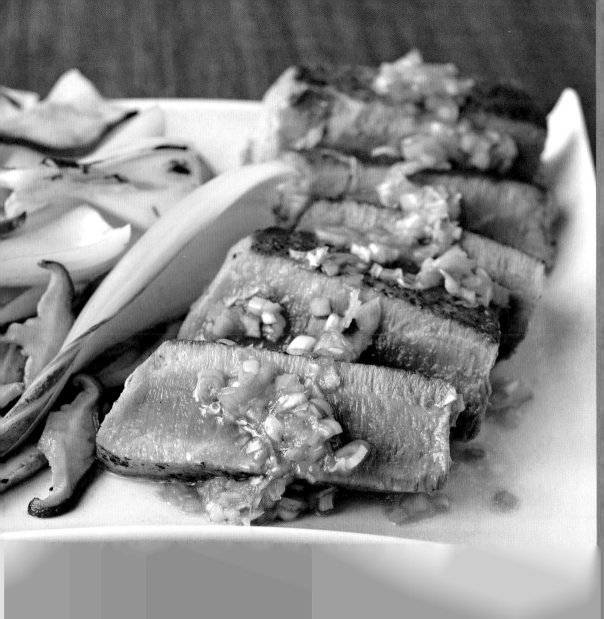

Cook This!
Chicken in Red Wine

Coq au vin, as it's known in France, is one of the world's great dishes and all it takes to create it is a whole chicken, half a bottle of wine, and a few vegetables. A slow cooker makes matters even easier, but a good old-fashioned pot will do, too.

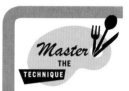

Master THE TECHNIQUE

Stovetop slow cooking

Don't have a slow cooker at home? Don't fret. Any recipe in this book that calls for a slow cooker can be executed in a pot on the stovetop or in a low oven. Rather than dump all the ingredients in the base of the slow cooker, simply combine them in a pot or pan large enough to fit them comfortably, then cover and simmer over very low heat or bake in a 250°F oven. Because slow cookers braise at such a low temperature, stovetop or oven cooking will always be faster—which may be exactly what you're looking for.

You'll Need:

- 2 strips bacon, chopped
- 1 whole chicken, cut into 8 pieces (or 1½ lb drumsticks and thighs)
- Salt and black pepper to taste
- 2 cups red wine
- 2 cups low-sodium chicken stock
- 1 bag frozen pearl onions
- 2 bay leaves
- 2 cloves garlic, peeled and smashed
- 8 oz button mushrooms, quartered
- 1 Tbsp butter
- 1 Tbsp flour

How to Make It:

- Cook the bacon in a wide cast-iron skillet or sauté pan until crispy. Reserve. Discard all but a thin film of the bacon fat from the pan. Season the chicken all over with salt and pepper. Add to the pan and cook for 7 to 10 minutes, until well browned all over. (Work in batches if you must; crowding will prevent it from properly browning.)

- Transfer the chicken to the base of a slow cooker. Add the wine to the skillet and use a wooden spoon to scrape loose any browned bits from the bottom. Pour the wine over the chicken, then add the reserved bacon, the stock, onions, bay leaves, and garlic, along with another good pinch of salt and pepper. Cook on high for at least 2 hours (or cook on low for most of the day), until the meat is falling off the bone. In the final 30 minutes, stir in the mushrooms and allow them to just cook through.

- When ready to serve, cook the butter and flour in a sauce-pan over medium heat for 1 minute. Ladle in 1½ cups of the cooking liquid and cook until it has thickened enough to coat the back of a spoon. Serve the chicken with the onions and mushrooms, then drizzle over the thickened sauce.

Makes 4 servings /
Cost per serving: $3.03

365 calories
11 g fat
(4 g saturated)
590 mg sodium

Not That!
California Pizza Kitchen Chicken Marsala
Price: $15.79

1,412 calories
15 g saturated fat
3,038 mg sodium

Save!
1,047 calories
and $12.76!

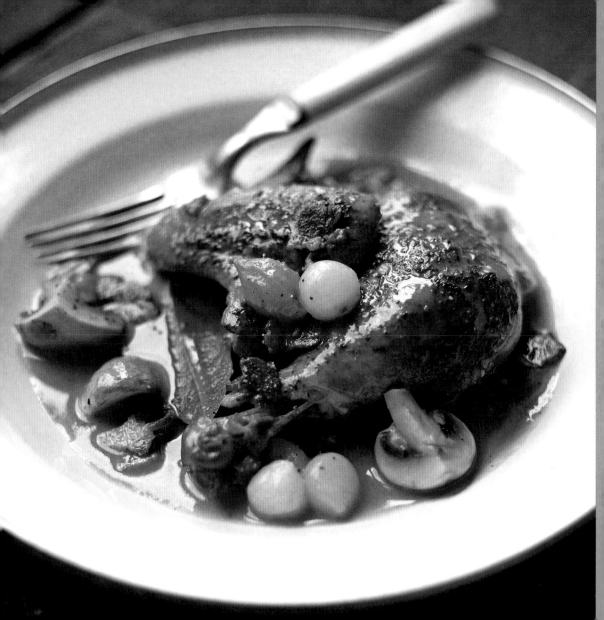

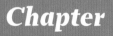

10-Minute Meals

The quickest, easiest, tastiest
meals for when you're short on time

Cook This!
Chicken Tacos with Salsa Verde

Tossed with a good dose of bright, mildly spicy salsa verde, rotisserie chicken is the perfect filling for tacos, burritos, and even enchiladas. Indeed, there might not be a better use of a supermarket rotisserie chicken. Even freshly grilled chicken breasts won't yield better results since it's hard to top the juiciness of a spit-roasted bird.

You'll Need:

- 8 corn tortillas
- 3 cups shredded rotisserie chicken (about three-fourths of a store-bought chicken)
- 1½ cups bottled salsa verde
- ½ cup crumbled Cotija or feta cheese
- 1 medium onion, minced
- 1 cup chopped fresh cilantro
- 2 limes, quartered

How to Make It:

- Heat the tortillas in a large skillet or sauté pan until lightly toasted. Combine the chicken with the salsa in a large mixing bowl, then divide evenly among the tortillas. Top with crumbled cheese, onion, and cilantro. Serve with lime wedges.

Makes 4 servings / Cost per serving: $2.33

Be sure to remove the skin first. As delicious as it may be, its finer points will be lost in the salsa-strewn meat itself, so you may as well save the calories.

$$(\Psi + \mathbf{I})^2$$

MEAL MULTIPLIER

This two-ingredient mixture is simply too delicious to confine to tacos. Here are a few other ways to let it sing:

- Make enchiladas by rolling it into warm corn tortillas. Top with more salsa and Jack cheese and bake in a 400°F oven for 20 minutes.
- Grill romaine hearts until lightly wilted and top with the chicken mixture, toasted corn, and chopped tomatoes.
- Follow this recipe, but top with a fried egg and eat with a knife and fork.

345 calories
12 g fat
(4.5 g saturated)
800 mg sodium

1,650 calories
76 g fat
(21 g saturated)
4,080 mg sodium

Not That!
Chili's Crispy Chicken Tacos
(flour tortillas)
Price: $8.99

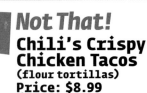

Save!
1,305 calories and $6.66!

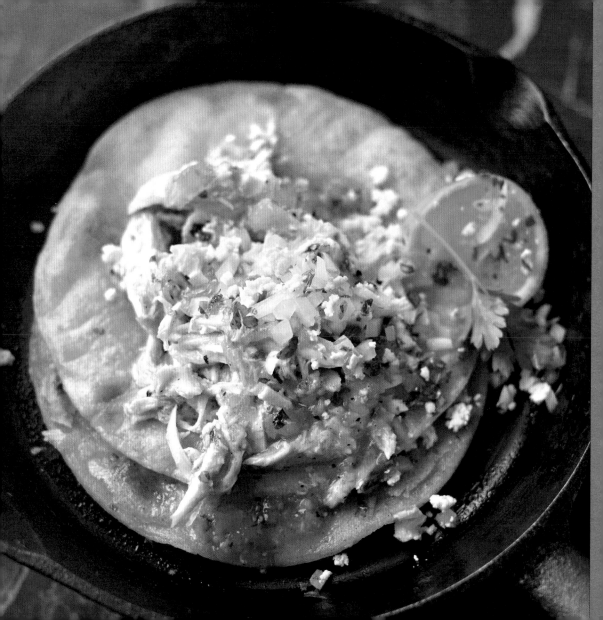

Coffee-Rubbed Steak

Coffee and steak might seem like an unlikely partnership, but the flavor of beef is actually heightened by the robust notes of java. This dish would be perfect with grilled vegetables and a side of black or pinto beans. Or heat up a few corn tortillas and pass them out so everyone can make their own little tacos. Either way, be sure to let the beef rest (even if it actually makes this 10-minute meal a 12- or 13-minute meal); cut into it too early and all the still-hot juices will bleed onto your cutting board, instead of being reabsorbed by the meat.

You'll Need:

- ½ Tbsp finely ground coffee or espresso
- ½ Tbsp chili powder
- Salt and black pepper to taste
- 1 lb flank or skirt steak
- Pico de Gallo (see page 307)
- 1 lime, quartered

How to Make It:

- Preheat a grill, grill pan, or cast-iron skillet. Combine the coffee grounds with the chili powder, plus a few generous pinches of salt and pepper. Rub the spice mixture all over the steak. Cook the beef for 3 to 4 minutes per side, depending on thickness, until slightly firm but still yielding.

- Let the steak rest for at least 5 minutes, then slice thinly against the grain of the meat. Serve with a big scoop of pico de gallo and a wedge of lime.

Makes 4 servings / Cost per serving: $2.41

Skirt and flank are among our two favorite cuts, but any steak—strip, tenderloin, ribeye—would benefit from this coffee treatment.

270 calories
15 g fat
(6 g saturated)
600 mg sodium

SECRET WEAPON

Odd couples

Steak and coffee isn't the only unconventional pairing that yields surprisingly excellent results. Try any of these tantalizing teams for a jolt to your taste buds:

- Watermelon and tomato, topped with crumbled goat cheese and basil
- Olive oil and ice cream, with a pinch of coarse sea salt
- Strawberries, balsamic vinegar, and black pepper
- Peanut butter, banana, and bacon between toasted bread (the King would approve)
- Mango, papaya, or pineapple chunks topped with lime juice and hot sauce

Not That!

On the Border Carne Asada
Price: $13.49

930 calories
35 g fat
(14 g saturated)
2,020 mg sodium

Save!
660 calories and $11.08!

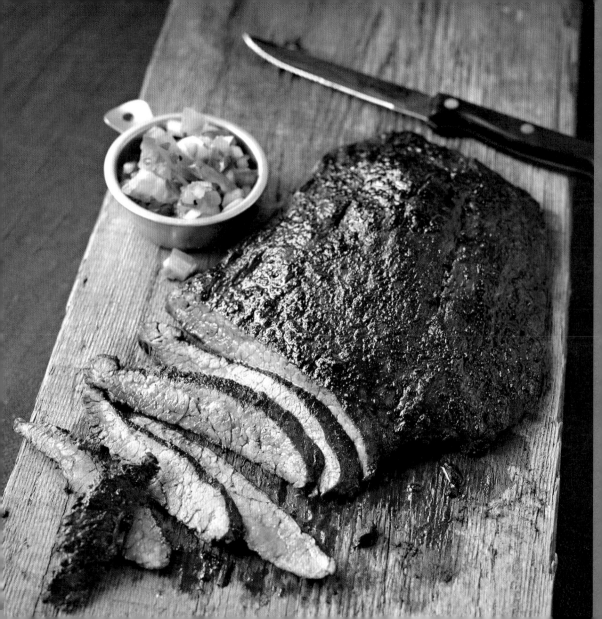

Sesame Noodles with Chicken & Peanuts

Italians might cringe in horror to hear it, but the noodle originally comes from Asia. In 2005, archaeologists discovered what they believe to be the oldest bowl of noodles on record, dating back some 4,000 years. (No word yet on what type of sauce they were dressed with.) The point being that sometimes a box of fettuccine is just as appropriate for an Asian-inspired meal as it is for an Italian repast. Think of this as a salad, with the noodles standing in for lettuce. Add some protein and as many or as few vegetables as you like, and toss the whole package with a light but powerful dressing. It's the culmination of four millennia of noodle knowledge. (Well, maybe not, but it's awfully tasty.)

You'll Need:

- 6 oz whole-wheat fettuccine
- 2 tsp toasted sesame oil, plus more for noodles
- Juice of 1 lime
- 2 Tbsp warm water
- 1½ Tbsp chunky peanut butter
- 1½ Tbsp low-sodium soy sauce
- 2 tsp chili sauce, such as sriracha
- 2 cups shredded chicken
- 1 red or yellow bell pepper, sliced
- 2 cups sugar snap peas
- 1 cup cooked and shelled edamame (optional)
- Chopped peanuts, sesame seeds, or chopped scallions (optional)

How to Make It:

- Bring a large pot of salted water to a boil and cook the pasta according to package instructions. Drain the pasta and toss in a large bowl with a bit of sesame oil and rice wine vinegar to keep the noodles from sticking.
- Combine the lime juice, water, peanut butter, soy sauce, chili sauce, and sesame oil in a microwave-safe mixing bowl. Microwave for 45 seconds, then stir to create a uniform sauce.
- Add the sauce to the noodles and toss to mix. Stir in the chicken, bell pepper, sugar snaps, and edamame if using. Top individual servings with peanuts, sesame seeds, or scallions if you like.

Makes 4 servings / Cost per serving: $2.05

The sugar snaps work perfectly fine raw in this dish, but if you prefer them cooked, toss them in with the pasta 2 minutes before it finishes cooking. You can do the same with green beans if you can't find sugar snaps.

340 calories
11 g fat
(2 g saturated)
400 mg sodium

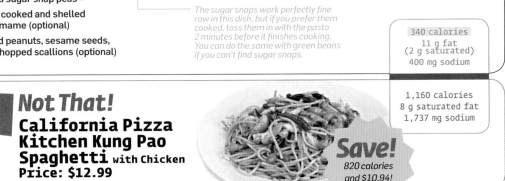

1,160 calories
8 g saturated fat
1,737 mg sodium

Not That!
California Pizza Kitchen Kung Pao Spaghetti with Chicken
Price: $12.99

Save!
820 calories and $10.94!

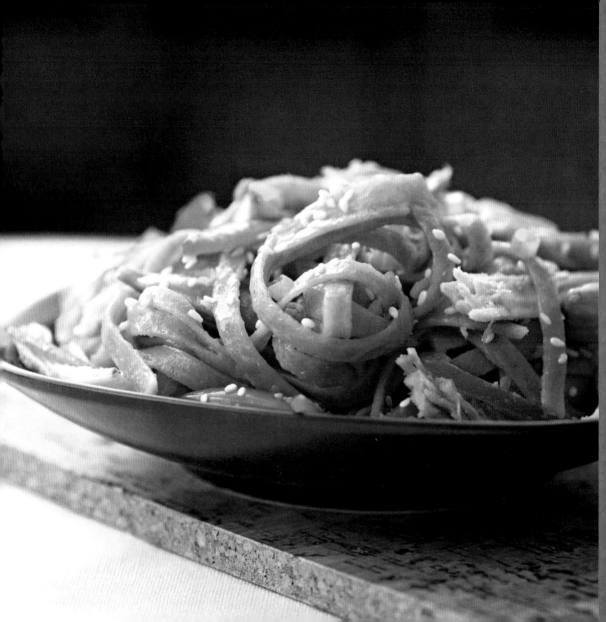

Chicago Dog

Chicagoans take hot dogs pretty seriously. So seriously, in fact, that the actual order in which you apply the ingredients is of paramount importance (at least as they tell it). We'll cut them some slack because, after all, they make the best dogs in the country (sorry, New York), and the fact that they come so loaded with produce ("run through the garden," as they say) means that what could be a snack for some quickly turns into a surprisingly reasonable meal.

You'll Need:

4 reduced-fat all-beef dogs (we like anything from Applegate Farms)

4 poppy seed hot dog buns

Yellow mustard

Relish

1 small yellow onion, minced

1 large beefsteak tomato, cut into wedges

4 pickle spears

8 sport peppers •

Celery salt

These little light green chiles have an awesome spicy pop but are tough to come by. Pepperoncini, if need be, can fill in.

How to Make It:

- Bring a medium pot of water to boil. Turn the heat to low, add the hot dogs, and cook for 5 minutes, until heated all the way through. Alternatively, you can grill the dogs until lightly charred all over (which, while untraditional, is probably more delicious).

- Dump out all but a few inches of the water and place a steamer basket in the pot. Steam the buns until warm and very soft.

- Place a dog in each bun, then arrange the toppings in the following order: mustard, relish, onion, a few tomato wedges, pickle spear, two sport peppers, and a pinch of celery salt.

Makes 4 dogs / Cost per serving: $1.86

250 calories
9 g fat
(3.5 g saturated)
1,020 mg sodium

570 calories
35 g fat
(15.5 g saturated)
1,271 mg sodium

Not That!
Five Guys Hot Dog
with Mustard, Relish, and Onions
Price: $3.19

Save!
320 calories and $1.33!

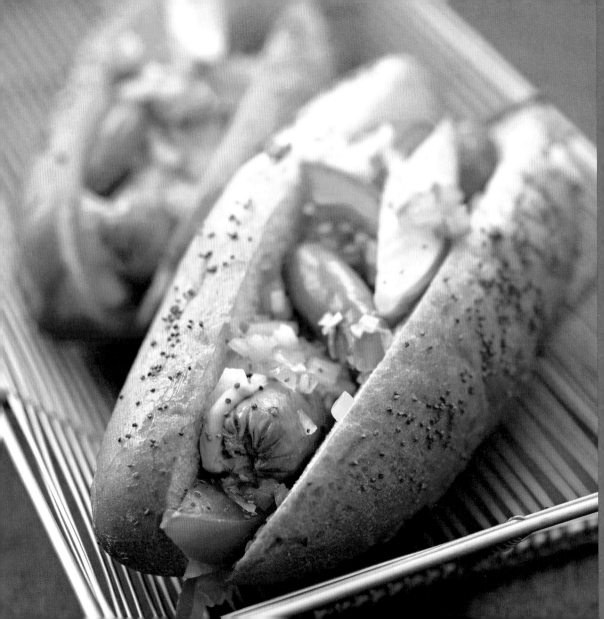

Chili-Glazed Salmon

This is the type of recipe that converts fish skeptics into bona fide believers, and all it takes is a glaze that you can whip up in a few minutes. The fattiness of salmon pairs perfectly with assertive spicy and sweet flavors, and this has both. Round this meal out with roasted broccoli (it can roast in the same oven as the salmon) and a side of couscous.

You'll Need:

- ¼ cup Asian-style sweet chili sauce
- 2 Tbsp low-sodium soy sauce
- 1 Tbsp grated fresh ginger
- 1 tsp sriracha or other spicy chili sauce
- 4 salmon fillets (4–6 oz each)

How to Make It:

- Preheat the oven to 425°F. Combine the sweet chili sauce, soy sauce, ginger, and sriracha in a mixing bowl. Place the salmon fillets on a foil-lined baking sheet. Use a brush or a spoon to lacquer the salmon with the chili glaze.
- Bake the salmon until the glaze has begun to lightly caramelize and the salmon flakes with gentle pressure, about 10 minutes, depending on the thickness of the fish.

Makes 4 servings / Cost per serving: $3.83

When possible, buy wild salmon. It may be more expensive, but it's lower in PCBs, toxins, and mercury than most farmed varieties. Plus, it just tastes better.

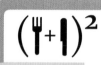

$$(\math{Y}+\math{I})^2$$

MEAL MULTIPLIER

Roasting salmon yields tender, moist fish every time, with no effort on your part other than turning on the oven. In addition to the chili glaze here, try one of these three easy variations to give salmon fillets a powerful flavor boost:

- 2 tablespoons hoisin, 2 tablespoons low-sodium soy sauce, and 2 tablespoons orange juice
- 2 tablespoons Dijon mustard, 2 tablespoons honey, and ½ tablespoon chili powder
- 2 tablespoons softened butter, 1 tablespoon canned chipotle pepper, the juice of 1 lime, and shaved Parmesan

330 calories
14 g fat
(2 g saturated)
560 mg sodium

790 calories
24 g fat
(4.5 g saturated)
3,000 mg sodium

Not That!
Applebee's Orange Glazed Salmon
Price: $13.49

Save!
460 calories
and $9.66!

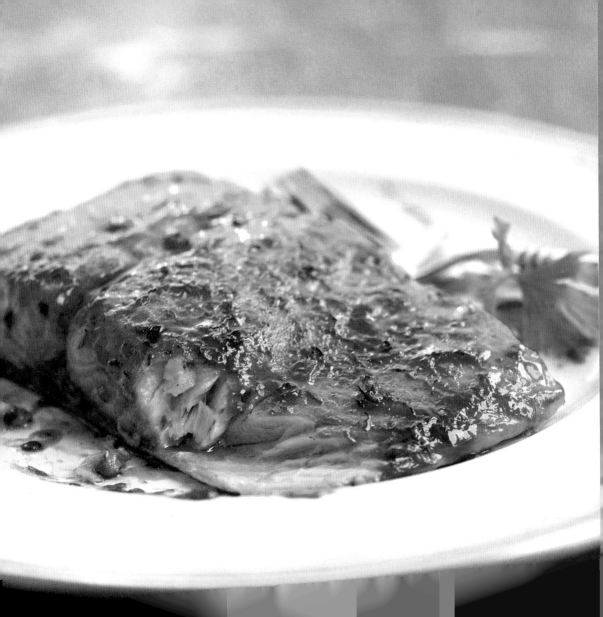

Cook This!
Chicken Fajita Burrito

Burritos have humble origins. During the early 20th century, Mexican workers would head out for the day with a bit of last night's dinner—some beans, a little meat, maybe some rice—wrapped in a tortilla to keep it warm until lunch. Many years later burritos have gone off the deep end. In particular, it's the combination of rice, beans, sour cream, cheese, and guacamole that lifts calorie and sodium counts into the thousands. This burrito is American in spirit, which is to say it's hearty and generously filled, but without the caloric excesses found at Chipotle Mexican Grill, Baja Fresh, and the country's other burrito barons.

You'll Need:

- ½ Tbsp canola oil
- 1 large onion, sliced
- 1 red bell pepper, sliced
- 1 poblano or green bell pepper, sliced
- Salt and black pepper to taste
- ½ can (14–16 oz) black beans, drained
- ¼ tsp cumin
- Juice of 1 lime
- Hot sauce
- 4 (10") whole-wheat tortillas
- 1 cup low-fat shredded Jack cheese
- 2 cups shredded chicken (about half a store-bought rotisserie chicken)
- Salsa (salsa verde is especially good here)

How to Make It:

- Heat the oil in a large skillet over high heat. Add the onion and red and poblano peppers and cook until browned, about 7 to 8 minutes. Season with salt and pepper.
- Combine the beans with cumin in a saucepan and warm through. Add the lime juice and a few shakes of hot sauce.
- Preheat a griddle, cast-iron skillet, or large nonstick pan over medium heat. Microwave the tortillas for 20 seconds, just enough so they're pliable. Building one burrito at a time, sprinkle on some cheese, top with some beans, onion-pepper mixture, chicken, and salsa. Roll into a tight package. Place the burritos directly on the skillet, cooking for a minute on each side until lightly toasted.

Makes 4 burritos / Cost per serving: $2.92

355 calories
13 g fat
(6 g saturated)
740 mg sodium

870 calories
30 g fat
(13 g saturated)
1,940 mg sodium

Not That!
Chipotle Grilled Chicken Fajita Burrito with Black Beans, Cheese, Sour Cream, and Tomato Salsa
Price: $5.85

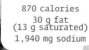

Save!
515 calories
and $2.93!

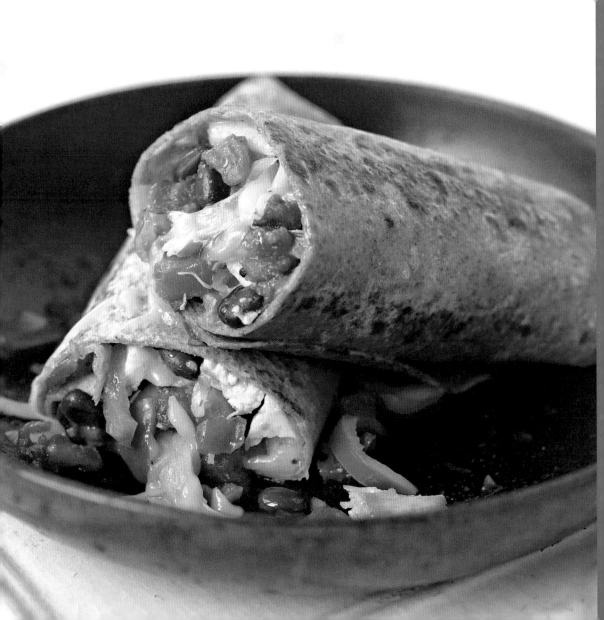

Cook This!
Blackened Tilapia with Garlic-Lime Butter

Ever eaten any blackened food that wasn't delicious (besides those steaks your dad scorches every year at the Fourth of July barbecue)? Neither have we. Consider it a bonus that blackening is actually an incredibly healthy way of cooking, giving the fish or meat a body armor of potent disease-fighting antioxidants in the form of tantalizing spices. Truth be told, the flavored butter here is the icing on the cake; if you have a great fresh piece of fish, just coat it with a bit of blackening spice, follow the cooking instructions, and maybe squeeze a lemon over the top.

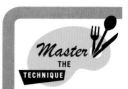

Master THE TECHNIQUE

Blackening

You can blacken fish or meat on the grill, but the best—and most traditional—way to get the full sear you want is in a scorching-hot cast-iron skillet. Heat a thin film of oil in the skillet over the highest possible heat (and turn on the hood or kitchen fan). When wisps of smoke begin to rise from the oil, carefully add the fish or meat. Don't touch it—whatever it may be—for at least 2 minutes; you want a dark crust to set in over the protein, and fiddling with the food will prevent this from happening. Cook for 75 percent of the time on one side, then flip and finish on the other.

You'll Need:

- 2 Tbsp butter, softened at room temperature
- 2 Tbsp chopped fresh cilantro
- 2 cloves garlic, finely minced
- 1 tsp lime zest, plus juice of 1 lime
- 1 Tbsp canola oil
- 4 tilapia fillets (6 oz each)
- 1 Tbsp Blackening Spice (see page 305)

How to Make It:

- Combine the butter, cilantro, garlic, lime zest, and lime juice in a small mixing bowl and stir to thoroughly blend. Set aside.
- Heat the oil in a large cast-iron skillet or sauté pan over high heat. Rub the tilapia all over with the blackening spice. When the oil in the pan lightly smokes, add the fish and cook, undisturbed, for 3 to 4 minutes on the first side, until the spice rub becomes dark and crusty. Flip and continue cooking for 1 to 2 minutes, until the fillets flake with gentle pressure from your finger.
- Transfer the fish to 4 serving plates and immediately top each with a bit of the flavored butter.

*Makes 4 servings /
Cost per serving: $2.32*

300 calories
14 g fat
(6 g saturated)
510 mg sodium

640 calories
27 g fat
(14 g saturated)
1,520 mg sodium

Not That!
Denny's Lemon Pepper Grilled Tilapia
Price: $12.59

Save!
340 calories
and $10.27!

286

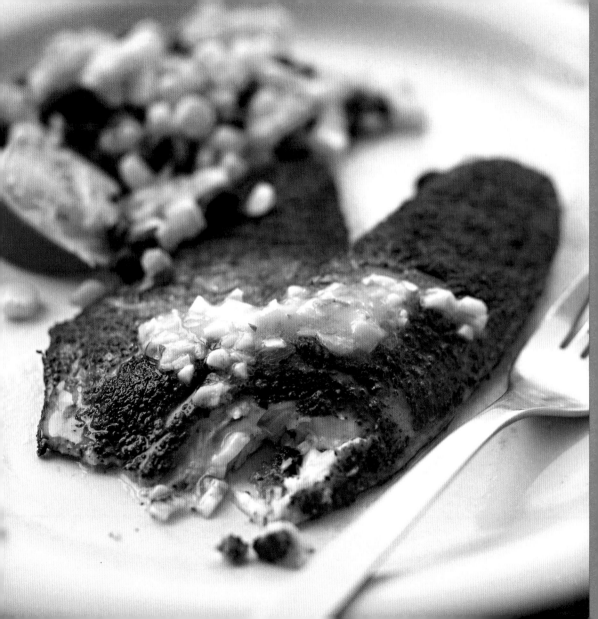

Spicy Thai Chicken with Basil

The cuisines of Southeast Asia—Thai, Vietnamese, Malaysian—deliver more flavor per calorie than any other on the planet and make for a refreshing break from the cartons of Chinese takeout that clutter so many American refrigerators. This Thai classic (called *gai pad grapow*) gets its flavor from chiles, garlic, and fresh herbs—nutritional powerhouses known to boost metabolism and fight cancer. Together, they also make for a full-throttle flavor experience that trumps nearly any Chinese stir-fry in the health department. Adjust the heat to your liking, but if it's not at least somewhat fiery, then it's not Thai.

You'll Need:

- 1 Tbsp peanut or canola oil
- 1 medium red onion, thinly sliced
- 2 jalapeño peppers, thinly sliced (or more if you really like your food fiery)
- 4 cloves garlic, minced
- 1 lb boneless skinless chicken breasts, cut into small pieces
- 2 Tbsp fish sauce
- 1 Tbsp sugar
- 1 Tbsp low-sodium soy sauce
- 2 cups fresh basil leaves (preferably Thai or holy basil, but you'll only find those at specialty markets)

How to Make It:

- Heat the oil in a wok or large skillet. When hot, add the onion, jalapeños, and garlic and stir-fry for 2 minutes, using a metal spatula to keep the ingredients in motion. Add the chicken and cook for 2 to 3 minutes, until the meat is beginning to brown on the outside. Add the fish sauce, sugar, soy sauce, and basil and cook for 1 minute more. Serve over rice.

Makes 4 servings / Cost per serving: $1.67

If you absolutely can't find fish sauce, you can substitute with more low-sodium soy sauce and a dash of Worcestershire, which is actually made in a similar manner as fish sauce.

SECRET WEAPON

Fish sauce

Made from fermented oily fish, fish sauce tends to pack a stiff aroma. But this funky condiment forms the backbone of much of Southeast Asian cuisine and, despite it's strong nose, adds a pleasantly salty, sweet punch of flavor to a variety of dishes and sauces. Find a bottle in large grocery stores or Asian markets. We find that Thai Kitchen brand is the easiest for fish sauce newbies to enjoy.

190 calories
6 g fat
(1.5 g saturated)
890 mg sodium

849 calories
39 g fat
(6 g saturated)
2,121 mg sodium

Not That!

P.F. Chang's Dali Chicken
Price: $13.50

Save!

659 calories and $11.83!

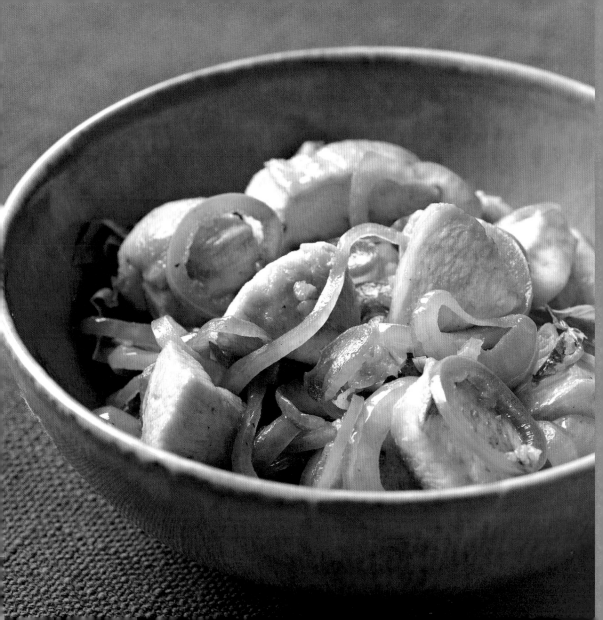

Cook This!

Seared Tuna Tacos

Taco night in the average American home generally means ground beef, crunchy shells, and shredded cheese. Nothing wrong with that, but other meat and fish can deliver more flavor for a fraction of the calories. Exhibit A: ahi tuna. Not only does the combination of silky rare tuna and creamy avocado fit a boatload of healthy fat into the palm of your hand, but the flavors are tough to beat, especially when crowned with a spicy slaw and the tang of a few pickled onions. Forget the fried version: This is your new fish taco.

You'll Need:

- 4 cups shredded red or green cabbage
- 2 Tbsp olive oil mayonnaise
- Juice of 1 lime, plus lime wedges for serving
- ½ Tbsp canned chipotle pepper
- Salt and black pepper to taste
- ½ Tbsp canola or olive oil
- 12 oz fresh ahi or other high-quality tuna
- 8 corn tortillas
- 1 ripe avocado, pitted, peeled, and sliced
- Pickled Red Onions (see Quick Pickles on this page)
- Hot sauce

How to Make It:

- Combine the cabbage, mayo, lime juice, and chipotle in a large mixing bowl. Season with salt and pepper. Set the slaw aside. (This is best done at least 15 minutes before cooking so that you allow the flavors to marry.)

- Heat the oil in a large cast-iron skillet or stainless-steel sauté pan over medium-high heat. Season the tuna with salt and plenty of black pepper. When the oil is hot, add the tuna and sear for 2 minutes on each side, until a nice crust has developed but the inside of the tuna is still rare.

- While the pan is still hot, heat the tortillas until lightly crisp on the outside.

- Slice the tuna into thin planks. Divide among the tortillas and top each with avocado slices, slaw, and pickled onions. Serve with lime wedges and hot sauce.

Makes 4 servings /
Cost per serving: $3.40

330 calories
13 g fat
(2 g saturated)
460 mg sodium

Master THE TECHNIQUE

Quick Pickles

Vegetables such as onions, cucumbers, and peppers pick up a perfect vinegar bite when soaked in a pickle brine. Combine equal parts warm water with apple cider or rice wine vinegar, plus a good spoonful of salt and sugar. Stir it all up, then drop in the vegetables for at least 10 minutes before serving. They keep covered in the fridge for up to a week.

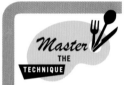

Not That!

On the Border Grilled Mahi Mahi Tacos
with Creamy Red Chile Sauce
Price: $9.99

1,210 calories
61 g fat
(13 g saturated)
3,030 mg sodium

Save!
880 calories and $6.59!

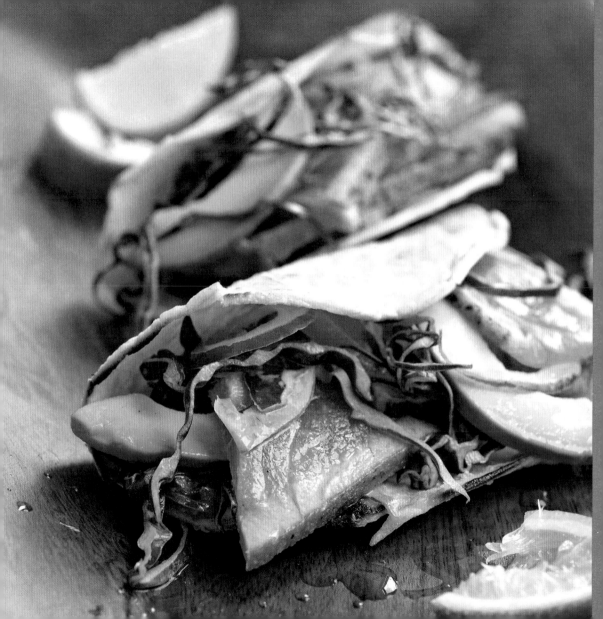

Cook This!

Steak with Blue Cheese Crust

Steak and blue cheese are a perfect match—the rich funkiness of the cheese intensifies the big beefiness of the steak. Mixed with bread crumbs and herbs, blue cheese forms a crunchy, melty crust on top of beef, which may be guilt-inducing in its deliciousness but ultimately contributes only about 40 calories to the dish (compared to Outback's blue cheese crust, which adds about 400 calories and 30 grams of fat to the Victoria's Filet). Tenderloin—or filet mignon—works best here, but if you're looking for great results for half the price, sirloin is just fine.

You'll Need:

- ½ cup bread crumbs (preferably homemade, see page 226) or panko
- ¼ cup crumbled blue cheese
- 2 Tbsp chopped fresh parsley
- 1 tsp chopped fresh rosemary or thyme
- 1 Tbsp olive oil
- 4 sirloin or tenderloin steaks (4–6 oz each)
- Salt and black pepper to taste

How to Make It:

- Preheat the oven to 450°F. Combine the bread crumbs, cheese, parsley, and rosemary in a mixing bowl and set aside.
- Heat the oil in a large cast-iron skillet, grill pan, or stainless steel sauté pan over high heat. Season the steaks all over with salt and plenty of black pepper. Sear the first side of the meat for 2 minutes, until well browned.
- Flip the steaks and top each with a quarter of the bread crumb mixture, using your fingers to gently press it into the meat. Transfer the steaks to the oven to finish cooking (ideally in the pan if it's oven-proof, but if not, a baking sheet or dish will do). The steaks should be done in 5 to 6 minutes, when they feel firm but still springy to the touch (an internal thermometer should read 135°F for medium-rare). This should happen at the same time that the bread crumbs have browned nicely and formed a crust. Let the steaks rest for a few minutes before serving.

Makes 4 servings / Cost per serving: $3.13

330 calories
17 g fat
(6 g saturated)
600 mg sodium

947 calories
78 g fat
(37 g saturated)
865 mg sodium

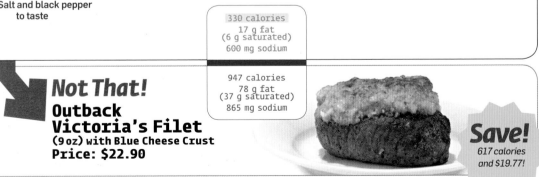

Not That!

Outback Victoria's Filet
(9 oz) with Blue Cheese Crust
Price: $22.90

Save!
*617 calories
and $19.77!*

292

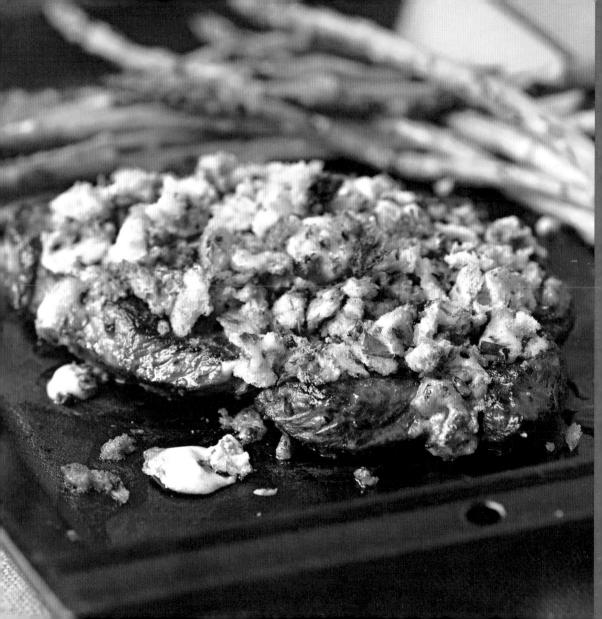

Sides, Snacks & Sauces

Little foods
that make a
big difference

12 Hunger-Squash

1

Warm toasted nuts: Toss a combination of nuts—pecans, almonds, peanuts, cashews—with chili powder, black pepper, and a pinch of cayenne. Roast in a 400°F oven for 10 minutes, until warm and toasty.

3

Boil a few cups of frozen edamame until tender. Drain and toss with a light coating of sesame oil, red pepper flakes, and kosher salt.

Spread the inside of a pita half with plenty of hummus and top with sliced tomato, onion, and lettuce.

2

ANTS ON A LOG: Slather celery with smooth or chunky peanut butter. Dot with raisins.

4

Make your own souped-up trail mix: Combine 1 cup almonds, walnuts, or cashews (or a mix of all three) with ½ cup sunflower seeds and 1½ cups dried fruit: raisins, apricots, apples, prunes, and/or banana chips.

5

6

Stuff cherry peppers or bottled Peppadew peppers with soft goat cheese or mini balls of fresh mozzarella.

ing Snacks

7

Lay a slice of Swiss cheese on a cutting board. Top with a slice of deli turkey and a spoonful of hummus or guacamole. Wrap like a jelly roll and eat.

9

Pop a bag of popcorn. While it's still hot, toss the popcorn with a half cup grated Parmesan and a good amount of chopped fresh rosemary.

11

Pop a bag of popcorn. While it's still hot, toss with a tablespoon of melted butter, then 2 tablespoons of sugar and a teaspoon of cinnamon.

Combine a can of tuna with your favorite salsa. Use Triscuits for scooping.

10

12

Pave a slice of toasted wheat bread with peanut butter and banana slices. Top with a drizzle of honey.

8

Cut fresh mozzarella into ½-inch cubes. Skewer on toothpicks with pitted green olives and sundried tomatoes.

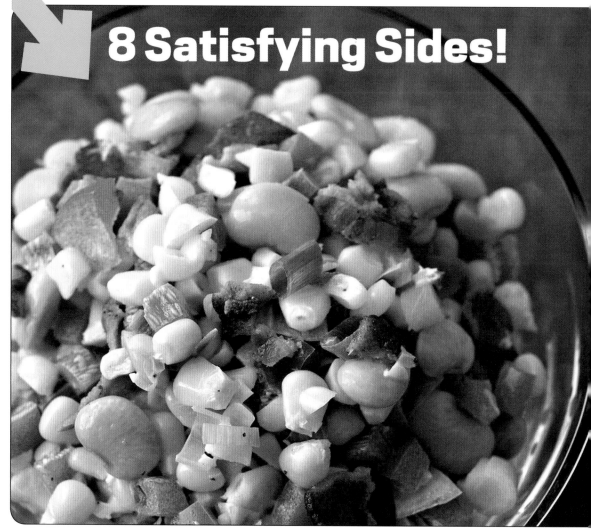

8 Satisfying Sides!

Succotash

There is hardly a piece of meat or fish—grilled, roasted, or pan-seared—that wouldn't benefit from a heaping scoop of succotash cuddled up next to it. Even better than its ability to improve most any plate is succotash's overall adaptability: If it's peak summer season, use fresh corn and green beans and zucchini to make it. If winter has set in, frozen vegetables will still give you a pretty amazing side. One constant, though: bacon. Even this tiny amount of bacon (one portion here is half a slice, for about 30 calories) adds a tremendous amount of smoky depth to the dish, which would be a shame to give up.

You'll Need:

- 2 strips bacon, diced
- 4 scallions, chopped, greens and whites separated
- 1 red bell pepper, chopped
- 2 ears corn, husked, kernels removed from cob
- 2 cups frozen baby lima beans, thawed
- Salt and black pepper to taste
- ¼ cup half-and-half

How to Make It:

- Cook the bacon in a large sauté pan over medium heat until brown and crispy, about 5 minutes. Remove and reserve.
- Add the scallion whites and bell pepper and cook until the vegetables soften, about 3 minutes, then stir in the corn and lima beans. Cook for another 3 to 4 minutes, stirring, until the corn is lightly toasted. Turn the heat down to low, season the vegetables with salt and pepper, then add the half-and-half. Gently simmer until most of the liquid has evaporated and coats the vegetables, about 3 minutes. Stir in bacon and scallion greens.

Makes 4 servings

It's the smokiness you're really after here, so look for either double-smoked or applewood-smoked bacon. Two strips of either is plenty to infuse this whole dish.

Balsamic Zucchini

A great example of how one ingredient can take a dish from average to excellent. Balsamic vinegar not only heightens the sweetness of the zucchini, but the acidity adds a lovely counterpoint as well. For a bit of textural contrast, try a handful of toasted pine nuts.

You'll Need:

- 1 Tbsp olive oil
- 2 lbs zucchini, sliced into ¼" coins
- 2 cloves garlic, minced
- 2 Tbsp balsamic vinegar
- Salt and black pepper to taste
- Fresh mint, chopped (optional)

How to Make It:

Heat the oil in a large sauté pan over medium heat. Add the zucchini and garlic and sauté until the zucchini is tender and lightly browned, about 7 to 10 minutes. Add the balsamic and cook until the liquid has thickened and clings to the zucchini, about 3 to 4 minutes. Season with salt and pepper, and stir in the mint, if using.

Makes 4 servings

190 calories
5 g fat
(2 g saturated)
270 mg sodium

80 calories
4 g fat
(0.5 g saturated)
190 mg sodium

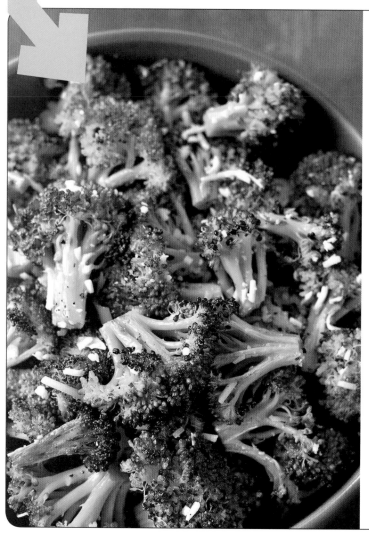

Parmesan-Roasted Broccoli

This simple roasting technique can be applied to any of a dozen different vegetables: asparagus, cauliflower, Brussels sprouts, red potatoes. Of course, the times will vary depending on the vegetable of choice (asparagus will be done in less than 10 minutes; potatoes will take closer to 30), but the results are uniformly satisfying.

You'll Need:

- 1 head broccoli, cut into florets, bottom part of the stem removed
- 1 Tbsp olive oil

Salt and black pepper to taste

- ¼ cup grated Parmesan cheese

How to Make It:

Preheat oven to 450°F. Toss broccoli with olive oil, salt, and pepper and spread out evenly on a baking sheet. Roast in the oven until the broccoli is tender and lightly browned, about 12 minutes. Remove from the oven, toss with the cheese, and serve.

Makes 4 servings

100 calories
5 g fat
(1.5 g saturated)
220 mg sodium

Roasted Garlic Mashed Potatoes

Mashed potatoes are the perfect canvas for big flavors. Consider this a base recipe (even without the garlic)—an infinitely mutable mash ready for whatever heady embellishments you can dream up. Some of the best: fresh chopped rosemary or thyme, caramelized onions, crumbled goat cheese, pesto, lemon (juice and zest) with olive oil (instead of butter), artichoke hearts with sundried tomatoes, and pretty much anything else you can imagine.

You'll Need:

- 1½ pounds Yukon gold potatoes, peeled •
- 1 cup low-fat milk
- 2 Tbsp butter
- 5-6 cloves Roasted Garlic (see page 307)
- Salt and black pepper to taste

How to Make It:

- Place the potatoes in a large pot of salted water and bring to a boil. Cook until a knife inserted into the flesh meets no resistance, about 25 minutes. Drain.
- While the potatoes boil, combine the milk, butter, and garlic in a small saucepan and heat until the butter is melted. Keep warm.
- Use a potato masher or a large wooden spoon to break up the large chunks of potatoes in a rough puree. (If you have a potato ricer, use it—nothing yields smoother mashed potatoes.) Slowly add the hot milk mixture to the potatoes, using a wooden spoon to beat continuously. Season with salt and black pepper.

Makes 4 servings

Red potatoes and russets both do the trick, but Yukon golds, with their smooth, buttery taste and texture, make for the best mash.

Pickled Cucumber Salad

This recipe resides in that small but happy space between side dish and condiment. It's good enough to eat on its own, but it's also the type of punchy, assertive salad that can be served over a piece of grilled salmon or chicken or tucked into a wrap or sandwich.

You'll Need:

- 1 large English cucumber, sliced into thin rounds
- 1 small red onion, very thinly sliced
- 1 Tbsp sesame oil
- ¼ cup rice wine vinegar
- 1 Tbsp sugar
- 1 tsp salt
- 1 tsp red chili flakes

How to Make It:

Combine all the ingredients in a mixing bowl and toss. Let sit for at least 15 minutes before eating. This will keep covered in your fridge for up to 5 days.

Makes 4 cups

180 calories
8 g fat
(5 g saturated)
360 mg sodium

60 calories
3.5 g fat
(0.5 g saturated)
480 mg sodium

Cook This!

Crispy Rosemary Potatoes

Of the dozens of different ways to prepare potatoes, none gets better results for less effort. Rough chop some potatoes (red are best, but any kind will do), toss them with olive oil, rosemary (fresh is best, but dried will do), salt and pepper and cook at a high temp until brown and crispy. Any questions?

You'll Need:

- 1½ lbs red potatoes, cut into ¾" chunks
- 1 Tbsp olive oil
- 1 Tbsp chopped fresh rosemary

Salt and black pepper to taste

How to Make It:

Preheat oven to 425°F. Toss the potatoes with the oil, rosemary, and a generous amount of salt and pepper and spread out evenly on a baking sheet. Roast until brown and crispy on the outside and tender inside, about 30 minutes.

Makes 4 servings

150 calories
3.5 g fat
(0.5 g saturated)
330 mg sodium

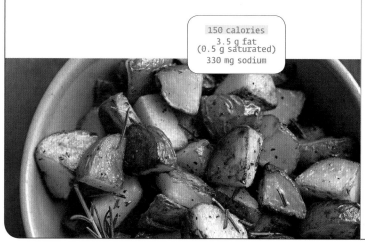

Honey Roasted Carrots

Roasting teases out the inherent sweetness in vegetables. As a vegetable's water content evaporates, its natural sugars are concentrated, making for something considerably more enjoyable to eat than, say, a raw carrot.

You'll Need:

- 8 medium-size carrots, tops removed, peeled
- 1 Tbsp olive oil
- 2 Tbsp honey
- ½ Tbsp fresh thyme leaves (optional)

Salt and pepper to taste

How to Make It:

Preheat oven to 400°F. Toss carrots with olive oil, honey, thyme leaves (if using), and a generous amount of salt and pepper. Spread out on a baking sheet and cook in the oven until brown on the outside and tender all the way through, about 35 minutes.

Makes 4 servings

110 calories
3.5 g fat
(0.5 g saturated)
285 mg sodium

Sweet Potato Fries

French fries can be boring. Tell someone you're serving sweet potato fries, though, and watch eyebrows rise in anticipation. Beyond being healthier than white potatoes (loaded with vitamin A and fiber), the sugars in sweet potatoes make them the perfect candidate for a superior fry.

You'll Need:

- 2 medium sweet potatoes, peeled and cut into wedges
- 1 Tbsp olive oil
- Pinch of cayenne
- ½ tsp smoked paprika (optional)
- Salt and black pepper to taste

How to Make It:

Preheat the oven to 425°F. Combine all the ingredients, plus a generous amount of salt and pepper, on a baking sheet and toss to coat evenly. Bake until the sweet potatoes have browned on the outside, are crisp to the touch, and are tender inside, about 25 minutes.

Makes 4 servings

80 calories
3.5 g fat
(0 g saturated)
230 mg sodium

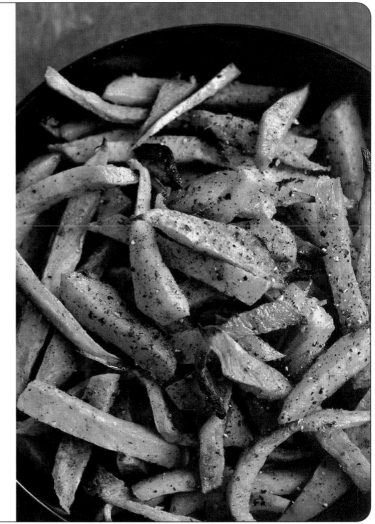

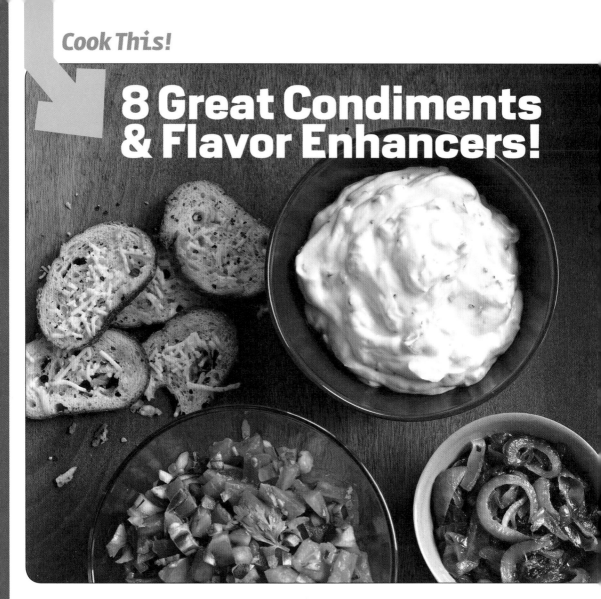

8 Great Condiments & Flavor Enhancers!

The whole point of a con-di-ment is to complement a dish and simultaneously take it to a height it wouldn't be able to achieve on its own. Yet, the condiments we turn to most frequently—mayonnaise, full-fat ranch, honey mustard—do more to elevate calorie counts than they do to elevate flavors. In fact, the tide of oil, salt, and sugar that defines so many packaged dressings, dips, and spice mixtures works against dishes, obscuring flavors rather than enhancing them.

Not the case here. These recipes may be the shortest in the book, but in many ways, they're the most vital. That's because it's the little things—the harmony of a homemade vinaigrette, the bright punch of fresh-chopped salsa, the pop of a pickled pepper— that will take your cooking from average to extraordinary.

Blackening Spice

This is a basic blueprint for blackening spice, one that you should readily tweak to fit your taste buds. Don't like heat? Cut down on the cayenne. Want a smoky note? Try a bit of cumin. This makes more than enough for one recipe, but after blacken-ing one batch of fish or chicken, you'll be coming back for more in a matter of days.

You'll Need:

- 2 Tbsp paprika (smoked or sweet)
- 1 Tbsp salt
- 2 tsp onion powder
- 2 tsp garlic powder
- 2 tsp cayenne
- 1½ tsp black pepper
- 1 tsp dried thyme or oregano leaves

How to Make It:

Combine all ingredients in a sealable container. Rub up to 1 teaspoon of the mix on catfish, tilapia, or other flaky white fish before grilling or searing in a cast-iron skillet. The mix will keep for up to 6 months in your cupboard.

Makes about ⅓ cup

Caramelized Onions

Is there anything not made better by the addition of syrupy sweet slow-cooked onions? If there is, we haven't found it. You can cook these for as long as you like—they only improve with time. But if you do plan to cook these down to an oniony jam (a consistency that is achieved after about 45 minutes of cooking), add an extra onion or two (might as well, if you're taking the time to do this) and keep the flame really low. Don't have the time but want the sweetness? Add a splash of balsamic vinegar in the final moments of cooking.

You'll Need:

- 1 Tbsp olive oil
- 2 large red onions, sliced
- ½ tsp salt

How to Make It:

Heat the oil in a large saucepan or sauté pan (one that you have a lid for) over medium-low heat. Add the onions and salt, cover, and cook, stirring occasionally, until the onions are soft and beginning to take on a caramel color, about 20 minutes.

Makes about 1 cup

Cook This!

Balsamic Vinaigrette

Bottled dressing is okay in a pinch, but homemade vinaigrettes are so easy and affordable to make, there's really no reason why you shouldn't whisk up your own dressing as often as possible. This is a classic, the most versatile of all dressings, able to do wonders to pretty much any bowl of lettuce and toppings you dare to toss it with.

You'll Need:

- 2 Tbsp minced shallots (about 2 small)
- 1 garlic clove, minced
- 2 tsp Dijon mustard
- ¼ cup balsamic vinegar

Salt and black pepper to taste

- ½ cup olive oil

How to Make It:

Combine the shallots, garlic, Dijon, and balsamic in a large mixing bowl, along with a good pinch of salt and pepper. Slowly drizzle in the olive oil, whisking as you do. Alternatively, you can combine all the ingredients in a clean mason jar and shake like crazy for 20 seconds. Keeps for 1 week covered in the refrigerator.

Makes about 1 cup

Homemade Ranch

Most bottled ranch is an abomination, little more than an amalgamation of low-grade oils and powdered eggs. You might as well be pouring mayonnaise on your salad. This version, spiked with yogurt and fresh herbs, isn't just considerably healthier, it's also about twice as addictive (which can be a good thing and a bad thing).

You'll Need:

- ½ cup Greek-style yogurt
- ½ cup olive oil mayonnaise
- ¼ cup chopped fresh parsley
- 2 Tbsp chopped scallions or chives
- ½ tsp garlic salt

Black pepper to taste

How to Make It:

Place all ingredients in a food processor and pulse until thoroughly blended. Keeps for 1 week covered in the refrigerator.

Makes about 1 cup

Ginger-Lime Vinaigrette

This is an excellent all-purpose Asian-style dressing, equally good for dressing a salad as it is for topping a fish fillet or goosing a grilled steak.

You'll Need:

Juice of 2 limes

- ½ Tbsp fresh ginger, peeled and minced or grated
- ½ Tbsp minced jalapeño
- 1 clove garlic, minced
- 1 Tbsp honey
- 1 Tbsp sesame oil
- 3 Tbsp canola or vegetable oil

Salt and black pepper to taste

How to Make It:

Combine the lime juice, ginger, jalapeño, garlic, and honey in a mixing bowl. Slowly drizzle in the oils, whisking constantly. Season with a good pinch of salt and pepper.

Makes about ½ cup

Pico de Gallo

The most versatile of all salsas, this chunky mix of fresh produce can be scattered on tacos or nachos, folded into eggs and salads, strewn on sandwiches, or eaten with a batch of homemade tortilla chips and chased with a cold beer. You really can't lose.

You'll Need:

- 4 Roma tomatoes, chopped
- 1 small red onion, diced
- 1 jalapeño, minced
- 1 handful cilantro, chopped

Juice of 1 lime

Salt and pepper to taste

How to Make It:

Combine the tomatoes, onion, jalapeño, cilantro, and lime juice in a mixing bowl. Season with salt and pepper and mix to thoroughly combine. Keeps covered in the refrigerator for up to 1 week.

Makes about 3 cups

Pickled Jalapeños

Don't limit these chiles to Mexican food; try them on sandwiches and burgers, stir-fries, pizzas, or anything that would benefit from a sharp, spicy-sweet kick. This basic pickling technique can be applied to a variety of vegetables and fruit, from sliced red onions to parboiled green beans to sweet hunks of cantaloupe and watermelon.

You'll Need:

8-10 jalapeños

- 1 cup rice wine or cider vinegar
- 1 cup water
- 1 Tbsp salt
- 1 Tbsp sugar

How to Make It:

Cut the jalapeños into thin slices. If you like your peppers hot, cut all the way up to the stem; for a milder batch, stop a ½ inch before. Combine the vinegar, water, salt, and sugar in a saucepan and heat just enough so that the salt and sugar dissolve. Allow the liquid to cool briefly. Place the jalapeños in a sterilized jar or small mixing bowl. Pour the liquid over them, then cover, letting them soak for at least 10 minutes before using. Will keep for a week covered in the refrigerator.

Makes about 2 cups

Roasted Garlic

When roasted until sweet and nutty, garlic has more in common with butter than it does with the raw, pungent stuff we're all used to. Except, of course, that roasted garlic is nearly calorie-free and packs a host of cancer-fighting, heart-strengthening compounds. Roast a whole head and use a few cloves to spike mayonnaise, blend into a salad dressing, or stir into potatoes. Or serve the whole head, hot from the oven, with crusty bread, soft cheese, and a knife for spreading.

You'll Need:

- 1 head garlic
- ½ Tbsp olive oil

How to Make It:

Preheat the oven to 400°F. Use a knife to cut off the top ¼ inch of the garlic head, barely exposing the top part of the individual cloves. Place the garlic in the center of a piece of aluminum foil and drizzle the olive oil on top. Cover the garlic with the foil and fold the ends to create a sealed packet, then place in the oven and roast for 35 to 40 minutes, until the cloves are very soft. Keeps in the fridge for up to a week.

Makes 1 head

Desserts

Insanely decadent
post-dinner delights

The Milk Shake Matrix

Short of drinking melted butter through a straw, there are few worse foods you could put in your body than a milk shake made outside the house. It's the last part that is key, because shake-making at home gives you full control of the ingredients and portioning, meaning you can crank out a decadent drink in a minute that has fewer than a quarter of the calories of its restaurant or ice cream shop equivalent. Here's how:

CHOOSE A BASE

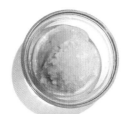

FROZEN YOGURT

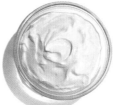

GREEK YOGURT

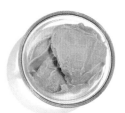

RASPBERRY SHERBET OR SORBET

CHOOSE FILLINGS

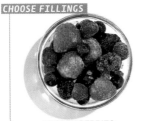

FROZEN BERRIES

FROZEN MANGO

PEANUT BUTTER

CHOOSE A LIQUID

Why not have a little caffeine buzz with that sugar surge? Coffee has been shown to boost metabolism, a benefit you'll need in the milk shake aftermath.

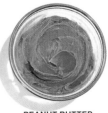

COFFEE

MILK

Four Super Shakes

Milk shakes don't need to be 1,000-calorie calamities. Choose a base, complement it with one or two fillings, and add just enough liquid to bring it all together. Insert straw. Enjoy.

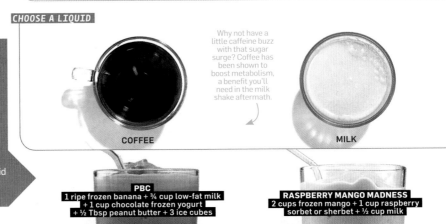

PBC
1 ripe frozen banana + ¾ cup low-fat milk + 1 cup chocolate frozen yogurt + ½ Tbsp peanut butter + 3 ice cubes

RASPBERRY MANGO MADNESS
2 cups frozen mango + 1 cup raspberry sorbet or sherbet + ½ cup milk

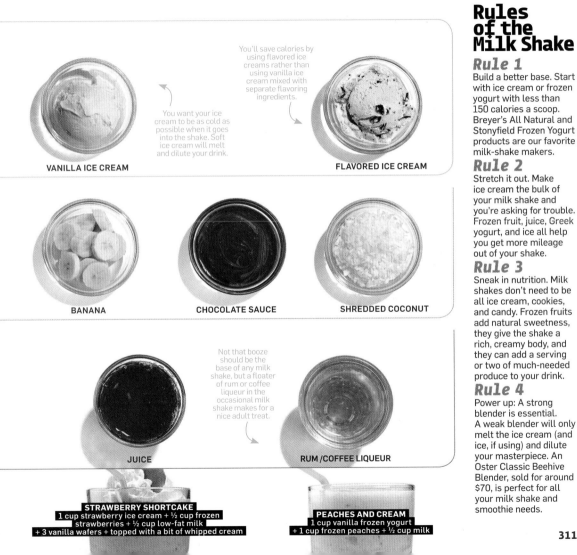

You'll save calories by using flavored ice creams rather than using vanilla ice cream mixed with separate flavoring ingredients.

You want your ice cream to be as cold as possible when it goes into the shake. Soft ice cream will melt and dilute your drink.

VANILLA ICE CREAM

FLAVORED ICE CREAM

BANANA

CHOCOLATE SAUCE

SHREDDED COCONUT

Not that booze should be the base of any milk shake, but a floater of rum or coffee liqueur in the occasional milk shake makes for a nice adult treat.

JUICE

RUM /COFFEE LIQUEUR

STRAWBERRY SHORTCAKE
1 cup strawberry ice cream + ½ cup frozen strawberries + ½ cup low-fat milk + 3 vanilla wafers + topped with a bit of whipped cream

PEACHES AND CREAM
1 cup vanilla frozen yogurt + 1 cup frozen peaches + ½ cup milk

CHAPTER 12

Rules of the Milk Shake

Rule 1
Build a better base. Start with ice cream or frozen yogurt with less than 150 calories a scoop. Breyer's All Natural and Stonyfield Frozen Yogurt products are our favorite milk-shake makers.

Rule 2
Stretch it out. Make ice cream the bulk of your milk shake and you're asking for trouble. Frozen fruit, juice, Greek yogurt, and ice all help you get more mileage out of your shake.

Rule 3
Sneak in nutrition. Milk shakes don't need to be all ice cream, cookies, and candy. Frozen fruits add natural sweetness, they give the shake a rich, creamy body, and they can add a serving or two of much-needed produce to your drink.

Rule 4
Power up: A strong blender is essential. A weak blender will only melt the ice cream (and ice, if using) and dilute your masterpiece. An Oster Classic Beehive Blender, sold for around $70, is perfect for all your milk shake and smoothie needs.

Tiramisu

Tiramisu is like guacamole and pizza: It's hard to have a truly bad version of it. The basic composition is so fundamentally delicious, even an ill-prepared rendition is still pretty damn satisfying. Unfortunately, that rule doesn't hold true for nutritional virtue, which tends to suffer in inverse proportion to the deliciousness of a given tiramisu. This version bucks that trend, ditching the high-cal constituents—egg yolks and mascarpone—in favor of a lighter treatment of beaten egg whites and whipped cream cheese, an approach that yields an ethereal, but still rich and satisfying dessert.

You'll Need:

- 3 egg whites
- ¼ cup confectioners' sugar
- ½ cup whipped cream cheese, softened at room temperature
- ½ cup strong espresso (or 1 cup strong coffee)
- ½ cup coffee liqueur such as Kahlúa or Tia Maria
- ½ (7 oz) package ladyfingers or 4 cups cubed angel food cake
- 1 oz dark chocolate, finely shaved

Espresso grounds or cocoa powder (optional)

How to Make It:

- Beat the egg whites until they form soft peaks. Add the sugar and lightly beat it into the whites. Place the cream cheese in a large bowl and fold in half of the whipped whites. Once fully incorporated, lightly fold in the remaining whites.

- Combine the espresso and coffee liqueur. Place a layer of ladyfingers (or angel food cake, if using) in the bottom of 4 wine or martini glasses. Spoon enough of the coffee mixture over them to soak the ladyfingers thoroughly. Divide the cream cheese mixture among the glasses, then top each with a good pile of dark chocolate shavings. Garnish with a dusting of espresso grounds if you like.

Makes 4 servings / Cost per serving: $2.02

Ladyfingers, short, stubby sponge cakes, are traditional here, but angel food cake provides a similarly soft, absorbent base and keeps the calorie count a touch lower.

260 calories
6 g fat
(4 g saturated)
23 g sugars

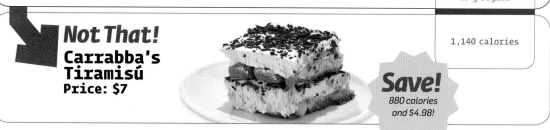

Not That!
Carrabba's Tiramisú
Price: $7

1,140 calories

Save!
880 calories
and $4.98!

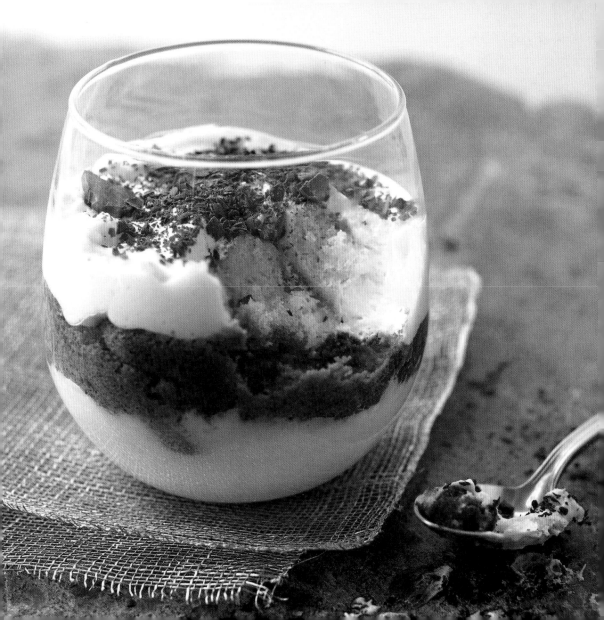

Cook This!
Apple Crumble

Though "as American as apple crumble" might not have the same ring to it, it does have the same spirit behind it. These individual dishes of tart, sweet roasted apples and crunchy cobbler topping make for a deeply satisfying end to a meal. What makes this one so special is the topping: Not only do the oats and almonds give this dish a shot of fiber, healthy fat, and antioxidants you wouldn't find in a standard flour-based crumble, the crunchy texture of the topping makes for a more rewarding contrast to the soft cooked apples.

You'll Need:

- 2 **Granny Smith apples,** peeled, cored, and cut into wedges
- ½ **cup apple juice**
- 4 **Tbsp brown sugar**
- ¼ **tsp cinnamon**
- ¼ **tsp nutmeg**
- 1 **cup rolled oats**

Pinch **salt**

- 2 **Tbsp chilled butter,** cut into small pieces
- ¼ **cup chopped almonds**

Whipped cream or crème fraîche

How to Make It:

- Preheat the oven to 400°F. Combine the apples, apple juice, 2 tablespoons brown sugar, ⅛ teaspoon cinnamon, and ⅛ teaspoon nutmeg in a large mixing bowl.

- In a separate bowl, combine the oats with the remaining 2 tablespoons brown sugar, ⅛ teaspoon cinnamon, and ⅛ teaspoon nutmeg, plus a good pinch of salt. Add the butter and work the mixture with your fingertips until it comes together in moist clumps. Add the almonds and work them in as well.

- Divide the apples among 4 ramekins and top with the oatmeal-almond mixture. Bake in the middle rack of the oven for about 25 minutes, until the apples are hot and bubbling and the crumble has begun to brown. (If the topping isn't significantly brown, you can turn on the broiler for the last minute of cooking.) Let cool for a few minutes. Serve with a generous dollop of whipped cream or crème fraîche.

Makes 4 servings /
Cost per serving: $0.94

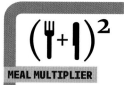

MEAL MULTIPLIER

This crumble topping—made from crunchy bits of almonds and fiber-rich oats—can be adapted to almost any fruit. It's best to follow the seasons, not only because the fruit will be more readily available and cheaper, but, more importantly, because it will be better. Three seasonal crumbles worth trying:

- Spring: Rhubarb and strawberries
- Summer: Peaches and blueberries
- Fall: Pears and cranberries

290 calories
12 g fat
(4 g saturated)
44 g carbohydrates

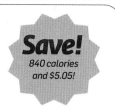

1,130 calories
44 g fat
(23 g saturated)
177 g carbohydrates

Not That!
On the Border Sizzling Apple Crisp
Price: $5.99

Save!
840 calories and $5.05!

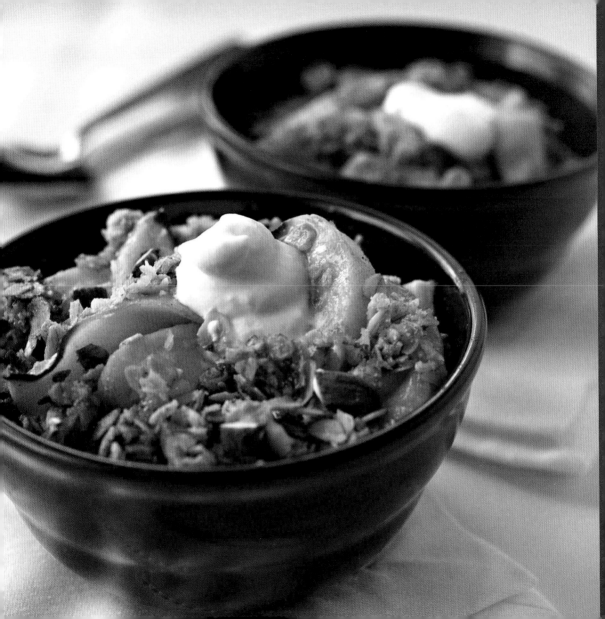

Cook This!
Banana-Nutella Crepe

It seems that crepes were invented for the sole purpose of housing fresh banana slices and chocolate—at least, that's what will be on your mind as you knife and fork your way through one of these. Truth is, dessert crepes of all stripes are special stuff, but nothing quite makes sense like this combination. Nutella, the Italian chocolate-hazelnut spread, is widely available in supermarkets, but even standard chocolate sauce will evoke fits of uncontrollable pleasure here.

You'll Need:

Butter for the crepes

½ recipe Crepe Batter (see page 258)

¼ cup Nutella

2 bananas, peeled and sliced

Confectioners' sugar (optional)

How to Make It:

- Heat a 10" nonstick pan over medium heat. Add enough butter to coat, then add 2 tablespoons of the crepe batter and swirl the pan to cover it in a thin, even film (use a rubber spatula to help, if needed).
- Cook on the first side for 3 to 4 minutes, until the bottom takes on a deep golden brown color. Flip and slather a tablespoon of the Nutella down the middle of the crepe, then top with a scant quarter of the banana slices.
- Cook for 3 to 4 minutes longer, until the bottom is golden brown. Fold the crepe sides over the filling and slip onto a plate. Top with a few slices of banana and a shake of confectioners' sugar if you like. Repeat to make three more crepes.

Makes 4 servings / Cost per serving: $0.74

Standard crepe batter is perfectly fit for desserts, but you can also sweeten it up with a tablespoon or two of sugar before cooking.

260 calories
12 g fat
(5 g saturated)
18 g sugars

Not That!
IHOP
Nutella Crepes
Price: $7.69

990 calories

Save!
730 calories and $6.95!

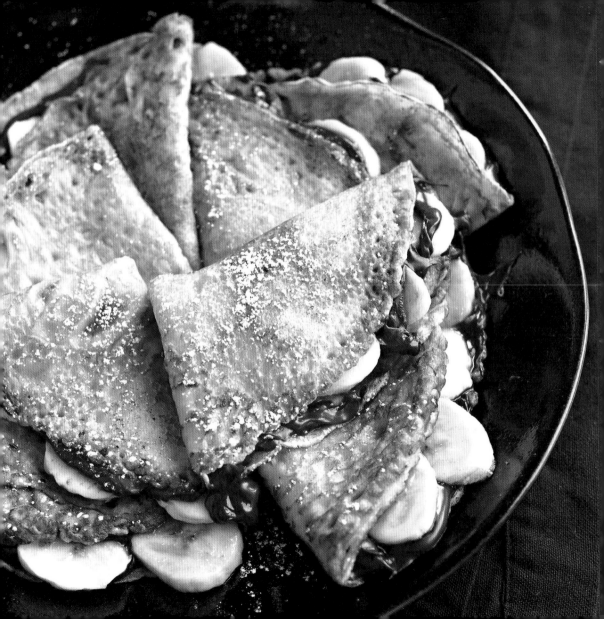

Sundae
with Grilled Pineapple & Rum Sauce

The banana may be the sundae fruit vessel of choice, but the standard split formula—one banana, three scoops ice cream—is a disastrous recipe for the discerning eater. Pineapple, on the other hand, holds one good scoop of ice cream perfectly, and its kick of sweetness and acidity—which is only intensified when it's grilled—matches nicely with the creamy vanilla. Add a swirl of rum sauce and some toasted coconut and it's like having a piña colada, minus the hangover.

You'll Need:

- 4 (½"-thick) slices fresh pineapple, core removed
- 1 Tbsp butter
- 2 Tbsp brown sugar
- 2 Tbsp dark rum
- 1 tsp vanilla extract
- 2 cups vanilla ice cream
- 2 Tbsp shredded sweetened coconut, toasted

How to Make It:

- Heat a grill, grill pan, or large sauté pan over medium heat (using a small pat of butter in the sauté pan). Cook the pineapple rings for 3 to 4 minutes per side, until caramelized all over.
- Cook the butter, brown sugar, rum, and vanilla in a saucepan over low heat, stirring occasionally, until the sugar fully melts and the sauce is a uniform dark brown. Keep warm.
- Place one slice of pineapple on each of 4 small plates. Top with a scoop of ice cream, drizzle on the rum sauce, then finish with the toasted coconut.

Makes 4 servings / Cost per serving: $1.10

Toasting the coconut is optional but highly recommended. To toast, spread on a baking sheet and bake in a 350°F oven for 12 minutes, until golden brown.

290 calories
11 g fat
(7 g saturated)
35 g sugars

Save!
720 calories
and $5.25!

1,010 calories
34 g fat
(20 g saturated)
125 g sugars

Not That!
Baskin-Robbins Classic Banana Split
Price: $6.35

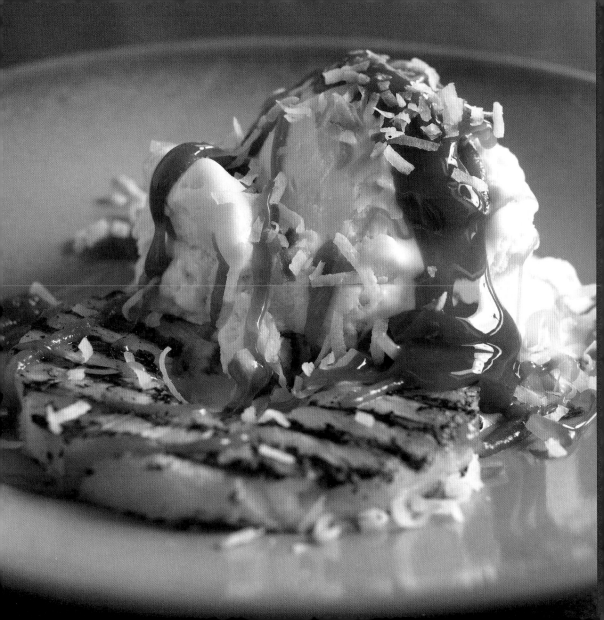

Cook This!
Chocolate Pudding with Olive Oil and Sea Salt

Packaged chocolate pudding contains more additives and fillers than actual chocolate, and purchased pre-made pudding contains more calories than one should ever consume with a spoon. What's a chocoholic to do? If you've made it this deep into the book, we'll assume you know the answer already. This homemade version skips the eggs, which doesn't just cut calories, but also saves you from having to slow-cook them in a double boiler or temper them with hot chocolate. What really makes this pudding special, though, is the final flourish. It might sound like a strange way to eat dessert, but the combination of chocolate, peppery olive oil, and crunchy little flakes of salt brings to mind a bag of chocolate-covered pretzels.

You'll Need:

- ¼ cup sugar
- 2 Tbsp cornstarch
- 2 cups low-fat milk
- 1 Tbsp unsalted butter
- 4 oz bittersweet or semisweet chocolate, chopped (or ⅔ cup bittersweet chocolate chips)
- 1 teaspoon vanilla extract
- Pinch of table salt
- Olive oil and coarse sea salt (like fleur de sel)

How to Make It:

- Combine the sugar and cornstarch in a medium saucepan over low heat. Slowly add the milk, whisking to blend. Bring to a bare simmer, then stir in the butter, chocolate, vanilla, and a pinch of table salt. Remove from the heat and continue stirring until the chocolate has melted uniformly. Pour into 4 small glasses or ramekins and place in the fridge for at least 2 hours.
- Before serving, drizzle the puddings with a bit of olive oil and top each with a pinch of sea salt.

Makes 4 servings / Cost per serving: $0.86

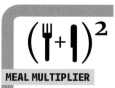
$$(\mathord{\text{\ding{"0238}}}+\mathord{\text{\ding{"0239}}})^2$$
MEAL MULTIPLIER

Three other ways to turn this very good chocolate pudding into something exceptional:

- S'mores pudding: Line the bottom of the glasses with crushed graham crackers. Top with marshmallows.
- PB&C: Whip together equal parts milk and chunky peanut butter. Divide among the glasses, then top with the pudding.
- Chocolate-covered strawberries: Cover the bottom of each glass with sliced strawberries or a heaping tablespoon of strawberry jam, top with a thin layer of ricotta cheese, then spoon in the pudding.

310 calories
19 g fat
(10 g saturated)
29 g sugars

900 calories
22 g fat
(14 g saturated)
130 g sugars

Not That!
Dairy Queen Chocolate Malt (medium)
Price: $2.99

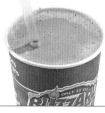

Save!
590 calories and $2.13!

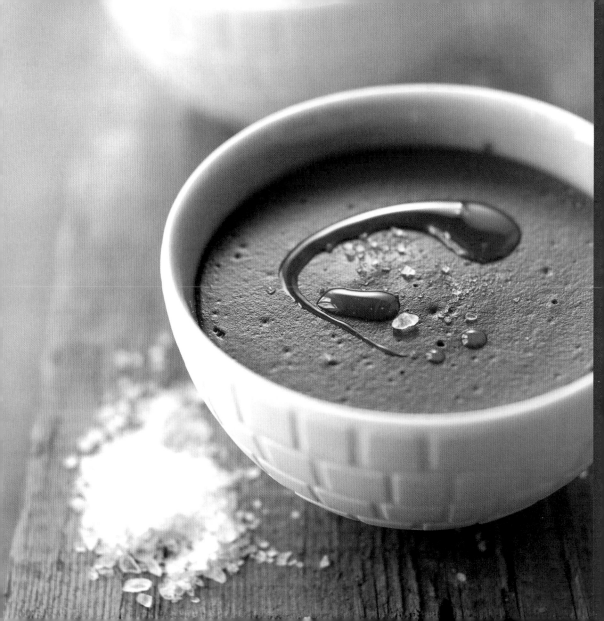

Cook This!
Key Lime Pie

This is the easiest pie in the history of baking. Mix, pour, bake, devour. Simple as that. If you can't find bottled Key lime juice (or fresh Key limes) in your local supermarket, you can have Amazon.com send you a 16-ounce bottle of Nellie & Joe's Key West Lime Juice for about $5. In a pinch, regular lime juice will do, even if the majority of south Floridians would cry foul.

You'll Need:
- 2 eggs
- 2 egg whites
- ½ cup Key lime juice
- 1 ½ tsp grated lime zest
- 1 can (14 oz) low-fat sweetened condensed milk
- 1 graham cracker crust (6 oz)
- 1 ½ cups low-fat whipped topping

How to Make It:
- Preheat the oven to 350°F. Beat the eggs and egg whites with a whisk or a mixer until blended. Stir in the juice, zest, and milk and beat until well-blended.
- Pour the mixture into the crust. Bake on the center oven rack for about 20 minutes, until the center is set but still wobbly (it will firm up as it cools). Allow the pie to cool on the counter, then cover with plastic wrap and refrigerate for at least 2 hours. Before eating, spread the whipped topping evenly over the filling.

Makes 8 servings / Cost per serving: $1.34

Key limes have an intense tart flavor that standard limes just can't match. If you do use regular lime, add some extra zest to intensify the citrus kick.

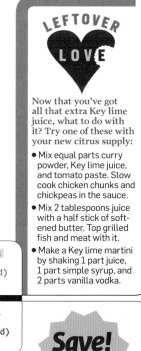

LEFTOVER LOVE

Now that you've got all that extra Key lime juice, what to do with it? Try one of these with your new citrus supply:
- Mix equal parts curry powder, Key lime juice, and tomato paste. Slow cook chicken chunks and chickpeas in the sauce.
- Mix 2 tablespoons juice with a half stick of softened butter. Top grilled fish and meat with it.
- Make a Key lime martini by shaking 1 part juice, 1 part simple syrup, and 2 parts vanilla vodka.

330 calories
10 g fat
(5 g saturated)
39 g sugars

620 calories
25 g fat
(14 g saturated)
66 g sugars

Not That!
Marie Callender's Key Lime Pie
with whipped cream
Price: $4.79

Save!
290 calories and $3.45!

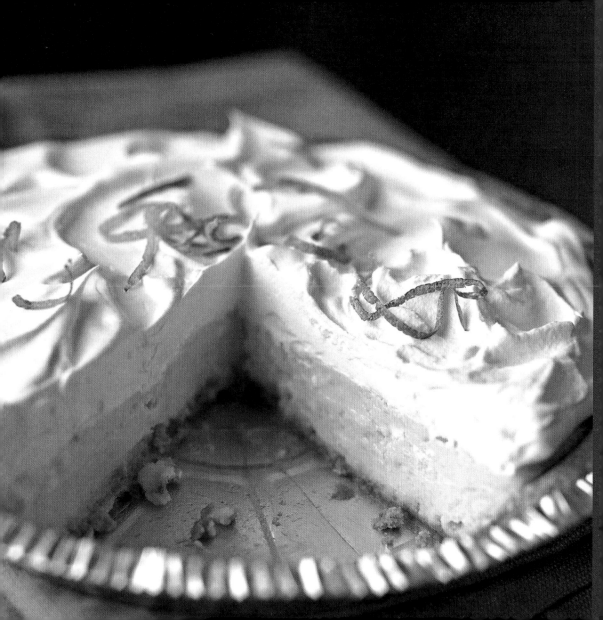

Molten Chocolate Cake

The idea of baking and frosting a multitiered chocolate cake is daunting for most, but these little self-contained parcels of joy are the lazy man's cake, the type of dessert that makes a non-baker feel like a pastry king when they emerge from the oven, pregnant with a tide of melted chocolate. Crack the middle and watch the flood of lava flow freely onto your plate—and eventually into your eagerly awaiting mouth. Did we mention these have only 360 calories?

You'll Need:

- 5 oz bittersweet chocolate (at least 60 percent cacao), plus 4 chunks for the cake centers
- 2 Tbsp butter
- 2 eggs
- 2 egg yolks
- ¼ cup sugar

Pinch of salt

- 2 Tbsp flour
- 1 tsp vanilla extract
- ½ Tbsp instant coffee or espresso (optional)

How to Make It:

- Preheat the oven to 425°F. Lightly butter four 6-ounce ramekins or custard cups.
- Bring a few cups of water to a boil in a medium saucepan over low heat. Place a glass mixing bowl over the pan (but not touching the water) and add the chocolate and butter. Cook, stirring occasionally, until both the chocolate and butter have fully melted. Keep warm.
- Use an electric mixer to beat the eggs, egg yolks, sugar, and salt until pale yellow and thick, about 5 minutes. Stir in the melted chocolate mixture, the flour, vanilla, and instant coffee if using.
- Pour the mixture into the prepared ramekins. Stick one good chunk of chocolate in the center of each ramekin. Bake the cakes on the center rack for 8 to 10 minutes, until the exterior is just set (the center should still be mostly liquid). The cakes can be eaten straight from the ramekins, but it's more dramatic to slide them on to plates (after letting them rest for a minute or two), where the molten chocolate can flow freely.

Makes 4 servings / Cost per serving: $1.20

360 calories
26 g fat
(13 g saturated)
34 g carbohydrates

1,070 calories
51 g fat
(28 g saturated)
143 g carbohydrates

Not That!
Chili's Molten Chocolate Cake
Price: $5.99

Save!
710 calories
and $4.79!

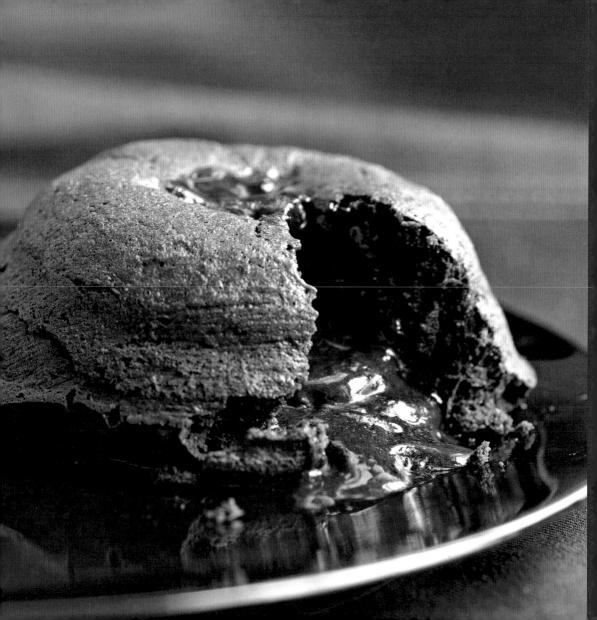

Affogato

Leave it to the Italians to come up with a two-ingredient dessert that satisfies as thoroughly as the most intricate cakes, pies, and pastries we normally find forced upon us at the end of a meal out. Affogato takes two traditional caps to a meal—ice cream and espresso or coffee—and combines them into one happy glass of gustatory joy. If you don't have an espresso machine, simply brew a brute-strength batch of coffee by using ¼ cup grounds and 1 cup water. Use the best beans you can find, though, since the intensity of the coffee magnifies both flaws and finer points.

You'll Need:

- 2 cups vanilla ice cream or gelato
- 1 cup hot espresso

How to Make It:

- Place one good scoop of vanilla ice cream or gelato in each of 4 small glasses (rocks glasses work nicely). Pour ¼ cup hot espresso over each scoop. Serve immediately.

Makes 4 servings /
Cost per serving: $0.94

Want to make excellent espresso without a $1,000 machine? The Bialetti Moka Stovetop Espresso Maker, at $25, brews top-notch shots.

The new wave of dessert "shooters" to hit restaurant menus like Chili's, Macaroni Grill, and Applebee's provides healthier alternatives to the regular dessert menu, but at 450 calories for a tiny portion, they're no bargain.

140 calories
7 g fat
(4.5 g saturated)
16 g carbohydrates

Not That!
Applebee's Chocolate Mousse Shooter
Price: $1.99

450 calories
31 g fat
(20 g saturated)
44 g carbohydrates

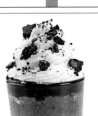

Save!
310 calories and $1.05!

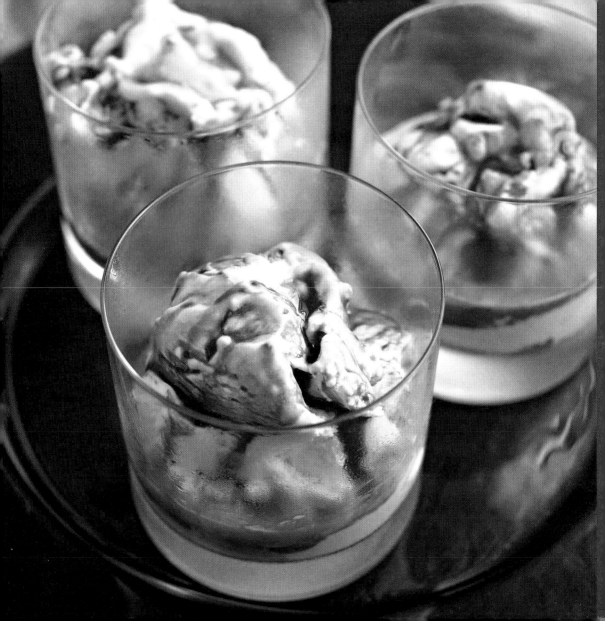

Paleta

We're predicting that the fruit-based frozen treats, called paletas in Mexico, will soon replace the overhyped, overly caloric cupcake as America's new dessert obsession. A welcome change, since each one of these packs close to a full serving of fruit. The type of fruit is up to you; if it can be thrown in the blender with a bit of sugar and pureed, then it's prime paleta material. This recipe is a dream for the kiddie cooks in the family.

Mango-Chile Paleta

You'll Need:

1 mango, peeled, pitted, flesh roughly chopped

Juice of 1 lime

2 Tbsp agave syrup or sugar

Pinch of cayenne pepper

Water

How to Make It:

• Place the mango, lime juice, agave syrup, and cayenne in a blender and puree, adding a bit of water if needed to help. Divide among 4 Popsicle holders and place in the freezer for at least 3 hours. (Do not cheat by checking along the way—the paletas won't freeze properly.) To easily release the paletas from the holders, run the bottoms briefly under warm water.

Makes 4 paletas /
Cost per serving: $0.69

Banana Paleta

You'll Need:

2 ripe bananas, peeled

½ cup low-fat milk

2 Tbsp sugar

2 Tbsp dark rum (optional)

Pinch of nutmeg

How to Make It:

• Place all the ingredients in a blender and puree, leaving the mixture slightly chunky if you like. Divide among 4 Popsicle holders and place in the freezer for at least 3 hours. To easily release the paletas from the holders, run the bottoms briefly under warm water.

Makes 4 paletas /
Cost per serving: $0.34

Strawberries & Cream Paleta

You'll Need:

2 cups fresh or frozen strawberries

¼ cup sugar

2 Tbsp heavy cream

Juice of ½ lemon or lime

How to Make It:

• Combine all the ingredients in a blender and puree. If you don't like seeds, strain them out through a fine sieve. Divide the mixture among 4 Popsicle holders and place in the freezer for at least 3 hours. To easily release the paletas from the holders, run the bottoms briefly under warm water.

Makes 4 paletas /
Cost per serving: $0.57

Save!
150 calories
and $0.68!

(average of all three)
80 calories
1.5 g fat
(0 g saturated)
15 g sugars

230 calories
12 g fat
(5 g saturated)
17 g sugars

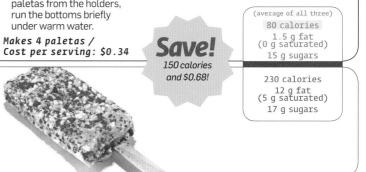

Not That!
Good Humor Strawberry Shortcake Bar
Price: $1.25

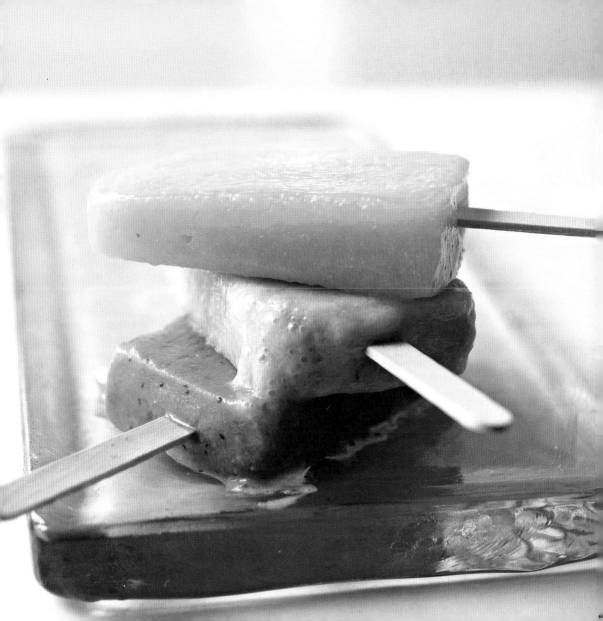

Index

Boldface page references indicate photographs.
Underscored references indicate boxed text.